# CONTENTS

# CONTENTS

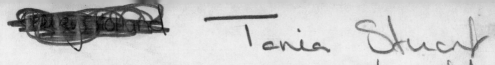

# HAIRDRESSING

## Theory, Science and Practice

# P CUTTING, R ROSS AND R HILL

**Second edition**

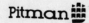
Pitman

PITMAN PUBLISHING
128 Long Acre, London WC2E 9AN

A Division of Longman Group UK Limited

First published in Great Britain 1988
Second edition first published in Great Britain 1991
Reprinted 1992

**British Library Cataloguing in Publication Data**

Cutting, P. (Peter)
 Hairdressing. – 2nd ed.
 1. Hairdressing
 I. Title  II. Ross, R. (Renie)  III. Hill, R. (Raymond)
 646.7242

ISBN 0–273–03457–X

Typeset by Avocet Typesetters, Bicester, Oxon
Printed and bound in Great Britain

# PREFACE

The aim of this book is to cover the competences (including the options) of the Hairdressing Training Board/City and Guilds National Vocational Qualification at Levels I, II and III. We have completely revised and extended the contents of the book to provide a single source of up-to-date and relevant information for people learning hairdressing.

The content is based on material tried and tested by our own students and on our own managerial experience. This has resulted in a generally student-orientated approach with the use of accessible language, emphasis of key points in bold, charts and diagrams and a glossary of terms (for quick reference). Each chapter ends with a summary, self-assessment questions and a practical assignment that students can complete without specialist facilities, in their own time if necessary. The practical procedures are listed step by step and illustrated to show key points. The themes of Afro-Caribbean hair styling, gowning clients and health hygiene and safety have also been introduced where appropriate.

The book is divided into four sections: **The Salon** – which includes reception, selling, payment, stock control, tools and equipment, basic safety, hygiene and first aid; **Hair and Skin** – which covers the basic structure of hair and skin, diagnostics, consultation and hair/scale treatments; **Actions and Reactions** – covering the hairdressing operations and **More Advanced Work** – which contains the Level III elements and options.

We hope people will find this book useful. Whether we have succeeded in meeting our aims only our readers can tell. If there are any comments you would like to make we would be glad to hear them.

December 1990

# ACKNOWLEDGEMENTS

We would like to thank the following:

North Manchester General Hospital for photographs of the scalp and skin conditions.

Mr Glen Jones for the use of his salon

Mrs Pat Roberts for her help with the photographic sessions

Mrs Sheila Jones for help with the photographic session, checking the manuscript and making suggestions for improvements

Mrs Susan Bain for permission to reproduce a 'Safety Policy' produced for her salon

Mrs Barbara Eden and Mrs E Middleton for their patience in proof-reading the manuscript

Ms Liz Hartley and Ms Rosemary Collyer of Pitman Publishing for their help

Mr Geoff M Armstrong for the photographs of salon procedures

Mrs Pam Young for her help with the initial illustrations and the wigmaking content

Mrs Barbara Egglestone and Mrs Connie Rorrison for typing the manuscript

To our families, who suffered long – again!

# SECTION 1
# THE SALON

# 1 RECEPTION

Hairdressing is a service industry, and as such it should be the major aim of every salon to provide a service which is:

- professional
- safe – it is taken on trust by the client that the service provided will be carried out with due regard to their health and safety.
- pleasant and relaxing to the client, so that their visit is enjoyable.

Each salon is a business, in a highly competitive field, and everyone earning money from the salon depends on the clients, regular clients being especially important.

It is sometimes difficult for younger members of staff to realise how easily a client can be offended or made angry by an off-hand remark or manner. Therefore, when a new apprentice/trainee joins the staff, it is in the interest of the staff and clients alike that the salon owner or manager, teaches not only the practical skills but also the equally important basic skills of attitude and behaviour in the salon. A client may not actually complain at the time, but will simply not come back. They will also tell their friends about the unsatisfactory service they received, so not just one client is lost, but many. A bad reputation is extremely hard to remove.

The reception will be the clients' first impression of the salon. A customer must always be greeted pleasantly, preferably by name, as soon as they enter the salon. A neglected client left waiting and ignored does not start their treatment in a happy frame of mind. Although not all salons can afford a receptionist, on busy days they are an asset and well worth their wages. They must be friendly and helpful and if a client does have to wait then they shoud be made comfortable and told approximately how long the delay is expected to be with a simple polite explanation. The client will then feel that they have been treated with consideration and will be less irritated by the delay.

Even if the salon employs a receptionist, all staff should be taught reception skills and how to deal with the salon's appointment and documentation system.

# Appointments

A booking should be entered in the appointment book in pencil so that it can be easily removed if the client cancels. The name of the client and the service required must be written **clearly** so that it can be easily read by all the staff; it is very embarrassing to call the client by the wrong name, therefore, if the handwriting is poor the information should be printed instead.

When booking an appointment, enough time must be allocated to each service otherwise the stylists become overbooked and clients have to wait, neither of which gives a good impression of the salon and causes frustration to all concerned. Different salons operate different systems, for example, some salons employ staff as specialists to carry out certain tasks such as perming or tinting etc. In this case, a client booking an appointment for a permanent wave followed by a semi-permanent colour and cut and blowdry may have more than three people working on their hair at separate times, and this has to be organised correctly in the appointment book. Thus, it is very important that all the staff know exactly what system is in operation in their own salon and how to dovetail bookings so that the salon runs smoothly and efficiently.

## Gowning

When an expected client arrives at the salon they should be greeted by name, then their name should be ticked off in the relevant appointment column to ensure that there is a record of which clients have attended.

It is often the duty of the receptionist or junior member of staff to gown the client after checking off their appointment.

Gowning is carried out before starting any hairdressing procedure. It is a means of protecting the client's clothing from chemical spillage or cut hairs. Adequate care *must* be taken when gowning the client as any damage to the client's clothing will be the responsibility of the salon and the client has every right to expect a replacement of any clothing which has been damaged through negligence.

The gowning of the client differs slightly before each type of service, therefore specific gowning procedures are dealt with in the practical areas within the relevant chapters.

# General behaviour in the salon

It is worth remembering that most people learn by 'copying' others, and it is therefore very important that all senior assistants set a good example when training new apprentice/trainees.

When dealing with clients, consider the following points:

1 attitude of staff
2 posture
3 personal appearance
4 non-verbal communication.

## Attitude of staff

The attitude of the staff towards the client and their work is very important. All members of staff should be pleasant, polite and helpful and show enthusiasm for their career. A sulky, sullen stylist makes the client feel unwelcome, uncomfortable and disinclined to return to the salon. Instead, it should be the aim of all staff members to give the client the best possible service and to ensure that a visit to the salon is an enjoyable experience.

Listed below are a few simple rules that should be followed if the salon is to maintain a good client/assistant relationship.

(*a*) Good manners. This involves showing respect to the client. Be polite at all times amd always make them feel welcome. Never be too familiar, nor too distant, as both of these attitudes can make the client feel uncomfortable.

(*b*) Never argue with other members of staff while working in the salon and *never* argue with the client; it is most unprofessional. Beware of argumentative subjects, e.g. politics and religion, as some people have very strong opinions and it is very easy to offend them, even unintentionally.

(*c*) Do not talk to other members of staff while dealing with the client, unless they are included and involved in the conversation.

(*d*) Never discuss or gossip about other people with the client.

(*e*) Always discuss fully the client's requirements. Apart from the obvious fact that you need to know this information before beginning any hairdressing service, it also helps to build up a strong client/stylist relationship which strengthens the trust that a client must have in the person who is dealing with their hair.

(*f*) Make sure that the client is comfortable at all times, particularly if they have to wait for their appointment.

(*g*) Never sit down, comb your own hair or apply make-up in the salon; it gives an unprofessional impression. Use the staff-room for this purpose instead.

(*h*) Never eat, smoke or drink in the salon. Again, use the staff-room.

(*i*) Remember that every client is paying for a service. They are entitled to courtesy and respect as well as the best possible service you can give them.

## Posture

Hairdressing may not seem like it, but it is a physically tiring profession and most hairdressers have to stand on their feet for a considerable length of time. Tired, irritable staff cannot give their best service to the client so it is very important that they stand and walk in such a way as to avoid too much physical strain on the body which will reduce the ability to work efficiently, and in some instances, could cause long-term problems, e.g. back strain.

Posture is the correct placing of the body in relation to the feet. If it is correct, staff will be able to work more efficiently and feel less tired. The major points for a good posture are:

(a) *Stand upright* – stooping causes backache, tiredness and makes it difficult to breathe correctly.

(b) *Balance* – the weight of the body should be evenly distributed on both feet. This reduces strain on the back and leg muscles.

(c) *Correct footwear* – shoes should be comfortable, attractive and heels should be a comfortable height. Avoid open toe shoes as hair fragments can enter under the skin and cause infection.

## Personal appearance

Personal cleanliness is extremely important in any walk of life, but particularly in the salon where assistants very often work physically hard, in warm surroundings (which increases sweating) and are also in close proximity to the client.

Body odour and bad breath can be offensive to both the client and other members of staff, therefore steps should be taken to ensure personal freshness at all times. Listed below are a few basic guidelines which can be adapted to suit individual needs.

(a) Assistants should bathe regularly and always use a deodorant when necessary – at least once a day.

(b) Regular brushing of teeth and correct diet are essential to prevent bad breath. It is also advisable to have a dental check-up every six months.

(c) Avoid eating food with an unpleasant odour, e.g. onions or garlic. They may taste delicious when eaten, but are very unpleasant second-hand!

(d) Assistants should always look neat and well groomed. Hair should be kept clean and well cut and if possible it should be coloured and permed, this encourages clients to do likewise. It is very difficult to persuade a client to have a permanent wave or a tint if none of the salon staff have had these treatments themselves! Stylists with long hair should keep it off the face, but in a fashionable style.

(e) Nails and hands should be well cared for. Where possible, use a barrier cream at night before going to bed; this will help to counteract the drying effect of degreasive shampoos and setting aids etc., and reduces the chances of developing dermatitis.

Nails must be kept clean and at a reasonable length to prevent scratching the client's scalp. If female stylists use nail polish it should be unchipped.

(*f*) Overalls or salon uniform must be spotlessly clean and fresh. Make use of tinting aprons to prevent staining when colouring or perming. Any clothes worn beneath the overall should not be allowed to show and woollen cardigans or jumpers should be avoided as these provide good conditions for skin bacteria to thrive.

The best type of overall is one made of cotton or of a cotton/polyester mixture. They are durable, easy to launder and do not increase perspiration. Nylon overalls do increase perspiration and can therefore be uncomfortable during busy periods.

(*g*) Avoid wearing jewellery, particularly jangling bracelets – they are disconcerting to the client and hinder efficiency. A watch or a ring can be worn, but they may be damaged if worn when shampooing so it is not usually worth the risk.

(*h*) Female stylists should wear make-up at all times in the salon and tights should be clean and unladdered. Male stylists should be close shaven or wear a neatly trimmed beard and/or moustache.

## Non-verbal communication

Non-verbal communication can be just as expressive as speaking. Postures, distances and the way in which we hold our bodies are all ways in which we express ourselves. Indeed many psychologists believe that a person's non-verbal behaviour can have more bearing on communicating feelings and attitudes than do their words. Thus, the client must always be treated in a pleasant and polite manner not only verbally but also by the body language that is used.

The main areas to consider are:

- distance
- facial expression
- body posture
- eye contact.

## Distance

Everyone requires their own 'space'. Touching and moving too near to the client can make them feel uncomfortable as usually only close relationships are allowed such close contact.

## Facial expression

An expressionless face which lacks emotion will appear 'cold' and hard. However, too much emotion can make the person appear neurotic! When working in the salon, try to maintain a positive facial expression e.g. smiling, so that the client feels that they are in a pleasant, happy environment.

## Body posture

This is believed by psychologists to provide clues as to what people really think or feel. Certainly, lounging around the salon in a slovenly manner does not create a businesslike impression and will make the client question your professionalism and therefore your practical ability even if this is unfounded.

## Eye contact

Eye contact with the client is extremely important as it is believed to be the basis of trust. Looking elsewhere when talking to the client will not only make him/her feel uncomfortable but will also make them doubt your sincerity.

# Use of the telephone

The telephone is an important link with the client but it must be remembered that the client hears only a voice which therefore must always be pleasant and helpful, no matter how busy the salon may be. Time must always be found to answer the phone – if staff are too busy to book an appointment at that particular second, the name of the salon should be stated and then, if necessary, the client could be asked to hold on for a moment. All staff must be trained to answer the telephone and to book appointments, even if the salon employs a receptionist. Bad telephone technique, like an abrupt reply or an unhelpful manner could lose many potential or regular clients.

In some salons, incoming telephone calls for members of staff are not allowed. Therefore, any rules regarding the receiving or ringing out of calls should be clearly indicated to all staff to prevent any unnecessary friction in the salon.

## Telephone services

There are now many operator sevices available for business use although not all of these services are suitable for the smaller hairdressing salon. New technology has meant that all communication services, including the telephone, are being expanded and updated at a bewildering speed. Consequently, it is often a useful exercise to become reacquainted with the facilities that are available approximately every 12 months or so.

The telephone is a vital link between the salon and the client so if the telephone is faulty in any way the fault should be rectified as quickly as possible to prevent loss of business. If the telephone is completely out of order then the fault should be reported immediately from elsewhere on a 'live' telephone.

# Using the emergency services

There are three or possibly four telephone emergency services: Fire, Police, Ambulance (and Coastguard in seaside locations), each of which consists of a highly skilled team used to dealing with all types of disasters.

An emergency usually involves an unusual or frightening situation so the most important thing to remember is to keep **calm** even though this may be difficult under the circumstances.

The correct procedure for contacting the emergency services is as follows:

1 Dial 999 or the emergency number shown on the number label.
2 When the **operator** answers, give the telephone number shown on the telephone.
3 Ask for the service you require.
4 When the **service** answers give the address where help is needed.
5 Supply any other information which may be of use.

NB Always try to speak **clearly** to prevent any misunderstandings and to enable the services to react immediately and bring help as quickly as possible.

# Use of the telephone directory

All the information needed for using the telephone is contained in the **phone book**. This is issued by British Telecom to all their subscribers free of charge and is written specifically for the area in which the subscriber lives.

The *phone book* contains far more information than just the names, addresses and telephone numbers of its subscribers. It also gives information on what services are available, how to use those services, the procedure for emergency calls, reporting faults and how to handle nuisance calls. It provides information on places of interest, call charges and usefull numbers within the subscribers locality and also gives guidance on how to find the number required and how to make Local, National and International calls.

All the information that may be required to make a telephone call is therefore contained within the *phone book*. However, some useful numbers to remember are:

100 **Operator Services** (including alarm calls, credit card calls, fixed time calls, freefone calls, personal calls, transferred charge and advice of duration and charge (ADC) calls)
151 **Faults**
192 **Directory enquiries**
999 **Emergency services**

## Types of call

There are four types of call, each of which requires a slightly different procedure.

*1 Own exchange call.* This is a call to within the same exchange area. In this case it is only necessary to dial the number.

*2 Own local area call.* This is a call made within the same local area but through another exchange. When trying to reach this number a **local code**, which is a code relating to the local call area only, must be dialled before the number.

*3 National call.* This is a call made outside the local area. Each village, town or city has its own **national code** which is fixed and applies from almost anywhere within the United Kingdom. To obtain a number outside the local area, the national code must be dialled before that number.

For example, a stylist in Bangor who wished to telephone a friend in Manchester whose telephone number was 4375293 then should dial the prefix 061, which is the national code for Manchester, before the number. Therefore the actual number that would have to be dialled would be: 061 4375293

*4 International call.* This is a call to a country outside the United Kingdom and can be made by International Direct Dialling (IDD) or through the operator. To dial a number in another country, the **international code** which is 010 must first be dialled. This is then followed by the **country code**, which is listed in the phone book, then the **area code** (if necessary) and finally the customer number.

The final set of numbers required when dialling abroad is usually very long, therefore to prevent costly mistakes it is a good idea to write down the complete number in full before starting to dial.

## Costing telephone calls

The cost of the telephone call will depend on where the call is to go to, how long the call lasts and when the call is made.

Obviously, the further away that the call is then the more costly it will be. Thus, an own exchange call will be cheaper per unit than an international call. The longer the call then the more it will cost so when using the telephone in a working environment, decide what needs to be said before dialling to make sure that it is used economically for messages and not for long and expensive chats.

There are periods during the day and night when it is substantially cheaper to make a telephone call, therefore considerable savings can be made by using the telephone during these cheap rate periods whenever possible. The three call rates are as follows:

**Peak**      This is the most expensive rate and is from 9 am until 1 pm Monday to Friday.

**Standard**  This is for calls from 8 am until 9 am and from 1 pm until 6 pm Monday to Friday.

**Cheap**     This is the cheapest time to use the telephone and is from 6 pm until 8 am Monday to Friday, and all day and night at weekends.

## Taking messages

Always **write down** a verbal message as it is often difficult to remember the correct information, particularly if the person who is to receive the message is not available at that precise moment. Writing down a message also has the added advantage of acting as a **reminder** to pass on the message at a later time.

The following facts should be included when writing down messages:

- date and time of message
- name of the person giving the message
- name of the person to receive the message
- exact details of the message.

When these details have been recorded, repeat the message back to the caller to make sure that it has been written down correctly.

# Career routes within the hairdressing industry

During the last few years there has been a movement away from the traditional 'time-serving' methods of training towards training to **levels of competence**, that is to say, once a trainee is competent in a particular area, they progress to the next stage. Thus, particularly talented trainees will require a shorter training period than their less competent counterparts.

However, some salons still recognise and operate a traditional 'apprenticeship' but there are also various other routes available to achieve 'qualified hairdresser' status. (*See* Fig. 1.1)

The first route is via a three-year indenture as an **apprentice** followed by two further years as a first and then second-year **improver**.

A second alternative route is to attend a college of further education (FE) until competence in all areas of the hairdressing craft ia achieved, after which time the trainee is usually employed by a salon as a junior stylist.

A third route is through **Youth Training** (YT) which offers full-time employment in a salon and if the **trainee** (i.e. the person who is being trained through YT) is suitable and enough work is available they can be retained by the salon as a junior sylist.

Most apprentices spend one day per week (for 36 weeks of the year) at an FE college while YT trainees also attend either a training centre or FE college for one day per week. This allows certification and provides skills testing through various examining bodies.

After the initial training period progression is to **chargehand**, then

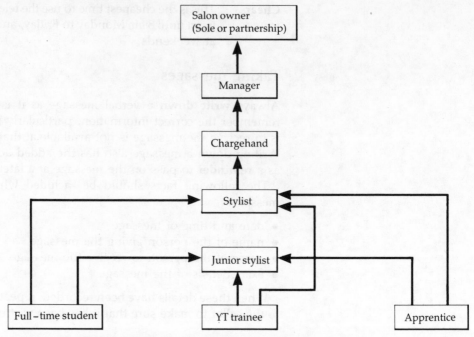

**Fig 1.1 Career routes within the hairdressing industry**

**manager** and then on to **owning** a salon, either solely or jointly with one or more partners. However, not every individual dreams of becoming self-employed and there are many other options available to the aspiring stylist once the initial training period or level of competence has been achieved. Indeed, if the trainee/apprentice is particularly talented and competent, it is often possible to progress to 'stylist' status very quickly.

# Career options

There are a variety of options available to the competent stylist and these can be divided into seven broad areas:

1 salon-based
2 theatrical
3 manufacturing industry
4 tricologist/consultant
5 teaching/technician
6 managerial
7 sales.

## Salon-based

For obvious reasons, the majority of career opportunities within the Hairdressing Industry are salon-based. However, salons are not

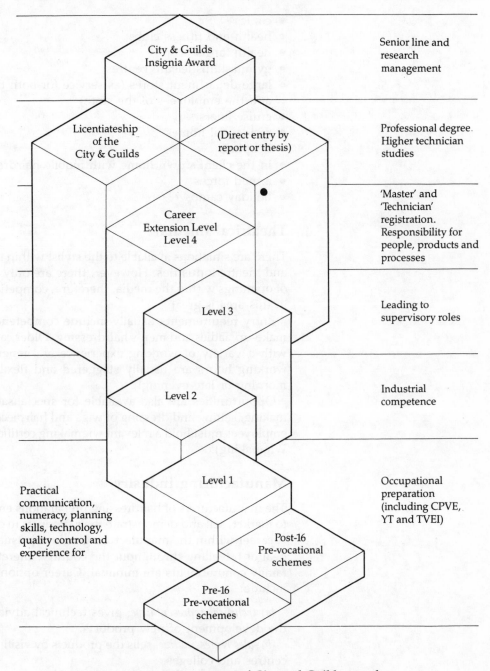

Senior line and research management

City & Guilds Insignia Award

Professional degree. Higher technician studies

Licentiateship of the City & Guilds

(Direct entry by report or thesis)

'Master' and 'Technician' registration. Responsibility for people, products and processes

Career Extension Level Level 4

Leading to supervisory roles

Level 3

Industrial competence

Level 2

Occupational preparation (including CPVE, YT and TVEI)

Level 1

Practical communication, numeracy, planning skills, technology, quality control and experience for

Post-16 Pre-vocational schemes

Pre-16 Pre-vocational schemes

**Fig 1.2 Progressive pattern of City and Guilds awards**

always situated on the 'High Street', they can be located in a wide variety of settings and the type of service they provide will reflect the needs of a particular clientele. Hairdressing services are often required in:

● hotels (both at home and abroad)

- clinics
- health and fitness clubs
- health farms
- gymnasiums/leisure centres
- large department stores (as service for both the general public and the employees of the store)
- cruise liners
- residential homes
- hospitals
- in the client's own home with mobile hairdressing
- armed forces
- holiday camps.

## Theatrical (media)

There are situations available to the stylist within the television, film and theatre industries. However, there are only a limited number of openings within the media, therefore, competition for a position in this area is great.

Entry requirements usually include competence in wigmaking, make-up, ladies and men's hairdressing. Older candidates (over 21) with a variety of working experience are generally preferred as working hours are usually staggered and flexible – often early morning or late evening!

Opportunities are also available for specialisation in the actual making, setting and dressing of wigs and hairpieces but prospective employees must hold a relevant wigmaking certificate (usually CGLI Wigmaking).

## Manufacturing industry

The manufacturers of hairdressing preparations employ hairdressers to market, sell and demonstrate their products to other hairdressers. A career within the manufacturing industry usually entails a great deal of travelling throughout the country; therefore, it is easier if family commitments are minimal. Career options within this area include:

(a) *technical representative*: gives technical advice and helps with the development of new products.

(b) *sales representative*: sells the products by visiting salons, training centres and colleges.

(c) *trade demonstrator*: demonstrates the uses of the products to hairdressers in salons, training centres and colleges.

(d) *tutor in manufacurers' own hairdressing school*: tutoring and giving advice to hairdressers who attend manufacturers' schools for specialised courses. The tutors also have to be prepared to work behind the scenes at the large, national shows and seminars. Other duties often include making videos and colour slides of new techniques that they have helped to develop.

## Tricologist/consultant

To practise as a registered tricologist the stylist must be an 'Associate of the Institute of Tricologists', which means that they have had a training period of three years which includes a **preliminary** year, an **intermediate** year and a **final** year. This qualification can be obtained through a correspondence course with the Institute of Tricologists or by attendance at a college of further education.

The Institute of Tricologists examination is very thorough and there is an entry requirement of four GCSE subjects (A, B or C grade or equivalent), one of which should preferably be a science subject.

The trained tricologist can practice within an existing hairdressing salon as a separate professional clinic to compliment the other hairdressing services or as a separate business enterprise.

## Teaching/technician

The teaching of hairdressing can be carried out in:

(*a*) private schools
(*b*) manufacturers' schools
(*c*) training centres/colleges of further education.

The qualifications necessary to teach vary depending upon the type of establishment. Often private schools train their own instructors who are chosen because of their proven hairdressing skills. Manufacturers' schools and training centres usually require their instructors to be experienced stylists with a sound knowledge of all aspects of the hairdressing craft both theoretically and practically, while colleges of further education demand the highest hairdressing qualifications available and preferably a recognised teaching qualification as well. Provision is usually made by the education authority for every college lecturer to obtain a university validated Teachers Certificate (if not already acquired) and lecturers are also encouraged to proceed to degree level, thus ensuring that they are suitably qualified to teach.

Technicians are employed in colleges of further education to give valuable assistance to the lecturers in the preparation and setting up of the teaching situation by organising stock, materials, equipment and audiovisual teaching aids. They play an important role within the college and work very closely with the teaching staff as part of a team.

## Managerial

This includes **salon ownership** either solely or with partner/s. However, there are also various other managerial options depending upon the size and type of salon and it is often advisable to gain managerial experience as an **employee** before becoming a salon owner.

Smaller salons may limit their higher management positions to either **chargehand** (with less responsibility) or **manager** but larger hairdressing salons, often require **artistic directors, educational directors** and **management staff** to market their salons and any courses they may run.

## Sales

This area involves the selling of hairdressing and beauty products. Potential opportunities in sales include employment as:

(a) *sales representative*: employed by the manufacturers to sell to the hairdressing trade.

(b) *sales person*: employed by large department stores to sell the products and give advice to their customers.

(c) *receptionist*: employed by the hairdressing/beauty salon and duties will include selling hairdressing/beauty products to the clients.

**Summary**

'Reception' involves a number of important operations.

- reception of clients
- booking appointments
- use of the telephone – an important link between salon and client
- message taking

In addition to these processes the general behaviour of staff in the salon is important in attracting and keeping clients. This behaviour involves attitudes, posture, personal appearance, and non-verbal communication.
The hairdressing industry has a structured training programme and a range of career opportunities for the trained stylist.

**Self-assessment questions**

1 List the four main areas involved in dealing with clients.
2 Which two topics should be avoided in conversations with a client?
3 Why is good posture important?
4 Why should open-toed shoes be avoided?
5 What action should be taken if a client has to wait?
6 What are the four main areas to consider for non-verbal communication with a client?
7 What is the procedure for contacting the emergency services by telephone?
8 When writing down a verbal message, what facts should be included?

**Practical assignment – Reception** _____

## Task

To help you to gain a greater understanding of the services which your salon has to offer, make a chart in the format set out below. You can obtain the information by *reading* the information contained in the packaging and instruction leaflets of the products, by *asking* the people who work with you and by *watching* the various services being carried out in the salon.

When it is complete ask if the chart can be put up in your staff room at work as a reminder while you are learning your reception duties.

| Service | Timing stylists | Timing client | Benefits and effects | Cost to client |
|---------|-----------------|---------------|----------------------|----------------|
| (a) | (b) | (c) | (d) | (e) |

In column (a) list all the services that your salon has to offer – you may be surprised at how long this list will be! Any large services, such as perming, should be subdivided into the different types as their benefits and costs will be different even if the timing is very similar.

In column (b) give the timings for the separate stages, particularly large tasks. This will help you to dovetail appointments in the future.

In column (c) find out the total time that the client will be in the salon.

In column (d) write down the benefits and effects of each service and look at the finished results in the salon. Why and how do you think their hair has been improved?

Use your own experience as well as other resources to complete this column. For example, if you have had your own hair permed or coloured, why do you think that it is better than before and why did you have it done?

Fill in column (e) by looking at the salon price list.

# 2 SELLING

Selling is an integral part of the hairdressing process. Many hairdressers however, think of selling as merely getting a client to buy a can of lacquer! This is not the case – hairdressing involves marketing – selling the salon image and experience as well as the other more obvious goods.

Selling is about offering goods which someone else is willing to buy, including both the salon services and the expertise of the staff. Never underestimate the power of perception (how people see things): if the client perceives you as an expert they will take your advice. However they will not wish to attend your salon or buy goods if they do not like what they see. First impressions are important and a prospective client/buyer can be encouraged to enter the salon by its smart and clean exterior and to keep returning because of its welcoming interior and the attitude of the staff employed there. Thus, selling with regard to hairdressing can be divided into three main areas:

- Selling the salon image
- Selling salon services
- Selling retail goods.

## Selling the salon image

As stated above, it is important to first attract the client to walk through the salon doors. New clients will attend the salon either because they have been recommended by someone else or because they like the look of the salon from the outside. This being so, the exterior of the salon must always project the salon image and the type of work that takes place within. It should always be kept clean and if there is a window display this must be regularly changed to attract attention.

The type and standard of work that is produced by the salon will also present a certain image. The standard of work should be as high

high as possible and can be improved by regular training nights for both junior and senior staff.

In addition, the appearance of the staff will contribute to the image of the salon, so looking neat, smart and professional is very important. For example, if you were to find yourself in hospital surrounded by nurses wearing shorts and 't'-shirts you would not be filled with confidence. This is because they would not be projecting the image of what you 'perceive' that a nurse should look like. While their attire will make no difference to the standard of their work, it will influence how capable *you* think that person to be. The same applies to hairdressing, if the staff look the part, then clients will believe them to be competent.

## Selling the salon services

Before you can sell any salon service you must have a thorough knowledge of what these services are, how they work and what benefits they will bring to the client. Often staff are reluctant to use or recommend new products as they are unsure of these points. However, most manufacturers have trained technical staff who will come to the salon to demonstrate and instruct the staff on any of their products. They will usually run short courses at their own training centres to give any tuition needed on their products. These courses are very useful as they also give background knowledge and usually offer ways in which to promote the products. Always remember that the manufacturers are also in business and it is in their best interest to help you as much as possible as the more of their products you use then the more profit they make!

A lot of stylists feel uncomfortable about recommending further treatments to their clients. This reluctance is, however, misplaced because the client relies on the experience of the stylist to make their hair look its best. Very often the client is totally unaware of the range of services available. While they may, for example, be aware that the salon does 'tints', they could be oblivious to the very many ways that colour can be used to create effects that range from dramatic to so subtle that the hair is given only a 'sheen'. It is the responsibility of the stylist, as the expert, to guide and advise the client as to what treatments would be the most suitable and beneficial. After all, the worst that can happen is that the client will say no. The conversation below gives an indication of how a treatment can be advised to the client without giving offence:

*Client:* 'I like my new haircut but the top keeps going flat. I know I should have a perm but I hate curls and besides the back is now too short to curl.'
*Stylist:* 'Your hair is rather fine so it really needs extra bounce. A body wave or root perm would be ideal as it will only give root lift and will not make it too curly. In fact, it will not give any curl at all but it will make the blowdry hold for longer and give your style

the height you like. I only need to wind the top so that the other hair will be unaffected.'

*Client:* 'That sounds ideal, I hadn't realised that it was possible to have a perm without curl and that I didn't need to have the whole head done. When can I book my appointment?'

Using a variety of techniques in the salon also creates interest, particularly if they are visually different from the norm. When clients see something unusual their curiosity is aroused and they will want to know all about it, for instance, when Molton Browner perm rods first came on to the market clients wanted a perm just to try the rods!

When selling salon services keep to the golden rule of knowing your products and what they are capable of. Never promise something that is impossible to achieve. If a particular product or service is unsuitable for the client's hair, tell them so and recommend something else. In time, when clients find that your recommendations improve their hair then they will learn to trust you and it is highly unlikely that they will take their custom elsewhere.

## Selling retail goods

When selling retail goods it is essential that the products are attractively displayed in a prominent place. Unless they are on show clients will not know exactly what is for sale. Large stores know the value of a good display stand where people can touch and try products. Remember; if a prospective buyer holds something they are more likely to buy it. The next time you go shopping look at how the goods are arranged and see what type of arrangement makes *you* stop and want to buy the products displayed.

The best place to display retail goods is in the reception area so that when the client is paying the bill they can buy the goods at the same time. Clients waiting in the reception area will also be able to look at what is displayed and people passing the salon can easily call in to purchase whatever they wish without having to go into the main body of the salon. For this reason it is a good idea to make sure that the retail display is visually attractive from the outside of the salon as well as inside.

All retail goods should be clearly marked with the price. Many people are put off buying products if they have to ask how much they are. The display should always be well-stocked and *clean*; it is surprising how dusty goods can become in a very short period of time and nothing is more off-putting to a prospective buyer than to see goods which look soiled or as if they have been on the shelf a long time. Human nature being what it is we believe that if nobody else wants them then they cannot be any good!

There are a multitude of products available for use on the hair and skin and it can be very confusing to be confronted by a vast range. Clients buying their hair products from other stores are often ignorant of what they should buy and this is where the stylists' expertise comes into its own. The stylist *knows* the clients' hair and can therefore recommend a suitable product. They also know the effects that the various products will have on the hair and these can then be explained to the client. If making a purchase at another store, the client must make a more *uninformed* choice as the assistants will not have the same amount of professional knowledge.

Often the best way to sell retail products is to use them in the salon, explaining their use when they are being put on the hair. For example:

*Stylist:* 'I am just going to put some wax on to the ends of your hair to make it fall into strands and give a more, tousled effect. I find that this particular wax is excellent for your type of hair as it counteracts any dryness and is very economical to use. In fact, we sell a great deal of this product and it is extremely popular with our clients.'

This stylist has covered several points here:

1 **introducing** the client to a new product – '. . . some wax.'
2 telling the client **where to apply** the wax for a certain effect – '. . . on to the ends of the hair.'
3 explaining to the client the **effect** it will have on the hair – '. . . make it fall into strands and give it a more tousled effect.'
4 **personalising** the product – '. . . excellent for *your* type of hair.'
5 giving some **benefits** of using the product – '. . . counteracts dryness and is very economical to use.'
6 **informing** the client that the wax is for sale – '. . . we sell a great deal of this product.'
7 **showing** that it must be effective because so many people buy it – '. . . it is extemely popular with our clients.'

Using the products in the salon has an added advantage in that the client has tried the product on their hair and therefore has an indication as to its benefits. In this way many of the products almost sell themselves.

Promotions are also an ideal way of boosting sales and there are many different ways that this can be done. For example, instead of promoting cheaper perms, why not keep the price the same but include a free specialised shampoo for home use? This will prolong the life of the perm by ensuring that the client uses the correct shampoo as well as introducing them to a new product. In addition, when the client requires more shampoo they will be more likely to purchase it from the salon than anywhere else. Other examples include selling small travel packs of the products during the summer months, or gift sets which are popular over the Christmas period. Selling two products together at a more reduced price than buying them separately or on a two for the price of one basis are also ideas for increasing sales.

## Selling techniques

If you look around your salon you will probably notice that some stylists make far more sales than others. Watch carefully how they deal with the client about what they are selling and believe firmly in the products. This brings us back to the point made earlier, that good product knowledge is essential and the best way to find out about the products is to use them yourself.

Some people seem to be born salespeople who are able to communicate easily and persuade others as if by magic. For those who find it more difficult there are certain strategies which can be used to help overcome any initial nervousness and ask questions in the most beneficial way.

To overcome initial nervousness make sure that you have enough product knowledge; this will give you confidence. Then take a deep breath and speak calmly. Remember to sound enthusiastic and positive when you talk – you will be surprised at how well the client will respond.

## Questioning

The following four types of questions are relevant to selling:

- *negative*
- *positive*
- *closed*
- *open*.

### Negative

These questions should be avoided if possible as they usually elicit a negative response from the client. For example:

*Trainee:* 'You didn't want a conditioner on your hair did you?'
*Client:* 'No.'

By saying 'You *DIDN'T* . . .' the trainee is inviting the client to say no; therefore there is no sale.

### Positive

These questions are asked in such a way as to elicit a positive response from the client. They are phrased so that it is very difficult for the client to say no. For example:

*Trainee:* 'I notice that your hair is very dry. Would you like me to use a conditioner to make it silky again?'
*Client:* 'Yes.'

In this case the client would have been unlikely not to wish to have silky hair again.

## Closed

A closed question is one which usually elicits a one word response from the client. For example:

*Trainee:* 'Is your hair dry?'
*Client:* 'Yes'.

## Open

An open question is one which will elicit a much longer response and will usually encourage the client to give a lot more information or an opinion. These types of questions are useful for finding out a lot of information about the client and their hair before making any decision as to which product to recommend. For example:

*Trainee:* 'What other treatments have you had on your hair over the past few months?'
*Client:* 'Now let me think a moment . . . it was permed before my holidays and tinted again when I got back . . .'

The client will then disclose more information to help the stylist to diagnose the hair condition and suggest a suitable treatment.

## Summary

Selling with regard to hairdressing can be divided into three main areas: selling the salon image; selling salon services; selling retail goods.

Selling the salon image concerns the visual appearance of the salon, both internally and externally, and the appearance and attitude of the staff.

Selling salon services requires a thorough knowledge of the services that the salon offers and their benefits to the client. Hairdressing manufacturers have trained, technical advisors who will demonstrate in the salon to enable staff to gain a thorough knowledge and keep up-to-date with the products used in the salon. Using a variety of visually different practical hairdressing techniques in the salon can also stimulate client interest and aid the selling process. Retail goods for sale should be prominently and attractively displayed to encourage clients to touch and smell etc. The reception area is an ideal location for the display of goods particularly if it can be seen from outside. The goods should be marked with the price and the display should be clean and well stocked, often the most effective way of selling retail products is to use them in the salon, explaining to the client their use, benefit and how they are applied. Promotions on certain products and services encourage clients to buy the goods.

There are four types of questions relevant to selling:

negative, positive, closed and open questions. Staff should avoid the use of negative and closed questions and try to concentrate on questions which are positive and open.

## Self-assessment questions

1 With regard to hairdressing, what three areas can selling be divided into?
2 How can the standard of work in a salon be improved and maintained?
3 Why is it important that salon staff look neat, smart and professional?
4 Why are staff often reluctant to use or recommend new products?
5 How can using a variety of hairdressing techniques in the salon, which are visually different, help/promote the selling of salon services?
6 What is the best place to display the retail goods and why?
7 What advantage does the stylist have over the shop assistant when selling products for the hair?
8 Name three ideas which could be used to promote and boost retail sales.
9 What strategies can be used to overcome nervousness when selling?
10 List the types of questions which are relevant to selling.

## Practical assignment – Selling

# Task

Design a poster 30 × 60 cm (12″ × 24″) to be used to promote a special offer in your salon. The special offer can be for either retail goods or salon services.

You may use any medium you wish to achieve your result, e.g. pastel, paint, crayon, ink, pictures and letters cut from magazines, stencils etc.

Sketch your ideas in rough before you start your final piece of work, it will help you to organise your ideas.

# 3 PROCESSING PAYMENTS AND STOCK CONTROL

Most salons will have their own system for keeping records of daily transactions. Computerised cash tills are now commonly used to balance stock control by allowing a constant and immediate check on any items that require reordering. Electronic cash registers (tills) have what are called **'clerk keys'** which will keep each stylists takings, and any other sundries such as sales, separate on the till roll which makes the totalling at the end of the day much easier.

However, salons without either of these systems have their own individual procedures which usually involve the checking of daily totals against the cash till receipts, client dockets, sales receipts and appointment book to ensure that there are no discrepancies.

Salons also have to have some form of **petty cash** to deal with any small items that may have to be purchased during the working day e.g. coffee, sugar etc. This may be in the form of a petty cash box or a book which lists any items purchased with a total at the end of each day. Whatever type of system is operated it is essential to keep a precise record, together with any receipts, of any cash used during the day, otherwise time can be wasted wondering why the day's takings do not add up correctly.

At the beginning of the day a set amount of small change and notes, known as a **float**, is put in the cash till. This is to make sure that there is enough change in the till should the client not give the exact amount for their service. The float must be subtracted from the days takings when 'cashing up' at the end of the day.

Remember that the handling of cash is always open to abuse by both staff and clients; therefore an efficient and effective system of cash control is essential to maintain a successful business.

## Cash transactions

All members of staff must be competent in operating the cash till, receiving cash, giving change and calculating any relevant VAT. It is also essential that staff are familiar with the varying procedures necessary to ensure the validity of client payments made by cheque, credit card, account card or gift voucher as errors in these areas can be extremely costly to the salon.

### Accepting cash payments

Great care must be taken when accepting cash from a client as mistakes can easily happen, particularly during busy periods. The short-changing of a client can cause ill-feeling and loss of future custom.

## Procedure for accepting cash payments

1 Inform the client of the charge for the service(s) they have received.
2 Check that the cash received is in the correct currency.
3 Ring up the correct amount on the cash till or computer. If the client requires change, place any paper money on the top before removing the change from the cash till to prevent any misunderstanding as to the amount given.

# Non-cash payments

Non-cash payments include cheques, credit cards and gift vouchers which are all legal tender but must be processed correctly to ensure that the salon receives payment for their services.

### Cheques

A cheque is usually paid directly into a bank account and is only transferable if the person to whom the cheque is payable signs the back of the cheque.

The writing on any cheque should be legible and must contain the following information, in ink, if it is to be accepted by the bank:

- correct date
- name of the person or salon to whom the cheque is to be paid
- amount to be paid in words as well as numbers
- signature of the person writing the cheque.

## Procedure for receiving a cheque

1 Ensure that the cheque contains the information listed above.
2 Ask to see the client's **cheque guarantee card**. This is a card issued by the bank, when used with a cheque, ensures that the bank will honour payment up to a certain amount even if the client does not have that amount in their bank account at that particular time.
3 Check that the signature on the cheque matches the signature on the guarantee card and that it is not past the expiry date.

4 Ensure that the bank name, bank code and account number is the same on both the cheque and guarantee card.
5 Write the guarantee card number on the back of the cheque.
6 Return the guarantee card to the client then place the cheque in the cash till.

## Precautions and considerations

Make sure that:

- the writing on the cheque is in ink
- the writing is legible
- any alterations are signed or initialled by the client
- the correct date has been entered
- the amount is made out in sterling
- it is not an 'open' cheque, i.e. it has the name of the person to whom it is payable written on it, otherwise it could be misused by someone else
- there are no spaces where other words could be added or altered
- the date on the cheque guarantee card is valid and not out of date.

## Credit cards

Some clients prefer to use this method of payment, particularly for large bills, as it allows them to spread payment over a period of time. However, not all salons accept credit cards, particularly smaller establishments, as a charge is made by the bank to the salon for the use of this facility. However, as with a cheque, the bank will honour the payment even if the client has insufficient funds in their account to cover the debt.

## Procedure

1 Use the imprinter and relevant voucher to duplicate the credit card details.
2 Using a pen, write in the date, description of goods, amount in words and numbers, your signature and the authorisation code.
3 The client must then sign the form in the space provided.
4 Check that the signature is the same on both the form and the credit card.
5 Check that the date on the credit card is valid.
6 Tear out the carbons then give the top copy to the client for their records and keep the remaining copies in a safe place.

## Electronic funds transfer cards (EFT)

These are the latest credit cards to come on to the market and fulfil the roles of both bank guarantee card and service card. The current account is debited electronically without the client having to write a cheque.

The card is drawn through a special terminal which then stores the details of the transaction. A two-part voucher is supplied which the client has to sign. One part is kept by the client as a record of the transaction and the other is retained by the salon. *Always* check that the signature on the voucher is the same as that on the EFT card.

### Gift vouchers

These are usually in multiples of pounds and are at their most popular during the Christmas season. Each salon will have its own system for processing gift vouchers but usually it is easier to deal with them if they are thought of as paper currency and treated as such.

### Value added tax (VAT)

Any salon with a yearly turnover of more than £25,400 must charge the client a tax, known as VAT, on all of its **services** (this does not include any sales, as retail items have any necessary VAT included in the price). This tax is then collected by the salon and returned, through certain procedures, to Governmental funds.

VAT can be included within the price of the service or may be added on to the bill at the end. At present, VAT is charged at 17.5% of the service, therefore a service costing £10.00 would incur £1.75 VAT, thus the client would pay a total of £11.75 for the service they had received.

# Banking procedures

### Paying money into an account

A **paying-in** slip is needed before money can be paid into an account. To fill in the slip correctly you will need to know the name and address of the bank holding the account, the sort code, account number, name of the account and the amount (money) to be paid in. Cheques and cash must be added up separately as well as together and the number of cheques entered in the box on the front of the slip. With this information money can be paid in at any bank and it will be credited to the account. However, if the bank is different from the one in which the account is held than a charge is usually made for the transaction.

Completing the paying-in slip before going to the bank saves time, as does dividing any coins into separate denominations e.g. 50ps; 20ps etc., then placing the correct amount of them into special bags provided by the bank. These bags can then be simply weighed by the cashier which is much quicker than having to count them.

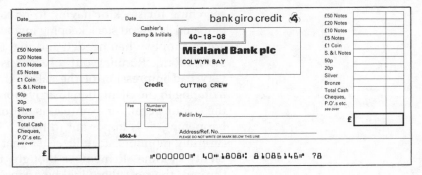

**Fig 3.1 Paying-in slip**

## Withdrawing money from an account

This can be done by using a cheque or withdrawal slip at your own bank. When withdrawing cash from any other bank, the cheque will have to be supported by a cheque guarantee card which usually has a limit of £50 or £100. Anyone with a current account can also use the Automated Teller Machine (ATM) which allows withdrawals outside banking hours and entails placing the cheque card in the machine then punching in a Personal Identification Number (PIN) before the required money is released. The amount which can be withdrawn each week is usually limited by the bank according to individual earnings.

Always keep a precise record of any withdrawals, writing down the date, amount withdrawn and to whom paid. The bank will send a statement, usually each month unless requested otherwise, and all transactions both in and out of the account should be checked. The banks are seldom wrong but they are not infallible. Make sure that there is enough money in the account to meet the amount which needs to be withdrawn. Most banks do not charge if the account remains in **credit** (i.e. has money in the account) but if it is in **debit** (i.e. has no money in the account) then the account will incur interest and handling charges. If the account is likely to be overdrawn (in debit) then arrangements must be made with the bank manager for an overdraft facility.

Mismanagement of money can be extremely costly, therefore, *always* keep very precise records of what is withdrawn and what is paid into the account. Getting used to managing money, and dealing with banks is also good grounding for future salon owners.

Mismanagement of stock can also reduce salon profits, therefore a comprehensive method of stock control which is fully explained to all the staff is necessary.

# How to ensure good stock keeping

To work efficiently in a well organised stock room with a good method of dispensing, staff should ensure that time is not wasted searching for stock or having to refuse a booking because of lack of materials. Good stock keeping involves checking that the products are in supply when needed and that they are easily located in the stock room. 'Running out' of stock is unprofessional and gives a very bad impression of the salon. In fact there is nothing more irritating to the client than to arrive for a treatment only to find that the colour/perm, for example, is out of stock. To help prevent this happening, it is important to have a system of stock control that carefully monitors stock levels so that materials can be ordered in plenty of time. Remember though, that when stock is ordered through the post there will be a lapse of several days before it is received. If stock is required immediately then it has to be obtained from a cash and carry store.

For security reasons stock that has been used is generally checked against both the appointment book and the till receipt, thus giving a double check as to when and where the stock has been used. When stock is ordered and delivered throught the post, the following system usually operates (*See* also Fig 3.2)

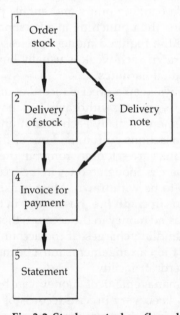

**Fig 3.2 Stock control – flow diagram**

1 New stock is ordered. A copy of this order must be kept for future reference.
2 The new stock is delivered. It is usual for the driver of the delivery van to ask for a signature to prove that the stock has been delivered safely. Before signing make sure that the merchandise is in good condition with no breakages. If there are any defects, send the whole order back and refuse to sign.
3 A **delivery note** will be found with the order when it is delivered.

The contents of this must be checked against both the **original order** and the *actual* stock delivered. This is to check that what was originally ordered has in fact been delivered.

4  An **invoice** lists the various products contained in the order, gives their price and also shows the amount of value added tax (VAT) payable. It may be included inside the order or it may be sent through the post separately. The invoice should be checked against the delivery note to make sure that the correct products are being charged for. Once checked the invoice must be kept in a safe place.

5  A **statement** is received separately and does not itemise the stock delivered: instead it simply gives the date and number of the invoice(s).

Once a statement has been received – and if there are no discrepancies between the stock ordered and the stock received – then the stock must be paid for.

The cross checking of an order in this way is very important as mistakes can often be made somewhere between the placing of the order and its actual delivery. If such a mistake should occur notify the supplier immediately otherwise all types of problems can arise over payment or deliveries etc.

When new stock has been checked it can then be entered in a stock book (if this is the method used) and then stored away. One important point is that stock must be used in rotation. Therfore the new stock should be stored in such a manner that the existing older stock is used first, otherwise some products could be unfit for use because they have deteriorated and outlived their 'shelf-life'.

## Summary

All salons have a system for keeping records of transactions, often helped by computerised cash tills. The 'float' is the amount of change put into the till at the beginning of each day which must be recorded. Petty cash must also be kept for buying small items and its use recorded.

Staff should be competent at all procedures of cash transactions. When accepting a cheque they should ensure that the date, name of the person or salon to whom payment is to be made, amount and signature are all correct and clearly written. When receiving payments by credit card they should ensure that the date is valid and that the signature on the voucher and card match. All details must be written on the voucher clearly and the top copy given to the client. Other methods of payment include electronic funds transfer (EFT) and gift vouchers. Larger salons will be required to charge clients VAT on services which may be added separately or included in the price.

When paying in money to a bank a paying-in slip must be completed. A cheque or withdrawal slip may be used to withdraw cash, or the Automated Teller Machine (ATM) may be used with a Personal Identification Number (PIN). Withdrawals must be recorded accurately; mismanagement can be costly.

Salons must also have an efficient system of stock-keeping. Stock levels must be maintained as 'running out' is unprofessional. When new stock is ordered, the order must be kept, and on delivery the contents must be checked against the original order. The invoice should be checked against the delivery note and then kept for checking against the statement. Stock rotation is important to prevent older stock from being left to outlive its 'shelf-life'.

## Self-assessment questions

1 What is the purpose of petty cash?
2 What is a 'float'?
3 What is the procedure for accepting cash payments?
4 Give eight precautions/considerations when receiving a cheque from a client.
5 If a bank account is in **debit** what does this mean?
6 What information do you need to know before you can fill in a **paying-in** slip correctly?
7 What are EFT cards?
8 Why is it necessary to check each invoice against the delivery note?

## Practical assignment – Banking

# Tasks

1 Paying cash into a bank. Your employer is extremely busy and asks you to go to the bank with the day's takings after completing a bank paying-in slip with the following amounts:

Cheques for £41.20p, £15.00, £25.80, £35.00, £7.50 and £18.00; £30.00 in £1 coins; £115.00 in £5 notes; £60 in £10 notes; £20 in Silver; £1.50 in Bronze.

On the paying-in slip below and top right show how you would

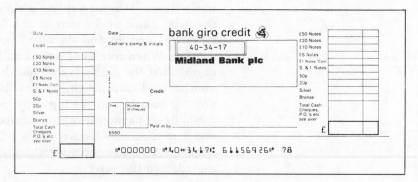

Fig 3.3 Front of a paying-in slip

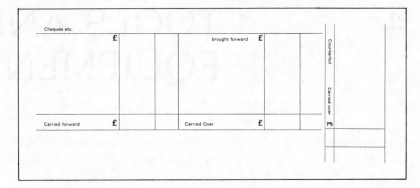

**Fig 3.4 Reverse of a paying-in slip**

enter the above amounts both on the front and reverse sides of the slip. What is the total amount to be paid into the bank?

2 Writing a cheque. You have to pay a telephone bill of £162.98p to British Telecom plc. Fill in the cheque below with all the relevant information.

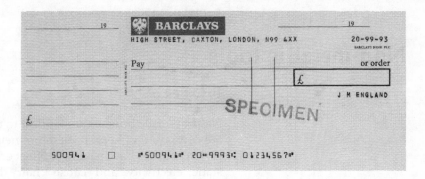

**Fig 3.5 Cheque**

# 4 TOOLS AND EQUIPMENT

Hairdressing tools should be chosen with care if they are to give good and lasting service. They can be separated into two groups:

- non-metallic tools
- metallic tools.

## Non-metallic tools

### Brushes

Natural bristle brushes are kindest to the hair. Both hair and bristle are composed of keratin therefore neither wears against the other. Nylon brushes have a harsher effect on the hair and tend to increase static electricity and cause 'hair fly' but they are useful in hairdressing because they are easily cleaned and sterilised, thus cutting down on the risk of infection between clients.

The bristles of any brush should have even tufts or rows to allow loose, shed hair to collect in the grooves without interfering with the action of the bristles. If the bristle tufts are spaced too close together they will not penetrate the hair meshes.

### Types of brushes

There are many different types of brushes and the choice depends upon the task the brush is used for and upon personal preference. The three main types are listed below:

1 *General purpose brush.* These are made in various shapes and sizes. They can be half, three-quarters or full round. Natural bristle is recommended because of its more gentle action. Used mainly when dressing the hair and for everyday brushing of the hair.

2 *Styling brush.* Used when blowdrying the hair, these can be obtained in various sizes and shapes depending upon the result

required. Nylon, bristle or a combination of both is the material used.
3 *Neck brush.* These are used to remove the loose hairs from the
face and neck after cutting the hair. Made from bristle, nylon or a
combination of both.

## Combs

There are a variety of combs that have been engineered to aid the
dressing, disentangling or setting of hair. Whichever type of comb
is used it should be made of a sturdy, durable material which will
not create static electricity and must also be easy to sterilise after
it is used. Vulcanite is the material used in the manufacturing of
most hairdressing combs as it fits all these requirements and is not
as expensive as some other materials such as ivory.

The teeth of the comb should have rounded points with a fine
taper and there should be adequate space between them where they
join the base. Combs with broken or irregular teeth should not be
used as they may scratch the scalp or tear the hair.

### Types of combs

Combs can be obtained in many shapes and sizes, the most common
of which are:

1 *Tail comb.* This comb has fine teeth. The tail part of the comb can
be made of the same material as the teeth or it can have a thin metal,
stiletto tail (known as a pin-tail comb). Care must be taken when
using a pin-tail comb as the tail is almost like a fine knitting needle
and if used carelessly it can stab either the client or the operator.

Tail combs are for sectioning, lifting or weaving the hair. Never
use the tail comb for disentangling the hair as the teeth are too fine.
2 *Dressing comb.* Dressing combs have a fine end and a rake end
and can be obtained in various sizes according to individual
preference. They are used for disentangling and dressing of hair.

The wide teeth of a dressing comb are usually used to smooth and
mold the hair into the desired shape. There are many sizes of
dressing combs to choose from and the stylist should choose
whichever is the most comfortable to handle. Very large dressing
combs are more difficult to use but are ideal when there is a lot of
volume and for backcombing in the hair as it smooths the hair into
shape very quickly and easily without flattening or removing too
much of the backcombing.

There are various other dressing combs available; some are
specially adapted to incorporate larger teeth at one end to smooth
the hair, and prongs at the other end to lift the hair if necessary,
thus incorporating the duties of both dressing comb and tail comb.
Other combs have been designed to aid backcombing by having
alternate long and short teeth.
3 *Cutting comb.* Smaller and thinner than other combs, it is more

pliable and allows the hair to be cut nearer to the scalp; for example men's graduation, short back and sides, shingle, etc.

4 *Setting comb.*  This comb also has a fine and a rake end, usually smaller than a dressing comb and can also be used by the stylist when finger waving.

5 *Afro comb.*  These combs are very thick with large teeth which are ideal for creating volume without frizz on extremely curly or Afro-Caribbean hair when the curl needs to be sustained throughout the style.

# Metallic tools

These include:

- scissors
- razors
- clippers
- styling irons
- hot brushes.

## Scissors

These may be obtained in a variety of lengths and weights. The choice of length and weight is entirely up to the individual but it is important that the scissors feel comfortable. When purchasing a new pair of scissors, test them first by holding between the thumb and the third finger, as this is how they should be held when cutting the hair – they should feel as if they are an extension of the fingers.

Hairdressing scissors should only be used for cutting hair. Using them for cutting string, paper etc., will blunt the blades very quickly and blunt blades will tear the hair. They should always be used by the same person and should not be dropped on the floor as this can alter the balance.

### Types of scissors

1 *Plain straight edged.*  Used for normal cutting including both club and taper cutting techniques. The longer blade lengths are used in men's haircutting. (*See* Fig. 4.1).

2 *Very fine serrated edge.*  These scissors are intended to be self-sharpening. They can be used for all cutting techniques except when 'slither cutting' the hair, e.g. taper cutting or slide cutting. In this case the finely serrated edge of the scissors tends to drag on the hair and does not cut it as cleanly as the straight edged scissors.

3 *Wide spaced serrated edge.*  These are known as aesculap scissors. Either one blade or both blades are serrated to allow a limited amount of hair only to be cut. This type of scissor is usually used to remove bulk or weight from the hair, i.e. thinning. However, there are many

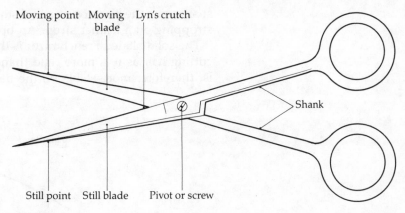

**Fig 4.1**

different types of aesculap scissors, some designed to remove far more hair than others. The choice of aesculap depends upon the required result and also the stylist's own personal preference. They must only be used on dry hair – if used on wet hair they can remove too much bulk as the wet hairs tend to stick together. (*See* Fig. 4.2).

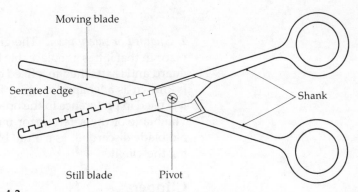

**Fig 4.2**

## Razors

Razors are used to cut wet hair.

## Types of razors

There are two types

- open
- guarded or safety razor

*1 Open razor.* An open, or cut-throat, razor requires far more attention than a safety razor and is more commonly used in men's hairdressing salons than in ladies'. The blade of the razor must be kept very sharp, by what is known as **razor setting**. This involves sharpening the blade on a special stone, known as a **hone**, and then stropping on a leather **strop**. An open razor is shown in Fig. 4.3.

The solid bladed French razor is the most suitable open razor for cutting hair as it is more rigid than the hollow-ground razor and is, therefore, more stable on the hair.

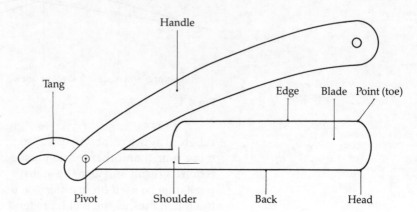

**Fig 4.3**

2 *Guarded or safety razor.* The guarded razor differs from the open razor in that it has a replaceable blade which is protected by a metal guard and is attached to a fixed or movable handle. It is either what is known as a 'shaper' razor or it is shaped like an open razor, and it is used in preference to the open razor by most present day salons. The blade of the safety razor must be changed frequently and the old blade discarded, as a blunt blade will tear the hair and is painful for the client.

## Clippers

There are two types of clippers: hand clippers and electric clippers. Both types consist of two blades with sharp edged teeth. One blade remains fixed while the other moves across it. The distance between the blade teeth determines the closeness of the haircut. Used in men's and ladies' haircutting to produce very short haircuts.

## Styling irons

There are two types: modern electrically heated and Marcel waving irons. Both types can be obtained in various sizes and are used on dry hair.

The Marcel types are marked 'A' to 'D'. 'A' is the smallest barrel size and 'D' is the largest.

Electrically heated styling irons include:
(a) *hair tongs* – round and usually obtained in small, medium and

large sizes and used to create curl or movement, e.g. after blowdrying, between sets, etc.

*(b) crimping irons* – specifically designed to produce a crimped effect on the hair.

*(c) straightening irons* – originally designed to temporarily straighten Afro-Caribbean hair but now also used on Caucasian (European) hair to produce straight or flattened results.

Both Marcel and modern irons are obtained already tempered. Tempering is done to harden the metal and to allow the irons to be more receptive to heat.

### Hot brushes

These work on the same principle and have the same use as round styling irons except that instead of just a smooth electrically heated barrel, the hot brush also has vulcanite prongs attached that act as a brush. Thus the hair can be combed and curled into position more easily.

### Pressing combs

There are two types of pressing combs: electrical and non-electrical. The comb has metal prongs (steel or brass) and a wooden or vulcanite handle. These are used to temporarily straighten afro-caribbean and extremely curly hair. The comb is heated then combed through the hair.

# Sterilisation of tools

Sterilisation means the destruction of all living things including the harmful micro-organisms that cause disease ('germs'). These can be passed from one person to another (transmitted) in the salon on tools and equipment particularly razors, scissors and clippers. There is some risk with *all* tools and equipment such as brushes, combs, clips, towels etc.

Sterilisation is only really possible by using an autoclave. Autoclaves work by using steam under pressure (like a pressure cooker) at high temperatures, 125°C for example, which is sufficient to kill *all* micro-organisms in about five minutes. Autoclaves have not been widely used in salons but their use is spreading as cheap automatic autoclaves enter the market.

# Disinfection of tools

Disinfection means reducing the chances of infection and techniques for this are widespread in hairdressing. They include:

- Chemicals
- Ultraviolet rays
- Heat – dry or moist

## Chemicals

These can either destroy or retard the growth of micro-organisms. A chemical which destroys micro-organisms is called a **disinfectant** (bacteriocide or germicide). The problems with disinfectants include:

- they rapidly go 'off' and cease to work efficiently
- they become 'overloaded' and cease to work efficiently
- some are poisonous to humans
- some attack tools, particularly metal tools.

If they are used for washing down walls, upholstery and surfaces, the best type to use are **alcohol** based but this can cause problems as alcohol is a *fire risk* as it is *inflammable*. Sterilising cabinets are still used in some salons but these suffer from all the problems listed for disinfectant.

Current thinking is that disinfectants are *not* recommended for reducing the risk of infection by tools.

## Ultraviolet rays

These are used in ultraviolet 'sterilisers' which do *not* 'sterilise' but only act as a disinfectant.

The cabinet contains a mercury vapour tube which is situated at the top of the cabinet enabling the ultraviolet rays that it gives off to fall and sterilise the equipment placed beneath them. As the rays cannot penetrate the equipment they must be 'turned' to ensure complete destruction of the bacteria.

Ultraviolet radiation can cause burns to the skin with continual exposure; therefore most of these cabinets have some form of lid that shields the hands of the operator when tools have to be removed from the cabinet.

## Heat

Very high temperatures are used in the **autoclave** which is the *only* current method of efficiently sterilising tools and equipment. Other methods which use lower temperatures to 'disinfect' rather than sterilise are:

*Dry heat* in glass bead sterilisers which are useful in the salon. The higher the temperature the shorter time tools need to be left in and the time to reach their operating temperature. Only the part of the tools covered by the beads will be treated and although good for tools such as scissors, they are less effective with clipper blades.

*Moist heat* is used in autoclaves and boilers/steamers. Autoclaves as explained on p. 39 work under pressure at high temperatures. Boiling or steaming works at 100°C and does not kill all micro-organisms. It is useful to reduce the chances of infection (disinfection) but not destroy all infection. Tools should be steamed or boiled for at *least* ten minutes.

# Care and maintenance of tools

## Non-metallic tools

### Brushes

Brushes should be kept as clean and sterile as possible. When not in use they should be kept in a sterilising cabinet.

*Method of cleaning*
1  Comb brush free from hair with a wide tooth comb and remove any other loose particles from the bristles and base of the brush.
2  Fill a basin with lukewarm water and add a cleaning fluid (do not use too strong a cleaning fluid as this can damage the brush).
3  With the bristles pointing downwards, swish the brush about on top of the water. Do not immerse wooden brushes in the water as it will crack the protective coating of varnish and split the wood.
4  Rinse carefully in clean water to which some disinfectant has been added.
5  Towel dry the handle and base of the brush and pat the bristles on a towel to remove excess moisture.
6  Leave the brush to dry face downwards on a clean towel.
7  When dry, place in an ultraviolet disinfecting cabinet.

### Combs

Combs should be thoroughly cleaned regularly to prevent loose flakes of skin and other debris lodging between the teeth of the comb at the base. When not in use and after use on each client, combs should be kept completely submerged in an antiseptic solution of the correct strength or in the sterilising cabinet.

*Method of cleaning*
1  Brush combs with either a nail brush or a special comb brush to remove loose debris.
2  Fill a basin with lukewarm water and cleaning fluid, as for cleaning brushes.
3  Immerse combs for several minutes to loosen any grease or oil particles.
4  Scrub combs on each side individually with a nail brush.
5  Rinse in lukewarm water to which some disinfectant has been added.

6   Dry thoroughly and place in sterilising cabinet or in antiseptic solution.

*NB* It is not always necessary to use disinfectant in the rinsing water if the brushes and combs are being placed immediately into the ultraviolet disinfecting cabinet.

## Metallic tools

### Scissors

These should be carefully looked after and always kept sharp. Remember the following points to ensure that they are always in good working order.

1   Always dry after use on wet hair.
2   Keep away from strong chemicals, e.g. permanent wave solution, bleach etc.
3   They should not be dropped as this can alter the balance and could loosen the pivot or screw.
4   Each pair of scissors should be used by only one person. If the same pair of scissors is used by everybody it blunts the blades very quickly.
5   Never use them for anything except to cut hair.
6   They should only be sharpened by experts.
7   Sterilise by wiping carefully with spirit then placing them in the sterilising cabinet for the recommended time.
8   The pivots should be treated with lubricating oil from time to time to prevent stiffness.
9   Store away from dust as this is a source of possible infection.

### Razors

For both safety and open razors:

1   Always dry after use, otherwise the metal will rust.
2   Keep away from permanent wave solution, bleach or any other strong chemicals.
3   Sterilise by placing them in a sterilising cabinet for the recommended time after wiping with spirit.

Open razors must be kept sharp by **stropping** on a leather strop, or by **honing** on a special stone known as a hone.
Safety razors must have the blades changed regularly to ensure that the razor is always sharp.

### Clippers

Both types of clippers are cleaned in the same manner but when using electric clippers check also for frayed wires, faulty plugs etc., before using.

*Method of cleaning*

1 Remove all loose hairs with a tissue or piece of flannel.
2 Remove any grease with surgical spirit.
3 Lubricate joints with a lubricating oil.
4 Place in a sterilising cabinet for the recommended time.

## Styling irons

Remove any grease or stains with surgical spirit then place in a sterilising cabinet. Electrical styling irons should be checked for frayed wires and faulty plugs.

*NB* Metal tools should not be left in a vapour-type sterilising cabinet for too long, as the chemicals used in these cabinets can cause corrosion.

**Table 4.1  Summary**

| Tools | Type | Use |
|---|---|---|
| Brushes | General purpose | For dressing and everyday brushing of hair |
| | Styling | When blowdrying the hair |
| | Neck | To remove cut hair from face and neck |
| Combs | Tail comb | Sectioning, lifting, weaving, never disentangling |
| | Dressing comb | Disentangling and dressing the hair |
| | Cutting comb | More pliable than other combs, used when cutting |
| | Setting comb | When setting and finger waving |
| | Afro comb | To style and dress curly hair, e.g. Afro-Caribbean |
| Scissors | Plain straight edged | For all cuttng techniques |
| | Very fine serrated edge | For all cutting exept slither cutting techniques |
| | Wide spaced serrated edge (aesculap) | To thin hair; used on dry hair only |
| Razors | Open | Used mainly in men's hairdressing to cut wet hair and in shaving |
| | Safety razor | Same use as the open razor but has changeable guarded blade |
| Clippers | Hand (manual) and Electric | In men's and ladies' hairdressing to cut hair close to scalp |
| Hot brush | | To temporarily curl dry hair |
| Styling irons | Electrically heated | To temporarily curl, straighten or crimp dry hair |
| | Marcel waving | When Marcel waving |
| Pressing combs | Electrically heated and non-electrical | To straighten Afro hair |

## Pressing combs

Rub the teeth of the comb with an emery board to remove any grease and stains then wipe over with surgical spirit. Check electrical pressing combs for frayed wires and faulty plugs.

**Self-assessment questions**

1 Which type of brush tufts are kindest to the hair?
2 What is the main disadvantage of brushes with nylon tufts?
3 Why are combs with broken or irregular teeth unsuitable for salon use?
4 What is the most suitable material for hairdressing combs;
5 What is the name given to a tail comb with a thin, metal, stiletto tail?
6 Why should a tail comb not be used for disentangling the hair?
7 Which type of open razor has a solid blade?
8 What is the name given to scissors with a wide spaced serrated edge?
9 Which type of razor has a guarded changeable blade?
10 Why is it unsatisfactory to leave metal tools in the sterilising cabinet for too long?

**Practical assignment – Tools**

Using the correct tools for a certain task is very important as it will enable you to work more efficiently. This assignment has been devised to help you to identify the range of available tools and equipment for use in the salon.

## Scenario

You are in the process of buying your own salon and need to choose the necessary tools and equipment.

## Tasks

1 Make a list of all the tools and equipment that are used in your work placement and/or training salon.
2 Collect illustrations or photographs of a selection of *each* type of tool and equipment including any extra or new equipment which may be available.
3 Cut out and mount the illustrations. Print a brief summary under the illustration, of the use of each.
4 Present your work neatly in the form of a folio.

# 5 SALON SAFETY, HEALTH AND FIRST AID

A large hairdressing salon on a busy day may have over one hundred clients using the premises. Most of those people will be concerned only with the finished style and few, if any, will give any thought to the possible *hazards* in the salon. The hairdresser needs to be much more aware of these so that whenever possible accidents or infections can be prevented. To some extent both the hairdresser and the client can be put at risk from a number of possible sources. These can be grouped into:

1  *Physical hazards* which include:
   (*a*) physical injury (e.g. cuts and knocks)
   (*b*) fire and heat burns
   (*c*) electricity (e.g. electric shock)
2  *Chemical hazards* which involve:
   (*a*) chemical burns (including chemicals on the skin and the eyes
   (*b*) storage and disposal of chemicals (e.g. hydrogen peroxide and aerosol containers)
   (*c*) dermatitis or eczema (e.g. from hair dyes).
3  *Biological hazards* which can be:
   (*a*) infections – caused by micro-organisms (germs), e.g. impetigo
   (*b*) infestations – caused by animal parasites, e.g. head lice.

Hairdressers have a responsibility to protect themselves and their clients in both a moral sense, in that it is wrong to cause pain or discomfort, and in a practical way, due to:

   (*a*) the **legal responsibilities** placed on the salon owner and worker;
   (*b*) the **bad publicity** which results from accidents or infections taking place in the salon.

An outline of the legal requirements for health and safety is given overleaf.

# The legal requirements for health and safety in the salon

This is a fairly complicated area and changes often take place. There are three main legal areas of importance to hairdressing. (A detailed treatment is beyond the scope of this book, but these regulations are summarised in *Croner's Reference Book for Self-employed and Smaller businesses*.)

## Offices, Shops and Railway Premises Act (1963)

This Act has a number of health and welfare provisions. These include adequate lighting, ventilation, toilet, washing and eating facilities. It requires that floors, passageways and stairs be uncluttered and that the floor covering is 'sound', i.e. will not cause people to trip. There is a general requirement for cleanliness, in that floors and steps must be swept or washed at least once a week and furniture and fittings must be kept clean. The temperature should be between a minimum of 16°C and a maximum of 19°C.

## Health and Safety at Work Act (1974)

This has partly, but not completely, replaced the 1963 Act above. It extends to virtually all working situations and sets out the responsibilities of both the employer and the employee in terms of:

1  general health and safety
2  first aid arrangements and reporting of accidents
3  enforcement of the Act.

## General health and safety

- The duties of the *employer* include:

  (*a*) care and maintenance of equipment
  (*b* prevention of risk in the storage and use of materials
  (*c*) instruction and training employees in safe practices
  (*d*) maintaining the place of work so that it is safe
  (*e*) with five or more employees, the employer needs to produce a written policy statement in terms of the general policy operated concerning health and safety. An example of one of these which was written for a hairdressing salon, is shown in Fig. 5.1.

- For the *employee* the duties are:

  (*a*) to take reasonable care for the health and safety of themselves and others who may be affected by their actions;
  (*b*) to co-operate with the employer (or others) to ensure health and safety at work.

### Statement of health and safety

**1  Objectives** – to:

1.1  Provide healthy and safe working conditions, ensure that working processes are carried out safely and involve staff in meeting these objectives.

1.2  Ensure compliance with changes in legal requirements

1.3  Train staff, so that safe working methods will be used within their own working environment.

1.4  Ensure that health and safety factors are fully taken into account when new machinery or processes are introduced, or any changes in existing premises are considered.

1.5  Ensure that first aid facilities are available.

**2  Specific arrangements**

2.1  Endeavour to eliminate environmental hazards and encourage hazard reporting by the staff.

2.2  Look into conditions and practices reported to be unsafe and investigate accidents.

2.3  Publish general safety rules.

2.4  Ensure employees receive adequate safety instructions.

2.5  Make provision for fire prevention, fire fighting and fire evacuation procedures.

2.6  Maintain an emergency evacuation system.

2.7  Insist on the wearing of protective clothing by staff where necessary.

2.8  Maintain accident reporting procedure, recording any statistics.

2.9  Endeavour to comply with Local Authority general safety documents.

**3 Responsibility – to all staff**

All staff can be reasonably called upon to share a responsibility for health, safety and welfare:

(*a*) to establish a safe and healthy environment throughout the salon;

(*b*) to establish and maintain safe working procedures among fellow workers;

(*c*) to teach safety where relevant;

(*d*) to create awareness, involvement and participation via consultation, so as to develop safety consciousness and self-responsibility.

Fig 5.1

While it is generally accepted that a sharing of responsibility is ideal, nevertheless, it is important to identify the different levels of responsibility.
These are as follows:

**3A Senior staff**
3.1  To aim at operating a safety awareness within the salon.
3.2  To ensure one is fully aware of safe working conditions and practices.
3.3  To instigate and participate in accident investigations.
3.4  To have authority to halt unsafe operations and practices in consultation with the proprietor.
3.5  To administer salon safety policy with the salon.
3.6  To have initial responsibility for ensuring the health and safety of the remaining staff.
3.7  To ensure clear instructions and warnings are given.
3.8  To provide safety guidance.
3.9  To follow safe working procedures personally.
3.10  To maintain the use of protective clothing, special safe-working rules and procedures.
3.11  To encourage safety participation and hazard reporting by staff.
3.12  To ensure safety, accidents should be reported and recorded and conveyed to the proprietor.
3.13  To make herself/himself and other users of the building aware of the action to be taken in the case of fire.

**3B Employees general**
3.14  To have personal responsibility for the health and safety of self, colleagues and others.
3.15  To observe safe standards of behaviour, dress, and protective clothing as required.
3.16  To use (and not wilfully misuse, neglect or damage, nor interfere with) the apparatus, equipment and protective clothing provided for their health and safety.
3.17  To participate in any safety training programmes.

**Fig. 5.1** *(cont'd)*

## First aid arrangements and reporting of accidents

The Act lists recommendations for **first aid kits** (*See* Table 5.1) and also requires:

(*a*) notification of serious injury, death or incapacitation for three working days, as a result of an accident and that a record be kept of these;

(b)  a written record be kept of all accidents in an **accident record book**, which list the sex, age and occupation of the victim and the nature of the accident and date of first absence from work (if this applies).

The Act also lists 'dangerous occurrences' and recommends that these must be reported and a record kept.

## Enforcement of the Act

Enforcement is carried out by Area Offices of the Health and Safety Executive by means of Health and Safety Inspectors. These have the right of entry to premises and the power to:

(a)  order improvements to be made
(b)  prohibit the use of apparatus or premises
(c)  seize, render harmless or destroy dangerous equipment.

## Control of substances hazardous to health (COSHH – 'cosh')

This regulation is concerned with **chemical** hazards. The main principles of these regulations (which took effect on 1st Jan 1990) are:

1  Assessment of risk from substances – much of this depends on information supplied by manufacturer.
2  Provision, use and upkeep of adequate control measure for chemicals – the main point is to prevent exposure if practicable or have adequate control.
3  Monitoring exposure of employees to potential hazards.
4  Health surveillance of employees – this means monitoring the health of people exposed to potential hazards.
5  Education and training of employees – for example, in terms of

(a)  purpose of personal protective clothing
(b)  how to avoid endangering themselves and others
(c)  storage and disposal
(d)  emergency procedures.

## Local bye-laws and other regulations

### Local bye-laws

These vary in different parts of the country but often:

(a)  involve registration of the salon with the local Environmental Health Department so that periodic checks by Environmental Health Officers can be made;
(b) overlap with other regulations in requiring adequate ventilation in toilet and washing facilities, general cleanliness etc.

## Other regulations

The regulations particularly important in the salon are:

● *Employers' Liability (Compulsory Insurance) Act (1969)* which requires employers to take out insurance on themselves and their employees for accidents to themselves and clients. The policies for hairdressing salons include a 'dyes' clause for staff or clients developing dermatitis due to exposure to the 'para' group of hairdyes. The Certificate of Insurance must be displayed in the premises.

● *Fire Precautions Act (1971)* which is enforced by the local Fire Authority, e.g. County Fire Brigade. This requires premises where more than twenty (or ten on one floor) people work at one time to be granted a fire certificate. For premises involving fewer people there is still a requirement that:

(a) room contents be arranged and doors left unlocked to enable a rapid exit in case of fire.

(b) fire-fighting equipment, suitable for the type of fires likely to occur, is in good repair and readily available.

## Routine hygiene practices and procedures

The salon should always be kept clean and tidy. Well-trained staff should automatically tidy any dirty areas. A salon which has hair all over the floor and dirty towels strewn about the place is very off-putting to the client and looks inefficient. A strict code of hygiene should exist, even during busy periods – bacteria thrive in the warm, moist atmosphere of the salon, and therefore risk to the client must be reduced to the minimum.

Training apprentices/trainees from the beginning to be neat and tidy, to clean up immediately and to keep equipment as sterile as possible produces an awareness of salon hygiene. These good habits will then endure through to when they are managers or salon owners themselves and this professional attitude can only be of benefit to the hairdressing industry in general.

Familiarity breeds contempt, and it is all too easy when working day to day in the same familiar surroundings not to notice that towels are becoming grubby and threadbare or that the salon requires redecorating. Try to take a detached or objective view of your surroundings, or get someone else in hairdressing to criticise the appearance and operation of the salon.

One point to be noted: a hairdresser works with hair and is therefore used to handling it and seeing it about. Clients feel differently – other people's hair in the wrong place can make them feel a little sick! Remember, try to see things from the client's point of view.

## Areas of cleanliness to note

(a) *Shop floor.* The floor should be swept and mopped each day and never left untidy. Cut hair should be swept up immediately. Check that all floor covering is sound. Any loose tiles, lino, carpet etc., can be dangerous to staff and clients.

(b) *Reception area.* This should be kept clean and tidy with a cloakroom or rack for the clients' coats, away from the main salon. If there is a retail sales area, the items for sale should be attractively displayed with the prices clearly marked and the display dusted regularly.

(c) *Work tops.* These should be kept free of litter, e.g. empty setting lotion bottles etc., and tidied up after each client. They should be wiped over regularly and kept free from dust.

(d) *Mirrors.* They should be cleaned every day and lacquer stains removed immediately with a lacquer solvent, such as methylated spirit or alcohol, e.g. surgical spirit. Back mirrors also need cleaning regularly to remove any lacquer stains or finger prints.

(e) *Towels and gowns.* Dirty towels should be placed in a linen basket after use and should not litter the salon. Clean towels only should be used on the client and any towels with holes in them are to be discarded or recycled as cleaning cloths etc.

Gowns should be laundered regularly and kept fresh and clean.

(f) *Rollers and brushes.* These should be washed and disinfected regularly to remove any stains from temporary rinses, flakes of dried skin, setting agents, etc. Any hair that has been caught in the rollers or brushes should be removed before washing.

(g) *Trolleys.* Trays and trolleys should be cleaned at the end of each working day and the feet of the trolleys should be checked to make sure that loose hair has not been caught in them.

(h) *Magazines.* Keep all magazines tidy and discard any that become 'tatty' looking. All magazines should be kept up-to-date and it is often a good idea to have a selection of hairstyle magazines for the clients to browse through.

(i) *Wash bowls.* Wash bowls and fittings should be kept cleaned and wiped over after each shampoo. Front wash bowls must be disinfected regularly to prevent unpleasant odours. Waste traps on the bowls prevent airborne germs from getting into the salon atmosphere. They should be checked once a week to prevent blockage and any trapped hair should be removed. The waste pipes can be treated with sodium carbonate (washing soda) and boiling water. Loose hair blocking the plug hole of the bowls is always a problem in salons, but special hair traps can be used to help prevent blockage. The hair should, however, be removed from these traps after each shampoo.

## Checking and maintaining equipment and tools

Properly maintained equipment can give long and good service.

- Every client should have a clean brush and comb used on their hair. Combs should be kept in antiseptic and brushes in a sterilising cabinet.
- Chairs should be kept clean and free from hair. A vinyl covering makes cleaning easier. They should be wiped down every day, including the backs of the chairs and the legs as these tend to get splashed with lotions. Any splitting or tearing of the material must be attended to immediately to avoid it getting worse.
- Light fittings should be kept clean. It is important that the salon is well lit from all angles.
- Dryers do long duty hours. If kept clean and dust free, the wear and tear on them is kept to a minimum. Regularly unscrew the top and remove dust and fluff from the fan, otherwise there is a real risk of fire. Arrange a yearly contract for servicing – there are firms that specialise in this service.
- Steamers and infra-red lamps should be cleaned after use. Always ensure that the water bottle on the steamer has enough water in it before use (distilled water should be used) and the steamer should be cleaned out regularly. Infra-red bulbs should be checked before use and any faulty bulbs replaced. Servicing once a year will prolong the life of this equipment and maintain its safety of use.
- Vapour and ultraviolet cabinets. Make sure that the vapour steriliser cabinet is checked each day and refilled with sterilising solution. Keep cabinets clean inside and out.

*Important points concerning electrical appliances:*

Always unplug all electrical equipment before cleaning. Never let junior staff begin to clean until all plugs have been checked as being out of their sockets.

Check all electrical equipment regularly for frayed wires and faulty plugs. All electrical equipment must be unplugged at the end of each working day.

Get apparatus professionally checked and maintained. This will prolong the lifetime of the appliance and the safety of its use.

(j) *Window display.* This is an important feature, as it can attract new clients to the salon. The glass must be kept clean inside and out and any display should be kept clean and changed regularly to attract attention.

## Safe practices in the salon

Safety is mainly concerned with preventing accidents, infections and infestations occurring in the salon. These may be caused by one or more of the following hazards:

- physical
- chemical
- biological.

Any account of safe practice has to be very much an outline, dealing with major points only and what follows deals with some of the common hazards and how to avoid them.

## Physical hazards

These can be divided into *three* main areas:

- physical injuries
- fire and heat burns
- electricity.

### Physical injuries

Include:

1  *Wounds caused by scissors and razors.*  By their design, scissors and razors are sharp. Scissors can cause **nicks** or **puncture** wounds if pushed in points first. Scissors should *always* be carried with the points inwards and razors should *never* be carried open. Both scissors and razors should be cleaned by wiping them in a direction away from the body. Make sure scissors and razors are out of the reach of children in the salon.

2  *Tripping and falling.*  There are two common causes for this:

- loose or broken floor coverings; these should be in good condition
- trailing electric flexes; you risk not only tripping over them but the tug of the flex can cause electrical faults. There is also the danger that the pull on the flex can cause the electrical appliance supplied by it to topple over and hurt someone.

3  *Knocks.*  These can be caused by a variety of reasons, often as a result of another accident, e.g. someone collapsing after an electric shock. They can also be due to:

- equipment collapsing onto a client, e.g. infra-red octopus or steamers, when someone bumps into them or trips over the flex.
- equipment being cleaned; there is a risk of pushing it over while cleaning it. Many salon driers have strong springs in their stands and if the drier is removed for cleaning and the spring released, the stand flies upwards with considerable force. This may strike someone cleaning the stand.

### Fire

There are two main causes of *fire* in salons: smoking and electrical faults.

Fires due to **smoking** can be caused by:

- lighted cigarettes falling on to the floor, into seating, etc.

- ashtrays with still smouldering cigarettes being thrown into rubbish bins.

There is also a risk of fire if people smoke near a client whose hair is being sprayed with lacquer. Never allow a client to smoke when using any kind of aerosol spray on their hair.

**Electrical faults** may result in cables or electrical appliances (or both) overheating – this happens particularly if the wrong size of *fuse* is fitted. Fuses work as a deliberate 'weak' link of thin wire in an electrical circuit. They are designed to melt and break the circuit if the flow of electrical current produces too much heat in the circuit they protect. If fuses with too thick fuse wire are used then these take longer to melt. This means that the heating effect on the electrical circuit is greater. If this is the case cable insulation can start to smoulder, plugs melt and electrical apparatus catch fire. It is very important for electrical safety that electric circuits, plugs, flexes and electrical equipment be regularly checked by an expert.

*NB* It is possible to arrange for a regular maintenance contract.

Faults develop even when apparatus is not in use, so it is important to remember to unplug electrical equipment at night.

*How to react in case of a fire in the salon*
A good exercise is to carry out fire drills in order to know what to do during a real fire alert. In the event of a fire you must:

- stay calm
- ensure everybody gets out of the salon
- send someone to ring the fire service
- depending on the nature and extent of the fire, decide whether to tackle it or not (if in doubt do not). Remember that aerosol spray cans and hydrogen peroxide containers will explode if sufficiently heated.
- try to turn off the main electrical supply. If this is not possible (or uncertain) do not use water to try to put out the fire. Water is a **good conductor** of electricity and electricity flowing through it could deliver an **electric shock**. It is best not to use water at all in the salon because of this problem. The salon should have at least one suitable fire extinguisher. Use it to put the fire out.

*Fire extinguishers*
These are produced in a number of forms, some of which are more suitable for salon use than others. The main types are:

- Fire blankets – which are thrown over a fire to smother it.
- Water and foam extinguishers – these work by carbon dioxide gas forcing water or foam from the extinguisher, through a nozzle which can be directed at the fire. These are not suitable for use in situations where the water or foam could come into contact

with electricity. Both could act as conductors and lead to electric shock.

- Carbon dioxide gas extinguishers – these consist of a cylinder of carbon dioxide gas under great pressure. When released the gas rushes out of a nozzle. The main problem is that once the gas clears, oxygen can get to any remaining smouldering material which could then burst into flames.
- Dry powder extinguishers – these are good for salon use. The carbon dioxide gas forces a fine white powder from the nozzle which coats the burning material and so prevents oxygen from reaching it after the extinguisher is switched off. The absence of foam or water means it can be used on electrical appliances.

## Heat burns

These can be caused by apparatus overheating and by fire but are more common in the salon when:

- using a blow drier too close to a client's scalp
- touching the skin with curling tongs or crimping irons
- touching the hot lamps of infra-red octopus lamps
- overheating steamers.

The only real prevention is to be aware of the risk and to be careful while using the apparatus.

## Electricity

People can be at risk for two different reasons:

- *Overheating* and possibly fire in cables and apparatus – the fitting of the correct fuse plugs and fuse boxes is important, as is regular and expert checking of plugs, cables and electrical equipment (*see* the section on fire on p. 54). It is important not to overload a circuit.
- *Electric shock,* which involves electricity flowing through a person's body. The amount of electricity and hence the severity of the electric shock depends on:

  (*a*) the **voltage** and **current** of the electrical supply involved
  (*b*) the **electrical resistance** between the person and the item from which they receive the shock.

The electricity supplied to and used in most salons has a voltage of 240 volts and a current of 13 amps. This is sufficient to produce a severe shock, especially if the electrical resistance between the person's body and the item causing the shock is low. A good example of this is when wet hands are used to plug in, switch on, or handle electrical apparatus. Water is a conductor of electricity and this lowers the resistance between a person and whatever they are touching. The water could also get inside plugs, sockets, switches and equipment and conduct (carry) the electricity into a person. Therefore, always use dry hands to plug in, switch on or handle electrical equipment.

A further factor in the amount of electricity received by the body is the **earthing** of equipment. In outline, the function of the earth (E) cable is to carry electricity from the metal outer casing of electrical equipment into the earth (or ground). This provides an easy route for electricity to flow and it will take this path rather than pass through the person's body and produce an electric shock.

Regular and expert checking is important to detect faults likely to cause electric shocks and to ensure that the earthing circuit is functioning properly.

## Background to electricity

Before looking at using electricity *safely* here is a little detail on some relevant background involving:

● static electricity
● conductors and insulators.

### Static electricity

This is not so much 'used' in hairdressing, but rather, causes a nuisance. Static electricity is produced by **friction**, i.e. materials of particular types rubbing together. This can happen for example when combing hair or removing a nylon overall from a client and a 'crackling' sound may be produced (and in dim light sometimes sparks are visible). In combing or brushing hair (especially fine hair) a further problem is **'hair fly'**, where the hair will not lie flat and is attracted towards the brush or comb. The reason for 'hair fly' and the sometimes encountered crackling or sparks is that the friction between certain materials, all non-conductors (of which hair is a good example) and other materials causes a transfer of electrons from one material to the other.

### Conductors and insulators

Electricity involves the movement of electrons and current electricity involves the flow of electrons. How easily these electrons can flow through something is measured by electrical resistance and this can be used to classify different materials into the following categories:

1   Those which have a low resistance, that is electricity can flow through them relatively easily, are called **conductors.**
2   Those which have a very high resistance, that will prevent the flow of electricity, are called **insulators.**
3   Those which fall somewhere between conductors and insulators in that they will allow the flow of electricity by have a fairly high resistance. This resistance causes some of the electrical energy to

turn into heat. The heating elements of steamers, driers, kettles and immersion heaters use this principle.

## Using electricity safely

In the UK electricity is supplied to consumers, including hairdressing salons, in quantities which can be very dangerous, either directly by electric shock or indirectly by fire. The terms fuses (or circuit breakers) and earth have already been referred to. These are deliberately placed in circuits for reasons of safety. Basically, fuses (or circuit breakers) help prevent fires and earthing prevents electric shock.

Many of the accidents that occur when using electricity are simply due to thoughtlessness, carelessness or downright bad practice. Some basic 'do's' and 'don't's' are listed below:

*Do*
- Make sure plugs are wired correctly and have the correct sized fuse for the appliance.
- Have electrical equipment checked on a regular basis or repaired, if necessary, or have changes made in the electrical supply by a competent electrician.
- Ensure that staff are trained to know what to do if a person receives an electric shock.

*Don't*
- Handle electrical appliances with wet hands or allow water to splash on to appliances.
- Overload sockets or other circuits by running too many appliances from it.
- Fit a larger fuse into a fuse box or plug if it keeps 'blowing'.
- Run flexes under floor coverings or place in a position where there is a chance of someone tripping over them.
- Pull out a plug by tugging on its flex.

## Wiring a plug

Fixing the wires from the flex of an appliance into a plug is a routine operation, as many appliances are supplied without plugs. It is very important that wires are connected properly in the plug and that the correct fuse is fitted. Failure to do so is dangerous.

The flex on an appliance has an outer insulation which has within it two or three wires, each with its own insulation. The insulation around each wire is colour coded as follows:

- brown (or red) is the live (L),
- blue (or black) is the neutral (N),
- green/yellow (or green) is the earth (E).

The earth (E) is only found in flexes with three wires (three-core flex) and is missing from those with two (two-core flex). The reason for the alternative colours (in brackets) is that older appliances follow this colour code, whereas new appliances follow the international colour coding.

Plugs are supplied in a variety of different forms, but modern circuits use **three-pin square** plugs. These are manufactured in a number of slightly different forms and are usually supplied with a 13 amp cartridge fuse in place. A typical square pin plug is shown in Fig 5.2(a) and (b).

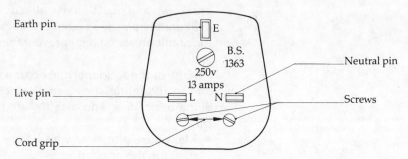

**Fig 5.2 (a)**

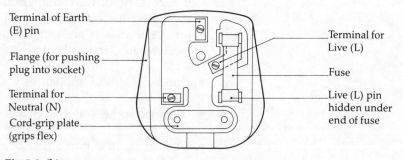

**Fig 5.2 (b)**

The larger single pin is the earth (E), and when viewed from the back (with the back removed), the left-hand pin is the neutral (N) and the right-hand pin (with the fuse) is the live (L). There is also a cord grip device of either a plate with two screws (as shown in (b)) or two plastic flanges, between which the flex is pushed. Both types prevent the flex from being pulled out of the plug.

*Basic steps to follow in wiring a plug*
Most appliances are supplied with flex with the outer insulation already stripped back, and the ends of the wires also stripped back.

1  Remove back of plug by unscrewing large central screw on underside.
2  Unscrew cord grip screws (if plug is of this type) and slide end of flex under plate, or insert flex between flanges of cord grip if of this type. In either case, make sure the outer insulation is held in the cord grip, not that around the wires. Check that the inner wires

are neither too long nor too short to reach screws in the pins of the plug (*see* Fig. 5.2 (*b*) ). If too short, then some more of the outer flex insulation needs to be removed. Use a special tool, available in most hardware shops for this use. If too long, the same special tool can be used to cut some of the wire away and strip back a little of the colour coded insulation.

3   Unscrew the terminals on the pins and slide the bare ends of the colour coded wires into them as follows:

- blue (or black) into the left-hand pin (marked neutral or N)
- brown (or red) into the right-hand pin (marked live or L), removing the fuse often helps in doing this.
- green/yellow (or green), if present in the flex, into the single large pin (marked earth or E).

Make sure in each case that all the bare wire is under the terminal. Screw down tightly.

4   Screw up cord grip tightly, or press wire down firmly between the flanges, depending on the type of plug.

5   Check that the fuse is correct for the appliances to which the plug is wired. Blow driers, for example, require a 3 amp fuse rather than the 13 amp usually supplied.

6   Screw top down firmly, making sure it is not obstructed. If it does not fit properly, remove and check why not.

*Points about plugs*
Square, three-pin plugs are manufactured in a variety of different types. The best have:

1   BS (for 'British Standard') 1363 and sometimes the BS 'kite' mark on them
2   Wide flanges around the bottom of the plugs for pushing it into the socket (*see* Fig 5.2 (*b*) )
3   Insulation covering about the first half of the two smaller pins where these leave the plug.

Both 2 and 3 helps prevent someone touching these pins when the plug is only halfway inserted into the socket.

*Correct fuse size*
Fuses act as a deliberately placed 'weak' part of the circuit. They are pieces of wire, much thinner than that in the cable or flex, which are designed to melt if the heating effect becomes too great. Because the thickness of the wire used (called the fuse size) is critical to this it is very important that the correct fuse size is fitted in the plugs. Those fuses protecting the whole circuit are usually found in the fuse box. Fuses are rated in amps; the higher the figure the thicker the wire used in the fuse. The larger the fuse, the thicker the wire, so the greater heating effect in the flow of electricity is needed to melt it.

In plugs supplied with fuses, it is usually a 13 amps fuse which would take longer to melt and break the circuit than the 2 amps fuse which should be used with the blow drier. The extra time needed for the 13 amps fuse to melt may cause damage to the drier, and possibly harm the hairdresser or client, due to the heat produced. In practice, a 2 amps fuse may not be available, but 3 amps fuses are available from most hardware shops and although this is slightly larger than actually required, it is still safer than a 13 amps fuse.

### Circuit breakers

These are fitted to modern commercial circuits, like those in hairdressing salons, and their use will probably become more widespread. They are really an automatic switch which switches the circuit off if the heating effect of the electrical flow becomes too great, or if a fault develops in the wiring or appliances. They have the great advantage of being very sensitive to electrical faults and will switch a circuit off in circumstances in which a fuse would not melt but a person using the appliance could receive an electric shock. They are also more 'tamper-proof' in that someone can deliberately or accidently put too large a fuse into the fuse box or plug, whereas circuit breakers have to be deliberately tampered with by someone with some knowledge.

Never tamper with circuit breakers or deliberately put a larger fuse into a fuse box or plug.

## Earthing

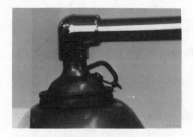

**Fig 5.3 (a) Earth connection**

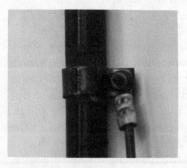

**Fig 5.3 (b) Earth cable connection**

In a three-pin plug the top single pin is described as the earth (E). This is used to carry electricity away into the ground or earth should a fault develop in an appliance or circuit (modern circuit breakers monitor this and are called 'earth leakage circuit breakers'). Some appliances, blow driers for example have only two wires in their flex. A live (L), with brown insulation and a neutral (N), with blue insulation. Other equipment, like hood driers, steamers and accelerators commonly have an additional third wire in the flex, this being the earth (E) wire with green/yellow insulation. The main reason for some appliances having just 'live' and 'neutral' and others having the extra third 'earth' is the material the appliance is made of in areas which can easily be touched. If these parts are good insulators, like plastic (in a blow drier for instance) then a fault within the appliance is most unlikely to produce a flow of electricity in the outer case.

A person's body has a large resistance to the flow of electrical current and the basis of an earth wire is to provide a low resistance route to earth and back to the power station. Thus, taking the route with least resistance, the electricity will flow from the faulty appliance into the earth and not through a person's body touching the appliance. Therefore, the end of the earth cable on a flex is usually firmly attached to the conducting part of the metal casing of an appliance. At the other end of the earth circuit, the cable is connected to the earth. Both these are shown in Fig. 5.3(a),(b).

## Salon lighting

Sufficient light to work by but without glare is extremely important in the salon. Light is also an important means of creating an image with work areas more brightly lit and waiting areas more softly. Modern salon design makes much use of light in order to create an 'atmosphere'.

The colour something appears to be depends on the type or quality of the light falling onto it. This is important in hardressing because the **artificial light** very often used does not have exactly the same colour mixture as daylight. This can alter the appearance of hair shades in the salon and how they appear outside in daylight. This is the same effect as when people take clothes near the shop window to see what shade they appear in natural light compared with the artificial light being used.

The two major sources of artificial light in the salon are **light bulbs** and **fluorescent light tubes** ('strip' lighting).

1   Light bulbs often contain a thin wire **filament**. The shape of the bulb varies depending on use. Spot-lamps and the infra-red lamps used in an 'octopus' array are flat across the top and often have a reflective coating on the inside of the bulb designed to reflect the light or heat in the desired direction.

The electrical resistance in the filament makes it become very hot when electricity passes through it and this produces the light. The mixture of colours in this light is slightly different from daylight in having more red and yellow and less blue light. This can alter the apparent shade of an object by enhancing reds and yellows and reducing blues.

2   Fluorescent light tubes (or 'strip' lighting) produce light by means of a gas inside the tube which glows or **fluoresces** when electricity passes through it. The radiation produced by the gas is mostly ultra-violet and this is converted to visible light by a substance coating the inside of the tube. The light produced is more like daylight than filament lamps but does tend to contain more blue, so these shades are enhanced and the reds and yellows reduced.

## Using mirrors

Mirrors are designed to reflect light efficiently with little scattering and so produce a clear image. A typical mirror consists of a sheet of glass coated on one side with a thin layer of reflective material called **silvering**. Mirrors are produced in many shapes and sizes but can be placed into three general groups.

1   *Plane mirrors* which are flat and produce a mirror image of actual size. The large mirrors at dressing stations and back mirrors used

to show the client the back of their scalp are of this type.

2 *Convex mirrors* – are curved slightly outwards. These produce a smaller than actual size image. This means that more area can be reflected from a smaller mirror. This type is used in powder compact lid mirrors and car driving mirrors.

3 *Concave mirrors* – are curved slightly inwards. These produce a larger than actual size image. This type is used in shaving and make-up mirrors.

## Ventilation

Routine activities in the hairdressing salon produce damp, warm, contaminated air, (stale air) which tends to rise to the ceiling as warm air is lighter than cooler air. The aim of a good ventilation system is to provide fresh air (i.e. less humid, cooler and with fewer micro-organisms) but *without* producing any draughts or low temperatures in the salon and therefore making conditions uncomfortable.

## Effects of bad ventilation in the salon

*On client and staff comfort*
The body cooling system depends on the evaporation of sweat from the skin. In conditions of high humidity (i.e. moist air) the evaporation process is reduced so the body tends to overheat very slightly. This produces feelings of drowsiness in clients and staff, or even feelings of being uncomfortably hot, if combined with warmth.

*On hygiene*
One type of micro-organism (germ) is a virus, some of which attack humans and are described as **pathogenic**, e.g. cold and influenza ('flu). These are mostly spread in tiny droplets of moisture which shoot out of a person's mouth and nose when they cough or sneeze. The more humid the air, the slower these droplets evaporate and the longer the viruses survive, thus increasing the chance of them being breathed in by other clients and staff.

Another type of micro-organism, bacteria, also thrives in damp conditions.

*On hair*
The major influence is due to the hair's ability to absorb water from the atmosphere, that is its tendency to be **hygroscopic**.

The more humid the air the more quickly this happens, so it is more difficult to carry out both wet and dry setting (both processes which involve drying some of the water from the hair) in conditions where the hair is continually reabsorbing the water from humid air.

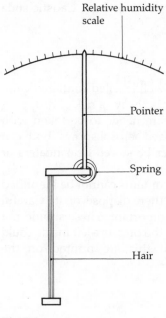

Relative humidity scale

Pointer

Spring

Hair

**Fig 5.4**

# Measuring humidity

This can be carried out using a **hygrometer** (note the *hygro*), this word is very similar to *hydrometer* which is a device for measuring the density of liquids and can be used to measure the 'strength' of hydrogen peroxide). A simple hygrometer is shown in Fig 5.4.

When air is humid the hair absorbs moisture and stretches, this allows the spring to move the indicator. When the air is less humid, the hair loses water and shrinks; this pulls the indicator in the opposite direction.

# Ventilation systems

This can be as simple as opening or closing doors or windows, or as complex as 'air conditioning'. Most salons operate a compromise between the two extremes. An extremely common ventilation method is to use an extractor fan. These have certain advantages:

- relatively cheap (can be positioned in windows or through walls)
- reliable
- produce good ventilation. Typical siting is fairly high up as the damp warm air tends to rise above cooler, fresher air.

There are a variety of other ventilation techniques. For example:

- louvred windows
- passive flow fans, set into windows which turn in air currents but are not driven by a motor.

# Chemical hazards

Hairdressing operations very often involve the use of chemicals on the hair and some of these are sprayed on to the hair using **pressurised containers**, e.g. hair lacquers. The chemical hazards in the salon come from three main sources:

- chemicals getting on to the skin or into the eyes
- storage and disposal
- dermatitis.

## Chemicals getting on to the skin or into the eyes

The main prevention here is to be aware of the risk involved in carrying out any hairdressing operation (even shampooing) that involves chemicals and to handle chemicals with care. Chemicals can be swallowed, especially by children, so care should be taken to put these out of reach.

Accidental spills can be avoided by replacing caps and stoppers on containers immediately after use.

Do not use **caustic soda** (sodium hydroxide) to clear blocked drains, get a plumber instead to clear the blockage. Caustic soda can cause severe skin burns.

## Storage and disposal

All salon reagents should be stored in well labelled containers and not put on to high shelves where there is always a risk of dropping when taking them down. Particular care needs to be taken with stored hydrogen peroxide and pressurised aerosol sprays. Both can explode if heated so they should never be stored near heaters or in direct sunlight.

If a container has lost its label or the contents cannot be identified with certainty for any other reason, then dispose of it. Careful disposal of empty pressurised cans is important. These should not be punctured or burned (incinerated) as the pressure left inside could cause an explosion. Warnings about this are printed on the container.

## Dermatitis (eczema)

Basically, this involves the body 'over-reacting' to a substance to which it has been exposed. Many of the chemicals used in hairdressing may cause dermatitis, but **paraphenylenediamine** used in some tints is strongly linked to people developing dermatitis. Both the hairdresser and the client are at risk, with the hairdresser at greatest risk due to their repeated and long-term exposure to hairdressing chemicals. The client can be protected agains 'para' dye dermatitis by carrying out a skin test before going ahead with the tint. The hairdresser can be protected by using rubber gloves for any hairdressing operation that involves chemicals, including shampooing.

## Biological hazards

These consist of infections and infestations both caused by living organisms.

They are either **infectious** or **contagious**; that is they can be passed between people or transmitted in the salon.

## Infections

These are caused by harmful germs or, more properly, **pathogenic micro-organisms**. Examples commonly encountered in the salon include:

- impetigo
- boils
- eye infections, e.g. conjunctivitis

- ringworm
- cold sores (herpes)
- some types of wart.

It is important to be able to recognise these conditions and distinguish between the infectious or contagious complaints and the non-infectious or non-contagious conditions. Also you should know which of these prohibit hairdressing operations. Of the examples listed above impetigo, eye infections and ringworm *definitely* mean that hairdressing operations should not start (or should *stop* if already started).

## AIDS and Hepatitis B

These are both very serious infections which can be transmitted by small amounts of blood or serum (clear liquid in blisters) from one person to another. The risk to hairdressers is *slight*.

There is a useful pamphlet produced by the government's Health Department with notes for guidance. Transmission of both diseases can be avoided by using simple and routine hygiene practices covered under the section on sterilization of tools and equipment (*see* p. 39) and prevention of infection or infestation (*see* below).

## Infestations

These refer to larger animal parasites living on the body and include:

- head and body lice
- flea
- itchmite (which causes scabies).

With head lice particularly, the hairdresser can be the first person to definitely detect the presence of these parasites. In *all* the examples above, hairdressing operations should not start (or should stop if already begun).

## Prevention of infection or infestation

To prevent any infection or infestation developing you must:

1 Be able to recognise which scalp conditions are infectious/contagious and know what to do if they are.

2 Carry out routine hygienic procedures in the salon, coupled with design considerations, like the choice of wall and floor coverings, upholstery, ventilation and temperature control.

Routine hygienic procedures include such practices as:

(*a*) *between clients:* washing your hands; sterilising personal tools and equipment; cleaning shampoo basins.

(*b*) *for each client:* preparing a clean towel (or towels) and neck strip; sterilising any tools accidentally dropped on to the floor; not keeping tools and equipment in pockets.

(c) *regular* washing down of walls, floors, work surfaces with an alcohol based disinfectant; sweeping up hair clippings and putting waste into a closed container.

(d) *personal routine:* not putting hair pins and clips in the mouth; wearing closed in shoes with low heels.

(e) *general:* not allowing animals in the salon; ensuring an adequate ventilation and heating system.

## First aid

First aid can be defined as 'the skilled application of accepted principles of treatment on the occurance of any injury or sudden illness, using facilities available at the time. It is the approved method of treating a casualty until placed, if necessary, in the care of a doctor or removed to hospital' (authorised manual of St John Ambulance, St Andrews Ambulance Association, British Red Cross Society).

The best thing to do with accidents is to prevent them. However, even in the best run salons, accidents will sometimes happen. There are also cases where events occur which are not under the control of anyone in the salon, a client suffering a heart attack for example. It is important to know what to do and the best method of learning this is to complete a first aid course. There are a number of these organised by the St John Ambulance, Red Cross, or at your local College of Further Education. It is an extremely good idea to have at least one trained first aider in the salon.

## Legal requirements

Under the Health and Safety at Work Act (1974), the requirement for 'low hazard' situations is one trained first aider for each 150 staff. There is therefore no obligation for a hairdressing salon to have a first aider, although it is a tremendous advantage to have one.

First aid boxes must be available and each employer must supply at least one. Each box should be clearly marked (preferably by a white cross on a green background). The boxes should contain the following items only (*see* Table 5.1). The quantities given are a minimum.

Soap and water and disposable drying materials should also be available.

## A brief outline of some first aid procedures

There is no real substitute for completing a proper first aid course. Here, for guidance, is an outline of what to do if someone suffers:

1 *Cuts*

- For **minor wounds** – cover the wound as soon as possible with a sterile dressing.

**Table 5.1**

| Item | Number of employees | | |
|------|:---:|:---:|:---:|
| | 1–5 | 6–10 | 11–50 |
| Card giving general first aid guidance | 1 | 1 | 1 |
| Individually wrapped sterile, adhesive dressings | 10 | 20 | 40 |
| Sterile eye pads, with attachment | 1 | 2 | 4 |
| Triangular bandage | 1 | 2 | 4 |
| Sterile dressing for serious wounds* | 1 | 2 | 4 |
| Safety pins | 6 | 6 | 12 |
| Sterile, unmedicated wound dressings: | | | |
| medium size | 3 | 6 | 8 |
| large | 1 | 2 | 4 |
| extra large | 1 | 2 | 4 |

* These should be provided if the triangular bandages are not sterile

- For **major wounds** – send for expert help immediately. Try to control the bleeding by pulling the sides of the wound together and hold firmly until the bleeding stops. Apply a pad of sterile dressings and hold in place (use disposable plastic gloves if possible). If these become soaked with blood add more dressings.
- For **blood spills** – pour neat bleach on to the blood. Leave for a few minutes. Put on disposable plastic gloves. Wash off with a large amount of hot water and washing up (or similar) liquid.

2  *Burns*

- **Heat burns** – cool immediately under cold water. If the person is seriously burnt, send for expert medical help. If the burn is widespread, cover it with loose dressings. Do not attempt to remove clothing sticking to the burnt area.
- **Chemical burns** – wash off with plenty of cold water. Remove any clothing which may have chemical on it. Apply a sterile dressing. Refer the person to expert medical help if necessary.

3  *Eye injuries*
These include:
  (a) object in the eye
  (b) chemicals in the eye.

- Attempt to remove the object with the moistened corner of a sterile dressing. If it cannot be removed or the eye is still painful after the object has been removed, cover with an eye patch and quickly send the person to a hospital or a doctor.
- If a chemical has run into the eye, wash out with a large amount of cold water. Force the eye open if necessary. Cover with an eye pad and either send the person to a hospital or a doctor or summon expert help depending on the injury.

## 4 *Collapse*

If a person collapses it could be due to a number of reasons, which include:

- electric shock
- heart attack
- epileptic fit
- fainting.

The person may be partly conscious or completely unconscious. In either case, talk reassuringly to them. They may also have knocked or cut themselves while falling.

- **Electric shock:**
  (*a*) Switch off the supply. If this is not possible then use an insulator (rug, clothing, paper or plastic) to pull the person away from the source of the shock.
  (*b*) If they are partly conscious keep talking and reassuring them. Keep them warm and if they do not recover within a few minutes send for expert medical help.
  (*c*) If they are unconscious then:
    (*i*) send immediately for expert help.
    (*ii*) check their heartbeat by trying to find the pulse in the neck.
    (*iii*) check breathing by either watching for breathing movements or by holding a mirror, e.g. compact lid mirror or watchglass, over their mouth and looking for 'misting'.
    (*iv*) if the heart has stopped, start external cardiac massage and/or if breathing has stopped, start mouth-to-mouth resuscitation (the 'kiss of life').
    *NB* To learn how to find the pulse and how to carry out cardiac massage and mouth-to-mouth resuscitation complete a first aid course!
    (*v*) Continue cardiac massage and/or mouth-to-mouth resuscitation until help arrives.
    (*vi*) Keep talking in a reassuring manner, even if they are unconscious.
- **Heart attack:**
  (*a*) If the person is partly conscious they will most likely complain of chest pains (often severe). They may have some medication with them. Loosen clothes; talk reassuringly to them. send for expert medical help.
  (*b*) If the person is unconscious treat them as for electric shock above.
- **Epileptic fit:**
  These can vary from a mild attack with only a brief loss of consciousness (much like fainting) to severe attacks involving the person becoming unconscious, going stiff and having convulsions, e.g. arms and legs twitching violently.
  Try to prevent them hurting themselves by protecting the head.

The attack will pass, again keep talking reassuringly.

● **Fainting:**

It can be partial or complete. If partial, the person will feel faint but will not be unconscious. Put their head between their knees, or lie them down with their feet raised above their head. Loosen tight clothing. Keep them warm and supply fresh air.

If they have fainted fully and are unconscious, lay them down with their feet raised above their head. Loosen clothing and keep warm. They should recover rapidly, but if they do not, summon expert medical help.

## Summary

**In a hairdressing salon, both the client and the hairdresser can be at risk from one or more of the following hazards:**

**1  physical – which includes physical injury, fire and heat burns and electricity.**

**2  chemical – due to chemical burns, storage and disposal of chemicals and dermatitis.**

**3  biological – such as infections caused by micro-organisms and infestations by larger animal parasites.**

**The aim of good hairdressing practice is to reduce the risk of injury to a minimum. There are legal responsibilities for both the hairdresser and the salon owner in this connection.**

**A large number of the possible events which can occur in the salon require some first aid. The best way to learn the basics of first aid is to complete a recognised course, such as those run by the St John Ambulance Brigade or the Red Cross.**

**Fires do occur in the salon, and it is important to know what to do and which type of fire extinguisher is most appropriate. The best is the 'dry powder' type, with carbon dioxide ($CO_2$) extinguishers as a good alternative.**

**The routine health hygiene and safety practices are also important and runs through all aspects of hairdressing.**

## Self-assessment questions

1  List the three major groups of hazards to which a client or hairdresser may be exposed.
2  Give two reasons for regularly cleaning the salon.
3  When should cut hair be swept up?
4  Why is it necessary to unplug electrical apparatus before cleaning?
5  What two types of accident are particularly linked to using electrical apparatus?
6  What is the first action if a chemical has run on to the skin or into the eyes?
7  What precautions need to be taken in the use, storage and disposal of aerosol spray cans?

8  What advantages does a 'dry powder' type fire extinguisher have over the water or foam type extinguishers?
9  What is the difference between infection and infestation?
10  How in particular can a hairdresser avoid dermatitis?
11  Name three dangers linked to trailing electrical flexes.
12  Outline the action which should be taken if a client faints.
13  What is the major aim of 'hygiene'?

## Practical assignment – Health and safety

Good hygiene and safety practices are essential in any working environment and great care must always be taken when dealing with any potentially hazardous tools, chemicals or equipment.

The following tasks have been devised to help you to be aware of any potential dangers and the precautions that can be taken to ensure that your salon is a safe place for both yourself and the clients.

## Tasks

1 (a) Use your work placement or training salon to identify any items/situations which could be a safety hazard.
(b) Make a chart listing the potentially hazardous items/situations together with any precautions which could minimise the risk to health and safety.

Use the following layout for your chart:

| Item/situation | Precautions |
|---|---|
| e.g. 1  Frayed electrical wires | Check all wires before using *any* electrical equipment. Rewire if necessary. |

2 Find out from your salon employment or work placement the procedure in case of fire on the premises.

Design a bright, noticable poster for display in the salon staffroom which illustrates the risks of fire and your own salon's procedure should a fire occur.

The poster should be on A5 size paper of any colour using whatever medium or combination of mediums that you consider suitable, e.g. paint, pastels, ink, collage etc.

# SECTION 2
# HAIR AND SKIN

# 6    THE HAIR AND SKIN

## Hair growth

Humans have as many hairs on their bodies as a chimpanzee, but we do not appear as hairy because most of the body hairs are fine, light coloured 'down' hairs which are much more difficult to see than the thicker, darker coloured scalp and body hair. Many new-born babies appear virtually hairless due to having only this type of fine hair. The fine 'down' hair is called **vellus** hair, and the generally thicker, darker hair on the scalp and body is called **secondary** (or terminal) hair.

The nails and scalp are some of the few parts of the human body which continue to grow even after the whole body has stopped growing. All types of growth, either the whole body, or parts of the body, depends on cell division. This process of cell division occurs fairly rapidly at the bottom of an actively growing hair.

## Hair structure

### Hair follicles

These are tiny pits in the skin (about 4 to 7 mm deep and 0.5 mm across) from which the hair grows. At one time it was believed that the shape of the follicle determined the natural wave or curliness of the hair. However, recent evidence suggests that the natural curl formation takes place in the dermal papilla, i.e. when the cell division (rates of mitosis) around the diameter of the hair is uneven it causes the hair to bend resulting in wavy or curly hair. The angle at which the follicles lie and their distribution (or 'pattern') on the scalp produces the natural direction of the hair growth and produces natural partings and crown on the scalp. The natural wave pattern of a person's hair is inherited from their parents (as is the colour). A diagram of a typical hair follicle is shown in Fig 6.1; the labels are numbered and these are used in the following description:

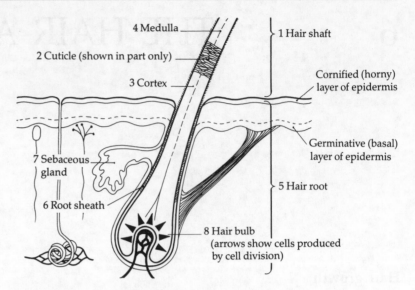

**Fig 6.1 Section through a hair follicle**

*1 Hair shaft* – the part of the hair which protrudes above the skin. The hair at this point is dead and is made up of:

- 70–80 per cent protein (mostly **keratin**)
- 3–6 per cent oils
- up to 1 per cent colouring pigments (**melanin** and **pheomelanin**)
- up to 15 per cent moisture (i.e. water)
- traces of carbohydrate and minerals.

*2 Cuticle* – is the outermost layer of the hair. It is made up of 7–11 overlapping flattened scales of keratin. It is virtually transparent, so light will pass through it as it would through glass in a window although it is not like 'clear' window glass, but more like frosted glass and the natural colour of the hair is seen through this layer; this is described as **translucent**. The cuticle holds the hair together but can be damaged by hairdressing processes (especially bleaching), and other factors such as the weather. Hair where the cuticle has been damaged is described as **porous** and hair where much damage has occurred is likely to split and fray.

*3 Cortex* – makes up about 90 per cent of the bulk of a hair. The fine detail of the cortex structure is show in Fig 6.2 but can be summarised (from largest units to smallest) as follows:

(*a*) Cortex 'fibres' (sometimes called cells) contain much keratin which is in the form of large numbers of fibres called **macrofibrils** held together by a 'cement'-like substance.

(*b*) Macrofibrils are, in turn, made up of bundles of microfibrils twisted together.

(*c*) Each microfibril is made up of 11 smaller fibres called **protofibrils.**

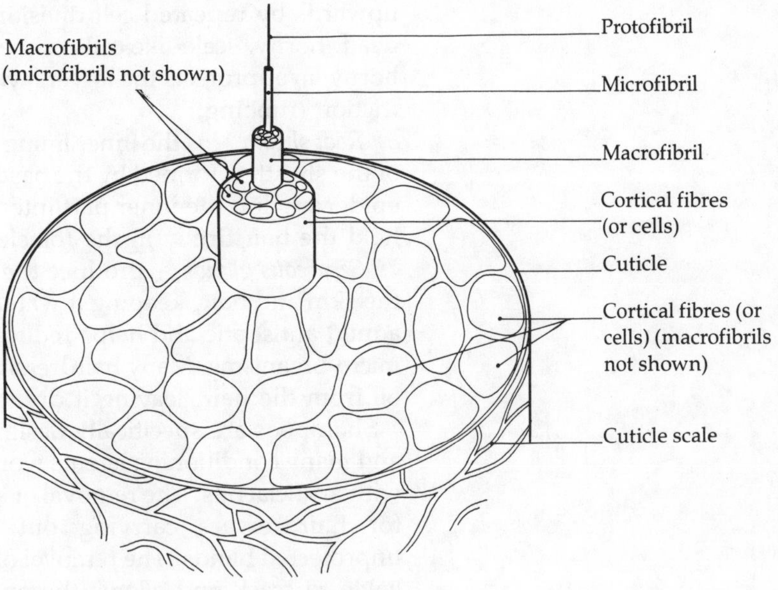

**Fig 6.2 Detailed structure of the hair**

(*d*) A protofibril consists of three very tiny polypeptide **chains** twisted together and held together by cross-linkages (broken and reformed in setting and perming hair).

(*e*) Each polypeptide chain is made up of **amino acids**.

This structure of fibres twisted together gives hair its tensile strength and elasticity. It is interesting to compare this natural structure with artificial products where tensile strength and elasticity are important: rope for example, where the same pattern of twisted fibres has been used.

4  *Medulla* – at one time this was considered to be a third, distinct layer of the hair, occupying the centre or core, of the cortex. Recent findings on the detailed structure of the hair have thrown some doubt on this and the present position is not clear. If the medulla can be counted as a third layer, it is certainly not found in all hair or along the whole length of a hair. When present it appears to be a spongy area containing air spaces.

5  *Hair root* – this is the part of the hair buried in the skin. As can be seen from Fig 6.1 the hair follicle extends down through the upper layer of the skin (the **epidermis**) into the lower layer (the **dermis**). The epidermis has an outer **horny** or **cornified** layer, made up of dead, flattened, scale-like cells filled with keratin, which are constantly flaking off the skin's surface. A person can lose up to one million of these tiny flakes in less than an hour. This loss is made up by the production of new cornified cells which begins in the lowest layer of the epidermis, called the **basal** or **germinative** layer. This layer of the epidermis is made up of living cells which carry out cell division. The new cells produced in this process are pushed

upwards by repeated cell division and gradually change into the dead, horny, scale-like cells of the cornified layer. The cornified or horny layer protects the lower layers of the skin from infection and friction (rubbing).

6  *Root sheath* – is the inner lining of the hair follicle. The outer part of the sheath is formed by the basal or germinative layer of the skin epidermis and the inner part interlocks with the hair cuticle which hold the hair firmly in the follicle.

7  *Sebaceous glands* – produce the natural oil, **sebum**, which coats the skin and hair, keeping it waterproof and supple. It also acts as a mild antiseptic and helps reduce the chance of skin infection by micro-organisms. Many hairdressing operations remove this natural oil from the hair, leaving it dry.

Shampoos are specifically designed to efficiently remove this oil and many conditioning agents work by replacing the natural sebum with artificial oils. The removal of sebum from the skin is a problem for hairdressers carrying out hairdressing operations with unprotected hands. The removal of the sebum makes the skin more liable to crack and allows the entry of chemicals that can cause **dermatitis** or infection by micro-organisms. Barrier or hand creams are designed to replace the sebum lost in this way. But the best protection is to use rubber gloves.

Sebum (with sweat) produces the **acid mantle** of the skin and hair (*see* Chapter 9, Hair and scalp treatments).

8  *Hair bulb* – is situated at the lower end of the hair follicle. It is a swelling in the hair follicle and it encloses a knot of **blood capillaries and fat cells** called the **dermal papilla**. In the hair bulb (or just above it) the following processes take place:

(*a*) **Cell division** which causes the hair to grow. This is because the new cells produced by cell division push the older cell upwards in the hair follicle so that the whole hair lengthens. Hair that had been artificially straightened or waved is gradually replaced by hair having its natural wave, unless the new growth is treated. The process of cell division requires a supply of chemicals.

These chemicals include **oxygen** and **glucose** (both used to produce energy), and amino acids (used to make proteins like keratin). All these chemicals are supplied by the blood flowing through the capillaries of the dermal papilla. In addition, living cells produce waste chemicals, like **carbon dioxide** and these are carried away by the blood.

(*b*) **Hair colouring** which is due to minute **granules** of the hair's natural pigments, i.e. melanin and pheomelanin which are almost entirely found in the hair cortex. In the hair bulb fine filaments from special cells called **melanocytes** extend into the hair. Melanocytes have the ability to produce the natural pigments found in hair (and in the skin) and when these are made they pass down the filaments from the cell into the hair and are then deposited there. Artificially changing the hair colour by bleaching or tinting only involves the hair shaft, so as the hair grows, the new hair produced has the natural colouring; this is called regrowth. Because of this, bleached or tinted hair has to be 'retouched' at intervals to maintain the artificial colour. If this is not done, the bleached or tinted hair eventually 'grows out'.

With age or sometimes as a result of hair regrowth, after alopecia areata (form of baldness) for example, hair grows with no pigmentation, a condition called **canities**. The mixture of unpigmented and normally pigmented hair produces grey hair. There are no partly pigmented grey hairs only unpigmented or normally pigmented.

(c) **Keratinisation** which takes place at the top of and just above the hair bulb. In this region the hair cells start to produce large amounts of the protein keratin. The production of keratin in the cells, coupled with the increasing distance they are pushed up the follicle and away from the supply of chemicals from the dermal papilla causes the cells to die. They then break down leaving the structure of the keratin in the overlapping scales of the cuticle and the fibres of the cortex.

The hair being dead at the time it reaches the surface of the skin means it can be cut, heated and chemically treated without discomfort. The living part of the hair follicle is connected by **nerve fibres** to the nervous system and these are sensitive to touch and pain. So movements of the hair in the follicle are 'felt' and pulling hair out, plucking eyebrows for example, hurts.

9 *Arrector pili muscle* – pulls hair upright when it contracts. It has no real function in humans and produces 'goose-pimples'.

## The hair growth cycle

Hair grows at about 1.25 cm (0.5″) per month due to cell hair division down at the hair root (as seen left). There are about l00 000 hairs on a full scalp of hair, and any one of these hairs lasts for one to six years. During the time it lasts (or its 'life expectancy') the hair passes through the three stages of the hair growth cycle i.e. *anagen, telogen* and *catagen* stages.

The details of these are summarised in Table 6.1 overleaf.

About 100 scalp hairs a day are normally lost and replaced by new hairs in the anagen stage. The common forms of **baldness** are caused by the lack of new hairs being produced in the follicle which ceases hair production.

## Types of hair

In physically mature people, hair varies in its diameter (thickness), density (the number of hairs per square centimetre), direction of growth and form (amount of natural curl). There are three different types of hair produced by hair follicles and these are:

**Table 6.1**

| Name of stage | Description | Duration of stage | % scalp at stage |
|---|---|---|---|
| anagen | hair growing due to cell division in hair bulb | 1–5 years | 80–90 |
| catagen | hair stops growing as cell division stops. By end of this stage follicle has shortened by about one third. End of hair has become separated from dermal papilla and forms a 'club' hair. | 2 weeks | 1 |
| telogen | hair 'resting', no growth. By end of this stage new hair has started to grow from papilla. Old hair falls out. | 3–4 months | 13 |

## Lanugo hair

This the first hair produced by the follicles of developing babies. This type of hair is very fine and is usually formed on the baby while it is still in the uterus (womb). It can sometimes be seen on premature babies.

## Vellus hair

This is the fine 'down' hair which covers the bodies of children and is often present on the scalps of newborn babies (although this varies).

## Secondary or terminal hair

This develops after vellus hair. It may be present on the scalp at birth or develop relatively soon afterwards. Some of the vellus hair on the body develops into the thicker, generally more pigmented (therefore darker) secondary hair, during the process of reaching sexual maturity. This occurs in the pubic region and in the armpits of both sexes but is generally more widespread in males and includes the face (beard), arms, legs, chest, etc.

The removal of hair is a matter of personal preference and opinion. The removal of facial hair is common in men by shaving, and the removal of body hair, especially on the legs, is common in females by depilatory or shaving. It is worth noting that hair removal does not increase the thickness or pigmentation of hair, so shaving legs does not make the hair grow back thicker or darker.

## Afro hair

The main difference between Afro hair and European (Caucasian) hair is that while European hair is either fine, medium or coarse textured, the texture of Afro hair varies along the actual hair shaft. This results in an uneven porosity along the length of each individual hair which creates special problems when chemicals are applied to the hair. Extra care and thought is essential before and during the treatment of Afro hair to prevent damage and/or breakage to the weaker and more porous areas.

The degree of curl in Afro hair also differs from that of most European hair. Afro hair has a very diffuse hair growth direction pattern which makes it difficult to manage as it does not fall in uniform waves. It is usually extremely dry and brittle which means that it can be easily broken during combing or when using heated appliances. Both the hair and the scalp should be kept well oiled and supple by the use of conditioners, oils and waxes. Because of the excess dryness, specialised products containing ingredients such as, e.g. protein, lanolin, natural and mineral oils, are more effective than the conditioning agents formulated for European hair.

The anagen stage of Afro hair growth may last only nine to ten months and the growth rate is also often slower, therefore, Afro hair is considered to be long if it is 18 to 20 cms (7 to 8"). However, because of its tightly coiled nature Afro hair usually appears shorter than it actually is. The amount of curl present in the hair will depend on hereditary and racial factors e.g. African hair is very curly whilst Guyanese hair is merely curly.

When permanently changing the shape of Afro hair (curling or straightening), the same structural alteration takes place as in European hair, i.e. breaking sufficient chemical bonds within the hair and rejoining them in a new shape. However, specialised Afro straighteners must never be used on European hair as they are too strong and could easily dissolve the hair.

## Procedure when testing hair for porosity

Slide the index finger and thumb down the hair shaft from the points to the roots. If there is only a small amount of resistance, this indicates that the cuticle scales of the hair are smooth, compacted, in good condition and have normal porosity.

If it is difficult to slide the fingers down the hair shaft, this is an indication that the cuticle is raised, in poor condition and is porous.

## Procedure for testing the hair for elasticity

This is done on wet hair, usually after shampooing. A few strands of hair are pulled gently between the index finger and thumb of each hand. If the hair stretches and then reverts back to its original length the elasticity is normal. If the hair stretches a great deal and then either breaks or does not spring back to its original length then the elasticity of that hair is impaired and further chemical processes, except those of restructuring or conditioning, should be avoided.

## Skin structure and functions

Skin covers the entire body (about 3.5 square metres, 40 square feet in an adult). On average it is only about 3 mm thick, yet it acts as a waterproof over-covering between the 'inside' and 'outside' world. People lose about 1 million tiny flakes of skin in only 40 minutes, (the majority of household dust is skin), so skin needs constantly to replace itself. It also has the ability to grow thicker where it is constantly rubbed, especially on the soles of the feet and the palms of the hands. It is elastic, which means it stretches as a person moves and returns to its original shape. As people age skin becomes less elastic. The outermost layer of the skin is kept supple by the natural oil called sebum. There are two basic skin types on the body:

- hairy skin – covers most of the body and has hair follicles and hairs
- non-hairy skin – found on the palms of the hands and soles of the feet, which has no hairs.

When a slice or section down through the skin is seen under a microscope, a number of layers and other structures can be seen. These are shown in Fig 6.3.

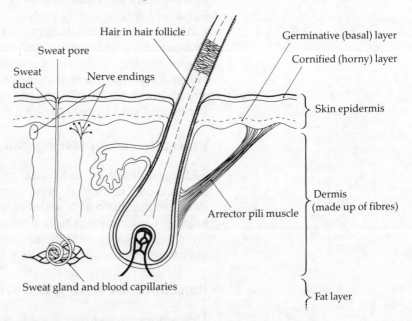

Fig 6.3 Simplified diagram of a section through the skin

## Layers of the skin

The outer skin of the **epidermis** has under it an elastic layer called the **dermis**. The outer epidermis is constantly being worn away (which is why stains on the skin 'wear off'). The epidermis has a lower layer called the germinative or basal layer, where the cells divide to produce new skin epidermis. As the cells produced in the germinative layer are pushed upwards by new cells produced underneath (a very similar pattern to hair growth) they produce keratin and have **pigment** laid down. By the time they reach the outer suface of the epidermis they are dead and scale-like and form the outer **cornified** or **horny** layer of the epidermis. This layer acts as the main barrier against water loss and infection. The epidermis is shown in Fig 6.3. The cornified layer is particularly thick in non-hairy skin and has ridges for better grip; on the hands these form fingerprints.

Under the epidermis is the **dermis**, which is made up of fibres (not cells) of elastic proteins called **collagen** and **elastin** which gives skin its ability to stretch.

## Pigments in the skin

Unless someone is an **albino**, (a person with no pigment in their skin), everyone has some of a pigment called **melanin** in their skins. The amount is partly inherited and partly due to a reaction to **ultraviolet** light reaching the skin. Ultraviolet rays are present in sunlight and can damage the sensitive cells of the germinative layer and other skin structures. Melanin absorbs these rays and protects the skin cells. If skin with relatively little melanin in it is exposed to ultraviolet rays from sunshine (or produced by a special lamp), extra melanin is made and laid down in the epidermis by special cells called **melanocytes**, and this results in a sun tan. Some people's melanocytes are not evenly spread on their skin but occur in clumps, which result in freckles, common to people with red hair and fair skins. These same pigment-producing melanocytes are responsible for depositing melanin into the hair as it grows up the hair follicle.

## The head and the face

Like other parts of the body, the head and face are made up of:

1  an underlying framework of bones, which provides support and some protection;
2  muscles, which cause movement;
3  nerves, which control muscles and take messages back to the brain, e.g. the pressure and touch nerve endings in the skin;
4  a blood supply to provide the living cells with the chemical they need to take waste chemicals away.

## Bones of the head and face

The bones of the head and face make up the **skull** and contribute to the **shape** of the face. Most of the bones are flattened and are 'plates' of bone. The main ones are:

1 the 'dome' or the **cranium** or the top of the head, underlying the **scalp**. This is made up of a number of **cranial bones**.
2 the **cheekbones**.
3 the **jaw bones** – the lower jaw is able to move but the rest of the bones are locked firmly together.

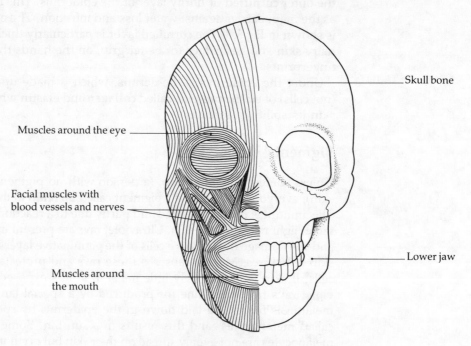

Skull bone

Muscles around the eye

Facial muscles with blood vessels and nerves

Lower jaw

Muscles around the mouth

**Fig 6.4 Muscles of the face**

## Muscles of the face

These are used in eating, talking and also in facial expression. Humans are thought to have the most expressive faces of any animal – we have over 200 muscles in our faces. The muscles contract and produce movements. Facial bones, muscles and underlying fat together produce the shape of someone's face.

## Nerves of the head and face

The large number of muscles in the face and the way they are used in facial expression means that the head and face are richly supplied with nerve fibres which carry 'instructions' from the brain. The scalp and face are also sensitive and nerve endings buried in the skin send 'messages' to the brain. Some parts are more sensitive than others, the lips for example, are very sensitive to touch.

## Blood supply

Blood is supplied to the muscles, bones and skin of the head and face by a network of **blood vessels**. The scalp has a rich supply and this is why scalp wounds bleed so much.

## Summary

Hair grows as a result of cell division in the dermal papilla of a hair follicle. The distribution and angle of the follicle in the skin produces the density and pattern of hair growth. The hair shaft consist of two layers, an outer cuticle made up of overlapping plates and inner cortex which consists of a large number of fibres held together by a 'cement'-like substance. The presence of a third layer, an inner medulla is not clear.

The follicle contains a root sheath which holds the hair in place and a sebaceous gland which produces sebum, the natural conditioner of hair and skin. Removal of sebum from a hairdresser's hands may be a factor leading to dermatitis.

In the hair bulb the cells making up the hair are alive but as they are pushed up the follicle they become keratinised and pigmented and thus die. During its lifetime a scalp hair goes through three main phases:
1  Anagen: where the hair is actively growing
2  Telogen: where growth stops and the base of the hair forms a 'club root'
3  Catagen: where a new hair eventually starts to develop and the old hair is pushed or falls out.

The types of hair encountered on an adult are vellus and secondary/or terminal hair

Skin covers the entire body and consists of two main layers: the outer epidermis and an inner dermis. The epidermis has as its outer layer the horny or cornified layer which waterproofs the body and acts as a barrier against infection. The cornified layer is made up of flattened scale-like dead cells containing keratin and pigments such as melanin. The skin pigments protect the underlying cells from ultraviolet rays in sunlight. The cornified layer is constantly flaking off so it is replaced by cell division in the basal or germinative layer of the epidermis. This cell division also gives skin the ability to repair itself. Under the epidermis is the dermis which consists mostly of elastic fibres which gives skin its elasticity. The head and face have the underlying bones of the skull on to which the muscles are attached. This is shown in Fig 6.4. The head and face have a rich blood and nerve supply.

## Self-assessment questions

1  Name the process which causes hair growth.
2  Where is sebum produced?
3  What are the average width and depth of a hair follicle?
4  What features of the scalp hair are influenced by the distribution of follicles in the skin?
5  What name is given to the part of the hair above the skin?
6  How is the hair cortex organised?
7  Why is there a risk of dermatitis with constant removal of sebum from the hands?
8  Where does keratinisation take place in the follicle?
9  Name the three stages in the growth of a hair. About what percentage of scalp hair will be in each stage and about how long does each stage last?
10  What is vellus hair?
11  List three main functions of the skin.
12  What is the proper name for the 'growing layer' of the skin?
13  Name three ways whereby the skin helps body temperature control.
14  Which rays in sunlight can trigger the skin melanocytes?
15  Name two sensations that can be felt from the hair.

## Practical assignment – Hair and skin structure

The porosity and elasticity of the hair has an effect on all hairdressing services. The following task has been designed to give you practice in identifying the degree of porosity and elasticity of various hair types.

## Tasks

1  Carry out a test for both elasticity and porosity on a variety of clients with the following types of hair:

(a)  Virgin
(b)  Tinted
(c)  Highly bleached
(d)  Strong, coarse, naturally white hair.

2  Take a hair cutting of each of the above hair types.
3  Attach the hair cuttings on to plain A4 paper. Label and state the degree of porosity of each hair cutting and categorise the degree of porosity as follows:

(a)  Extremely porous
(b)  Slightly porous
(c)  Normal
(d)  Resistant.

4  Describe the effect(s) of extremely porous hair on:

(a)  Setting and blowdrying
(b)  Permanent waving
(c)  Tinting.

# 7 DIAGNOSTICS

A client in a hairdressing salon is usually most concerned with the results of the styling carried out and the hair treatment by the salon workers. They seldom think of the potential hazards in the salon until something goes wrong and they, or someone else, are involved. A hairdresser needs to be aware of these potential hazards in order to prevent problems from arising both to themselves and the client. The potential hazards in the salon can be roughly divided into three categories. These are:

(a) **Physical** hazards – which are treated in detail in Chapter 5, and include, wounds, tripping, heat burns and electric shocks.

(b) **chemical** hazards – also treated in detail in Chapter 5, and referred to in many other parts of this book. These include chemical burns, skin reactions to chemicals, e.g. 'para' hair dyes and contact dermatitis, and the safe storage and disposal of chemicals and aerosol spray cans.

(c) **biological** hazards – which include the possible infections and infestations to which the hairdresser or the client may be exposed. This chapter concentrates on these.

## Body infections and infestations

Both infections and infestations are caused by parasites. These terms are explained below:

- A **parasite** is a living organism which lives off another living thing (called the parasite's **host**) but with only the parasite benefitting.
- A body **infection** is caused by a disease-causing, or **pathogenic micro-organism**, living on the body, feeding from it and producing the 'signs' or symptoms of the disease. These parasites (commonly called **germs**) involve many different sorts of living things, but they all share the characteristic of being too small to be seen with the unaided eye.

• A body **infestation** describes an invasion by larger animal parasites which are visible to the unaided eye and mostly live at or near, the surface of the body. A specialised use of the word 'infestation' refers to buildings where large numbers of 'unwanted' animals (e.g. rats and mice) are living.

## Transmission

Both pathogenic micro-organisms and the larger animal parasites need to be passed or transmitted from one person to another. This transmission may take place in two main ways, which are either by contact or through the air.

### Transmission by contact

'Contact' means that physical touching causes the transmission of the parasite. If a parasite can be passed in this way it is described as being **contagious**. This contact can be direct or indirect. Touching lips during kissing can transmit the micro-organism which cause **cold sores (herpes)** from one person to another. Touching heads allows the **head louse** to walk from one head to another. Both of these examples involve direct contact.

Indirect contact often involves inanimate objects which have been in contact with one person and are then touched by another; **cold sores**, for example, can be spread on damp towels, face cloths etc., which have been in contact with one person and then used by another. Head lice may be transmitted from brushes and combs from one person to another.

### Transmission through the air

This only involves the parasitic micro-organisms. If a parasite is passed from one person to another in this way it is described as **infectious**. The micro-organisms which cause the common cold and influenza ('flu') are spread by tiny droplets released by coughing and sneezing being breathed in by someone else. The micro-organisms which causes **ringworm (tinea)** is often spread in minute **skin flakes** released by an infected person (or animal) which settle on to someone else.

### Preventing the transmission of parasites in the salon

The prevention of transmission of infections and infestations depends on two main factors:

(a) general salon hygiene;
(b) the ability of the salon staff to recognise which skin and scalp conditions are infectious or contagious and which are not.

## Hygiene

The transmission of the parasites which cause infections and infestations can be limited by good hygiene in the salon. Good hygiene involves a number of things but these can be summarised as:

(a) the routine practice carried out by the hairdresser, e.g. sterilising brushes and combs, using a new neck strip, etc. for each client;

(b) salon management practice, e.g. regular laundering of uniforms and gowns, regular cleaning of surfaces, etc.; training staff to carry it out;

(c) salon design features which help hygiene, e.g. choice of wall and floor coverings, type of upholstery on seating, type of ventilation system, etc.

## Salon staff

The transmission of infections and infestations can also be reduced by the salon staff knowing:

1  how to recognise the various scalp and skin conditions and to know which of these are contagious (spread by contact), which are infectious (spread by the air) and which are neither infectious nor contagious these are covered later in this Chapter;

2  how to deal with the client if a scalp or skin condition is thought to be of an infectious or contagious type;

3  what steps to take in the salon to prevent this from happening.

1 *Recognition of skin and scalp conditions* – this is very much a job for an expert. Few hairdressers have the training or experience needed to be able to determine exactly what many skin or scalp conditions are. Some are relatively easy and hairdressers have an important role to play in often being the first to notice the condition and be in a position to advise the client. An infestation by head lice is a good example of this, where the client may have noticed the itching, but may be unaware of the cause. Other skin conditions involve rashes, skin scaling, crusting or weeping and these can be due to a variety of causes, some infectious or contagious and others not.

This chapter covers these in outline, but the rule should be:

**If in doubt do not start hairdressing operations (if they have started, then stop) and advise the client to see their doctor.**

2 *How to deal with the client* – the key word here is tact. The hairdresser is in a difficult position and there are no rules for dealing with the client. Here are some general points.

● Talk quietly to the client and, if possible, speak to them alone.

Find out whether they have seen a doctor about the condition. If they have not, strongly advise them to do so.

- If the condition has been identified, do not be too certain when discussing it with the client. It is far better that an expert confirms the nature of the condition.
- Stress that the condition is nothing to do with personal hygiene (this is particularly important with infestations) and that anyone can contract it.
- If hairdressing operations are not possible explain to the client the risk of infecting other clients (even if not sure which condition they have).
- Explain that if the condition is diagnosed by experts as non-infectious/contagious they will be welcome to return to the salon. If it is infectious or contagious, they will be welcome when it has been successfully treated.
- Stress that there are few hair or skin conditions which cannot be successfully treated.

3 *What to do in the salon* – if an infectious or contagious condition has been provisionally identified then:

- carefully sterilise any tools or equipment used on the client;
- take gowns, towels, etc., used on the client and soak in a strong disinfectant solution;
- wipe down chairs they have used with a disinfectant solution (and vacuum clean if possible);
- carefully sweep or vacuum up any hair clippings and dispose of them immediately outside the salon, by burning if possible.

## Infections caused by micro-organisms

For any infection to take place, the disease-causing micro-organism needs to invade (or infect) the body, i.e. the pathogen must pass the **body defence system** which operates in three parts:

(*a*) The outer defence is the skin and the lining of the lungs and digestive system. All of these act as a physical barrier to the pathogens. The skin, for example, has the outer cornified (or horny) layer which protects the living cells underneath. It is constantly flaking off and this helps remove micro-organisms living on the skin's surface. The natural oil, sebum, also helps control the number of skin micro-organisms, as it acts as an **antiseptic.**

(*b*) The blood contains **white blood cells** which may kill invading pathogens by **engulfing** them, i.e. taking the micro-organism inside the cell.

(*c*) The body also has the ability to produce **antibodies** which are special chemicals which help to destroy the invading pathogens.

If the pathogen is successful in invading the body and if it can survive the action of the body defence system, then it produces the signs or symptoms of the disease.

## Types of micro-organism

There are many types of micro-organism; the only feature they share is their small size which makes individuals invisible to the unaided eye. They can be grouped into:

(a) bacteria
(b) moulds and yeasts
(c) fungi
(d) viruses.

The vast majority of any of these groups are either neutral, i.e. not having any effect on humans, or useful, e.g. yeast in bread making and brewing wine and beer (neutral) and bacteria in cheese and yoghurt making and moulds in the manufacture of **antibiotics** (useful). Antibiotics are very useful chemicals which can be taken by mouth, applied as an ointment or injected into a person, where they kill most pathogens (the exception being viruses) without harming the individual. Only a relatively small number of micro-organisms are harmful in that they cause disease, and these are described as **pathogenic**.

## Skin and scalp conditons caused by bacteria

Bacteria can be found just about everywhere around us – on the skin, hair, clothing, in water and in the air. They can only be seen using a microscope, and when observed in this way, particular types of bacteria have characteristic shapes and cell clusterings. Others have tiny hairs, called **flagella**, which they use to move themselves about. Some of these different cells are shown in Fig 7.1. The shape of the cells are used to name types of bacteria, e.g.:

- rod-shaped cells are called **bacilli**, e.g. lactobacilli used in cheese making.

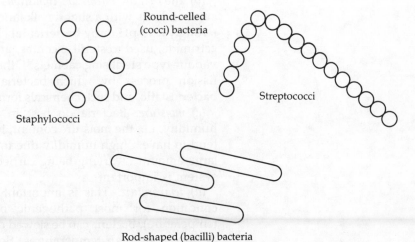

Round-celled (cocci) bacteria

Streptococci

Staphylococci

Rod-shaped (bacilli) bacteria

**Fig 7.1 Shapes of bacteria cells**

- round cells are called **cocci**, e.g. staphylococci on the skin;
- spiral cells are called **spirochaetes**, e.g. vibrios bacteria which cause cholera appear as spiral cells.

Most bacteria multiply by a process called **binary fission**, where one bacterial cell splits into two cells, which then grow and divide again. This process is shown in Fig. 7.2 and can produce very large

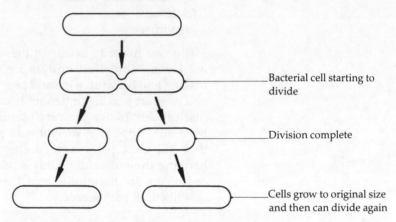

**Fig 7.2 Outline of binary fission in bacteria**

numbers of bacteria, from relatively few original cells, if conditions are favourable. Favourable conditions include:

(*a*) *a source of food*. Many bacteria feed on and cause the decay of dead organic material (this type of organism is called a **saprophyte**). Others feed on other living organisms and are called **parasites**. The pathogenic bacteria are all parasites when causing the disease, but many can also exist as saprophytes, which is the reason why dirt is an important source of pathogens.

(*b*) the right *chemical conditions*. Many bacteria thrive in surroundings with a slightly alkaline pH. They are destroyed at a strongly acid pH or by **bactericidal** chemicals in disinfectants, e.g. cetrimide, used to sterilise combs, and the sterilising fluid used in vapour-type sterilising cabinets. Other chemicals inhibit the binary fission process by which bacteria multiply, these are called **bacteriostatic**, and such chemicals form the basis of many antiseptics.

(*c*) *moisture*. Bacteria do best in damp conditions where the humidity, i.e. the moisture content, is high. As hairdressing salons tend to have a high humidity due to the use of hot water and the large amount of drying being carried out, an efficient ventilation system is important.

(*d*) *temperature*. This is important in that the most favourable condition for most pathogenic bacteria is 37°C (i.e. body temperature). Bacteria can be slowed down by low temperatures and destroyed by high temperatures. Some bacteria can form spores which act as tiny 'survival' capsules for the bacterial cell. These spores are very resistant to chemicals and heat and for this reason, bacterial spores are the last micro-organisms killed when something is sterilised (i.e. all the micro-organisms are killed).

Many skin and scalp conditions are caused by bacteria normally found living on the skin. Two groups in particular, staphylococci and streptococci, will turn up several times as the cause of bacterial skin and scalp conditions. Both of these can also cause wound infection (or **sepsis**) which involves reddening and inflammation (swelling) and pus formation. If this occurs, not at a wound, but at a hair follicle, it is described as **folliculitis**. The reddening and inflammation are caused by the body reaction to the activity of the bacteria. Pus is formed by the battle between the invading bacteria and white blood cells and consists mostly of dead white cells and dead bacteria resulting from the infection. But it also contains some living bacteria which can spread the infection to others if transmitted to them by direct or indirect contact.

In terms of skin conditions caused by bacteria, the following will be considered:

- impetigo;
- boils;
- barber's itch;
- folliculitis.

### 1 Impetigo (common type or impetigo vulgaris)
**Caused by:**
the skin bacteria staphylococci and streptococci.
**Major symptoms:**
blisters which contain a clear fluid and eventually form yellow crusts on the skin. Common on face and scalp, where the infection spreads rapidly. (*See* Fig. 7.3.)

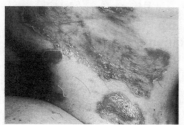
**Fig 7.3**

- Impetigo is commonly caused by bacteria invading skin broken by scratching, e.g. as a result of head lice or itchmite infestation. This is called **secondary infection**.
- It is very contagious and spread by both direct and indirect contact. Hairdressing operations should not be started, or if they have, the stylist should stop and take care to sterilise by disinfectant, tools and equipment used.
- A different form of impetigo occurs in children (called Bockhardts' impetigo) which is caused by staphylococci bacteria invading scalp hair follicles and causing them to become inflamed, i.e. producing folliculitis. The condition appears as small red spots in the skin at the base of the hair with a 'head' of pus (called a **pustule**). Hairdressers should treat it as impetigo above.
- The hairdresser should reassure the client that the infection often clears up completely fairly quickly, with no scarring.

### 2 Boils (furunculosis)
**Caused by:**
a staphylococci bacteria (often staphylococcus aureus) invading a

hair follicle or sebaceous gland and producing severe inflammation.
**Major symptoms:**
a red raised area of the skin, very tender, with a central 'core' containing pus.

- Boils are common where clothing rubs, e.g. back or side of neck in males, where shirt collar may rub. Staphylococcus aureus, which causes boils, is found living in the noses of between 10 and 30 per cent of the population. So it is possible to infect someone by coughing and sneezing. Sometimes a group of neighbouring follicles become involved, and this is called a **carbuncle**.
- Do not start hairdressing operations (or stop if already started) if a boil is in the area involved, e.g. scalp or beard. If the boil is not in such an area take great care not to touch it with the tools, equipment, towels, etc. This will be painful for the client and there is the possibility of picking up, and thus spreading, the bacteria.

*3   Barber's itch (sycosis barbae)*
**Caused by:**
staphylococci bacteria invading the hair follicles in the beard area in males.
**Major symptoms:**
inflammation and pus formation in some of the beard hair follicles (i.e. folliculitis). Pain and itching in these areas.

- Barber's itch can be spread by indirect contact on shaving brushes, razors and towels.
- If scalp operations are intended, take great care not to touch beard area involved with tools, equipment or towels and gowns. Sterilise all these items after use. Do not start shaving or beard-trimming.

*4   Folliculitis*
**Caused by:**
Staphylococci bacteria.
**Major symptoms:**

- Infected hair follicles producing yellow spot with hair in centre.
- Itching and scratching.

## Moulds and yeasts

These cover a wide range of micro-organisms, usually connected with decay of organic material. Moulds occur on the skin and are thought to produce 'natural' antibiotics, which help keep the skin bacteria under control. Yeasts have been found (with bacteria) under the flaking skin of scalps with dandruff. They do not cause the condition, but their growth is favoured by the damp, warm conditions under the flakes.

## Fungi

The fungi group ranges in size from mushrooms and toadstools down to microscopic varieties. Most live off dead organic material where they cause **decay**. Some microscopic types are parasites and cause skin and scalp conditions called ringworm in humans and animals. One characteristic of all fungi is that they are made up of tiny threads called **hyphae**. In a large fungus, e.g. a mushroom, there are millions of these bound together; in a microscopic fungus, there are relatively few. In parasitic fungi, these threads grow through the skin and hair shafts (if present).

*Ringworm (tinea)*
It can be found as:

(*a*) ringworm of the scalp (tinea capitis) – covered in detail below.

(*b*) ringworm of the body (tinea corporis) – similar symptoms to scalp ringworm but most often caught from domestic animals.

(*c*) ringworm of the foot or 'athlete's foot' (tinea pedis) – a common condition, where the fungus grows through the skin between the toes causing reddening and itching (and possibly skin cracking). Commonly contracted by indirect contact through wet floors, e.g. changing rooms and swimming pools. (*See* Fig 7.4.)

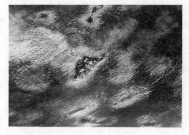

Fig 7.4

Ringworm of the scalp (tinea capitis) is:
**Caused by:**
the microscopic threads of the parasitic fungus growing through the cornified (horny) layer of the skin epidermis and through any hair shafts it encounters.
**Major symptoms:**
bald patches on the scalp with a stubble of broken off hairs (due to weakening of the hair shaft as the fungus grows through it). The bald patches are often circular and the skin inflammed.

- It is both highly contagious by indirect and direct contact and is infectious in that skin flakes breaking off from an infected person can land on another, and if they lodge for long enough they can grow from the flake into the other person's skin. It can be contracted from domestic animals.
- It is most common in children.
- Do not start (or stop, if already started) hairdressing operations. If operations have been started then disinfect tools, equipment gowns, towels and seating.
- Sweep up (or better, vacuum) any hair clippings; place in sealed plastic bags and preferably dispose of by burning outside the salon.

## Viruses

Viruses are the smallest of all the micro-organisms and unlike bacteria, moulds, yeasts and fungi, they cannot survive for long outside living cells, i.e. they are all parasitic. A common form of transmission of viral diseases is by **droplet infection**. When someone coughs or sneezes, hundreds of tiny droplets of liquid are blown into the air. These may contain living viruses which can survive as long as the droplet persists. In damp air (that is, air with a high relative humidity), the droplets evaporate slowly and this increases the chances of someone else inhaling the droplets and becoming infected. In dry air (that is, air with a low relative humidity), the droplets evaporate quickly and the viruses die. The common cold and 'flu (influenza) are spread in this way. Because of the large amounts of moisture entering the air in hairdressing salons (due to hot water being used, the large amount of drying etc.) the air tends to have a relatively high humidity, unless the ventilation system can cope with its removal. This is one reason why an efficient ventilation system is important in the salon.

The various skin conditions caused by viruses are cold sores (herpes simplex) and some types of wart.

### 1 Cold sores (herpes simplex)
**Caused by:**
a virus which lives in the germinative layer of the skin epidermis (present in about 90 per cent of the population) and develops when a person's general resistance is lowered, e.g. by another disease. (*See* Fig 7.5.)
**Symptoms:**
Often begins as a small crack in dry skin in the corner (or corners) of the mouth. It spreads rapidly with some blistering and develops into an oozing crust (like a soft scab).

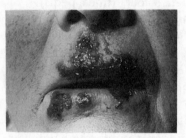

Fig 7.5

- It is very common, especially in children.
- It can be passed by direct or indirect contact; therefore, care should be taken to sterilise cups etc., used by clients or towels likely to have touched the face. If persistent, suggest the client sees a doctor. Often clears up spontaneously, but is 'carried' in the body until the next time conditions favour its growth.

### 2 Warts (verrucae)
**Caused by:**
a virus (called papova virus) which lives in the germinative layer of the skin epidermis, where it triggers a large amount of cell division in a small area. This produces the 'lumps' characteristic of common warts. On the feet the pressure causes the wart to grow inwards, which produces a plantar wart (commonly called 'verrucae').
**Symptoms:**
(*a*) raised warts – may be rough and rise some distance above the skin (common warts) or be smaller and smooth-topped (plane warts – common in children). (*See* Fig 7.6.)

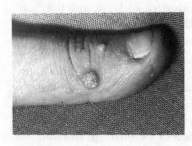

Fig 7.6

(*b*) plantar warts – grow into the skin on the feet, where the pressure caused by the weight of the body is greatest, e.g. on the 'ball' of the foot.

- Unless a client feels strongly that the size and position of the wart necessitates removal, they are best left alone. If removal is desirable, then recommend they see their doctor and do not use the proprietary 'wart removers' on the market.
- Warts often clear spontaneously as the body eventually becomes immune to the virus which causes them.
- They can be transmitted by direct or indirect contact, so take reasonable precautions.
- Plantar warts (verrucae) are spread by indirect contact in places with damp or wet floors, e.g. changing rooms and swimming pools.

*3 AIDS and Hepatitis B*
These are serious infections which could be passed on in the salon. The chances of this are very slight – they could be transmitted in blood spillage.

## Eye infections

These can spread rapidly by indirect contact with damp towels in the salon. The two main kinds are:

*1 Blepharitis (or 'styes')* – where staphylococci bacteria infect the eyelash follicles, causing soreness, reddening and swelling.
*2 Conjunctivitis* – which can have a variety of causes, e.g. bacteria like staphylococci and some viruses. Conjunctivitis is the inflammation of the outer, protective layer on the front of the eyeball and can be spread by indirect contact with damp towels; some forms are very infectious. Because of the high risk of transferring the micro-organisms on to towels, hairdressing operations should be stopped and the client advised to see their doctor.

## Infestations caused by animal parasites

These larger parasites are visible to the unaided eye and feed off the human body. Important examples in hairdressing are:

    (*a*) lice (especially the head louse)
    (*b*) flea
    (*c*) itchmite (which causes scabies).

A point to remember is that anyone can become infested and it is not a reflection on personal hygiene to have picked up these parasites. In fact, head lice prefer clean scalps to dirty ones.

Lice and fleas are insects and have six legs. Both have special jaws which can pierce the person's skin and then suck blood (the mouths work rather like the hollow needle of a hypodermic syringe used to take a blood sample at the hospital). When the person's skin is pierced, the animal injects a small amount of **anticoagulant** into the tiny wound to prevent the blood from clotting. It is this action that:

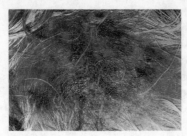

**Fig 7.7**

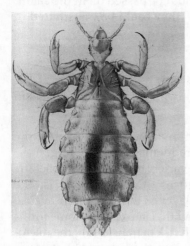

**Fig 7.8**

- produces the skin reddening and itching associated with lice and flea 'bites'. The scratching of these areas often breaks the skin surface and allows invasion by the skin bacteria, producing a secondary infection, e.g. **impetigo** (*See* Fig 7.7)
- can lead to other infections passed on by the parasite. This is unlikely in the UK, but fleas can pass on plague and lice, typhus.

Itchmites belong to a branch of the spider family and have eight legs. They are the smallest of the animal parasites with the female mite less that 0.5 mm long (the male is almost half that size). the female digs tunnels into the skin and in these lays her eggs. Chemicals released by the mites can cause intense irritation and itching and a common name for scabies is the 'itch'.

## Lice

There are three types of human lice and infestation of the body by lice is called **pediculosis**. The types are:

### Head lice (pediculus capitis)

This is the most important variety for hairdressers. About 4 per cent of the population have head lice at any one time and they are often first noticed by the hairdresser. A head louse is shown in Fig. 7.8. The adults are about 3 mm long and have flattened bodies. Each leg has strong claws at the end, used to grip hair shafts. The flattened bodies and the claws make it difficult to dislodge adult lice and any lice which fall out of untreated hair are dying (due to injury or old age).

Lice pierce the skin and suck blood, causing a certain amount of irritation (how much depends on the number of lice and the individual). Lice only have a life-span of about 30 days and events during this are outlined in Fig 7.9.

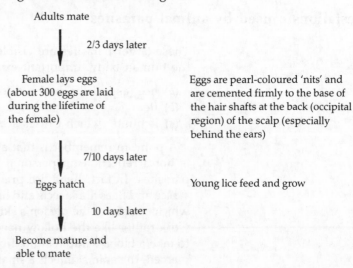

Adults mate

↓ 2/3 days later

Female lays eggs (about 300 eggs are laid during the lifetime of the female) — Eggs are pearl-coloured 'nits' and are cemented firmly to the base of the hair shafts at the back (occipital region) of the scalp (especially behind the ears)

↓ 7/10 days later

Eggs hatch — Young lice feed and grow

↓ 10 days later

Become mature and able to mate

**Fig 7.9**

Only a few of the eggs laid survive to maturity and a typical head infestation involves about 20 adult lice (although there can be more or fewer).

Head lice are contagious and can be transmitted from one person to another by:

(*a*) direct head to head contact, e.g. children get them while playing, which provides a chance for the lice to walk from one head to another. This is by far the most frequent method of transmission. *NB* Lice cannot jump or fly.

(*b*) indirect contact from pillows, towels, upholstery, etc., but this needs to happen fairly quickly as lice cannot survive for long off the scalp. Any seen off the scalp are usually dying, or dead.

**Symptoms:**
The client will probably have noticed some itching but may be unaware of its cause. The infestation is often first noticed by the presence of the eggs or **nits** glued to the bases of the hair shafts and sometimes the adults are visible.

- Reassure the client that contracting head lice is nothing to do with personal hygiene (many people are horrified when they are told) and that it is easy to eradicate (the Health Education Council produces a range of very useful pamphlets on body parasites, including the head louse and these are available free from your nearest office or Head Office).
- Do point out that others in the family are likely to be infected and that expert advice, e.g. doctor, health visitor or local health clinic should be sought.
- Because head lice are contagious, do not begin (or stop, if started) hairdressing operations. Take care to disinfect tools and equipment thoroughly, wipe down with disinfectant and vacuum clean the upholstery of chairs the client has used.
- The eggs or nits can sometimes be mistaken for flakes of dandruff. If in doubt, try to rub the flake off the hair. Dandruff flakes are easily removed, nits are not.

## The human flea (pulex irritans)

The human flea has a body which is flattened vertically to allow it to slip between hairs. Its long back legs make it very good at jumping and this is how it is transmitted from one person to another. It is possible for fleas to be carried into the salon by an infested client, but the infestation is unlikely to be large. The female flea lays her eggs on floors, carpets etc., and when these hatch they feed on organic material, e.g. skin flakes in dust. This is the vulnerable place in their lifecycle, because regular vacuum cleaning of floors and seating is very efficient at removing the eggs and juvenile fleas.

Adult fleas feed by sucking blood and the bites produce characteristic small red spots with surrounding pink patches. Another common feature of flea bites is tiny spots of blood on the clothing or bedding, corresponding to the bite in the skin.

## Itchmite (sarcoptes scabiei)

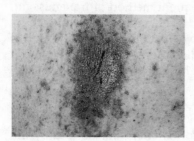

Fig 7.10

The itchmite causes **scabies** (or the 'itch') and about two per cent of the population is infected at any one time. The intense itching, which is often a characteristic of infestation, is due to the female mite **burrowing** into the skin. The mite burrows using its jaws and its front two pairs of legs, and the itching reaction is not so much due to the burrow itself as to chemicals released by the mite. The burrows are about 1 to 2 cm (½ to 1″) long and are dug mostly in non-hairy parts of the skin and particularly on the inside of joints, e.g. between the fingers and the inside of the elbow. The burrows are sometimes visible as red lines on the skin (*See* Fig 7.10) but are often obscured by scratching and secondary infections like **impetigo** are common.

The female digs burrows in the epidermis in order to lay her eggs in them; 10 to 25 eggs are laid along each burrow. The eggs hatch and the juvenile mites then move to hair follicles in which they lie until mature. When mature, they emerge onto the skin surface, mate, and then the females begin burrowing. Itchmites are very small (the female is only about 0.5 mm long) and only just visible to the unaided eye. On a first infestation, it may take six weeks (or three generations of mites) before the itching becomes noticeable. Thus, by the time someone realises that they have a problem, a considerable infestation can have taken place.

Itchmites can be transmitted by both direct contact, e.g. in bed at night, or by indirect contact with bedding, clothing and towels.

Because the face and scalp are rarely affected, it is unlikely that a hairdresser will detect this condition. If this does occur, refer the client to their doctor.

## Non-infectious/contagious skin and hair conditions

In addition to the infectious and contagious conditions (like impetigo, ringworm, warts, and infestation by head lice) there are a number of non-infectious/contagious skin and hair conditions.

Some of these are very common, e.g. split ends (**fragilitas crinium** where the hair at the points split lengthways. The only cure is to cut the ends off.

Other conditions are far less common such as:

- **trichorrhexis nodosa** – where hair is fragile due to splits along the hair shaft;
- **monilethrix** – a very rare condition where the hair shaft has a beaded appearance due to distorted growth.

Some conditions are caused by hair in areas that are normally vellus becoming secondary hair. Examples are hypertrichosis, where this happens in certain areas, and hirsutism, which is more general across the whole body.

These can be caused by external or internal factors. It is important to be able to recognise these and distinguish them from the infectious or contagious types of conditions. This is because the infectious or contagious conditions generally prevent hairdressing operations, whereas those in this section do not. Other problems include:

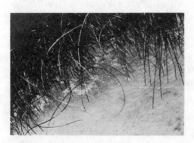

Fig 7.11 (a)

## Psoriasis

It is an inherited condition and, therefore, is commonly found amongst members of the same family. The cause of psoriasis is not known for certain, but it may be caused by a defect in the chemical reactions taking place in the germinative (or basal) layer of the skin epidermis.

**Symptoms:**
patches of thickened silver-coloured scales with the underlying skin appearing red. There is no hair loss or itching associated with the condition. (*See* Figs 7.11(a) and (b)).

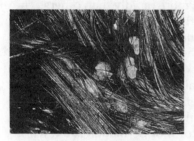

Fig 7.11 (b)

- The appearance and extent of psoriasis varies and scalp psoriasis, if extensive and severe, can be distressing to the client. They should be tactfully encouraged to seek expert advice and help.

## Dermatitis and eczema

Both the terms 'dermatitis' and 'eczema' are used interchangeably to describe an inflammation of the skin surface.

Distinctions can be made on the basis of:

(*a*) whether the condition is 'dry' or releases a fluid, i.e. 'weeps', where dermatitis is used for the 'dry' condition and eczema for the 'weeping' variety.

(*b*) what causes (or 'triggers') the development of the condition. Dermatitis is thought to be caused by both internal and external factors and eczema due to internal factors only.

The second distinction is analysed here, and contact dermatitis followed by eczema will now be treated in detail.

## Contact dermatitis

As its name suggest, 'contact' dermatitis may be produced in the skin due to contact with a chemical or chemicals. Some chemicals will produce a dermatic rash on first exposure and these are called **primary irritants** (examples are perm lotion and anti-perspirants, but many substances can be involved). The rash and other symptoms

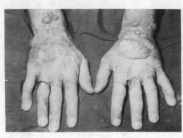

Fig 7.12

are due to the person's body 'over-reacting' to the contact with the chemical and this over-reaction can be called an **allergy**. People may be allergic to many different substances, a common one being pollen grains in the air, causing hay fever. All allergies involve the body defence system over-reacting to a substance.

Thus, the external factor involved is the contact with the chemical and the internal factors determine the person's reaction to that chemical. Other substances can produce dermatitis after a number of exposures. This is a major problem in hairdressing as the actual number of times a person needs to be exposed to a substance until they get dermatitis varies with different individuals. Substances which may eventually produce a reaction are called **sensitisers**, and a person **develops** a sensitivity to a particular substance. Why the number of exposures needed to provoke a reaction varies so much between people is not known but some people seem to have a **predisposition** to become sensitised more rapidly than others. The chemical in 'para' hair tints is a fairly common sensitiser and the reason for the skin test which should be carried out 24–48 hours before using such a tint is to check whether previous exposures have sensitised the client. As with primary irritants, the development of dermatitis depends on both external factors (such as the number and duration of exposures) and internal factors (how sensitised to the substance a person is). Many of the chemicals used in the salon can act as sensitisers. An extreme form of dermatitis is shown in Fig. 7.12.

**Symptoms:**

These are very variable, but include:

(a) inflammation of the skin surface;

(b) cracking of the skin and possibly 'weeping' of fluid;

(c) a certain amount of itching.

The risk to the hairdresser involves the hands in 90 per cent of cases. A hairdresser's hands are at risk due to two main factors:

(a) the regular use of shampoos on the client which removes the sebum (natural oils) from the hairdresser's skin. This natural oil acts as a waterproof barrier to many chemicals and if removed, this barrier is reduced. This makes it more likely that chemicals (including the detergent in shampoo) can penetrate to the living cells of the epidermis and produce a reaction.

(b) the frequency at which a hairdresser applies hairdressing preparations to the client. This means that the hairdresser is regularly exposed to chemicals which can produce dermatitis.

The risk to the client tends to be on the face. Dermatitis triggered by the 'para' dyes, for example, tends to involve the skin of the eyelids, ears and neck.

**Prevention:**

There is no cure once someone has developed a sensitisation to a substance, the only action is to avoid contact with it. If a hairdresser develops a high level of sensitisation to a commonly used hairdressing chemical, often the only course of action is to leave hairdressing altogether. The best prevention is protection, particularly by using rubber gloves for all hairdressing operations involving chemicals. Barrier creams offer some protection but are not as effective as a pair of rubber gloves.

Protection of the client involves taking care to prevent hairdressing products, especially those known to be sensitisers, from touching their skin.

## Eczema

Eczema is a condition more common in small children than in adults, but it may be encountered in the salon. There appears to be a link between eczema and allergies, in that eczema is often found in children (and adults) who suffer from hay fever and asthma, although the reason for the connection is not clear. Eczema seems to be triggered by internal causes and the severity of the condition varies between different individuals, and with the same person over time. A particular individual can develop the rash and then it disappears for a length of time, this is called a **remission**. The attack can be severe, in which case it is described as acute or less severe, but persistent; this is described as **chronic**.

**Symptoms:**

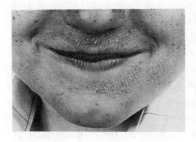

**Fig 7.13**

When severe (or acute) the skin is red and puffy. The rash develops **small cracks** which ooze a clear fluid (this is sometimes described as 'wet' eczema). In children, the rash is common on the face, where it can cover the whole area (apart from around the nose, mouth and eyes). In adults, the rash is more likely to be in small **patches**, with small red lumps in the skin. In all cases, **itching** is intensive and can be triggered by a change in skin temperature, or a change of mood, or contact with clothing. Because of the intense itching, **scratching** is very common (even while asleep) and consequently, there is the risk of a secondary infection, e.g. impetigo, through the broken skin.

When less severe (or chronic), the rash is less widespread, there is little or no cracking and 'weeping' and the itching is less intense (this is sometimes described as 'dry' eczema). (*See* Fig 7.13)

## Differences between contact dermatitis and eczema

The main differences are described in Table 7.1.

**Table 7.1**

| Feature | Eczema | Contact dermatitis |
| --- | --- | --- |
| Extent of rash | Widespread (especially in children) | Localised |
| Itching | Can be intensive | Less intensive |
| Chemical irritants involved? | No | Yes |

## Seborrhea

Seborrhea is the general name for the overproduction of sebum by the skin's **sebaceous glands**. The surplus of natural oil makes the hair greasy and the skin oily. This condition is common in people at **puberty**, where the sudden rise in the level of **sex hormones** in the blood triggers the overproduction of sebum.

Seborrhea is involved in the development of **acne** and in some kinds of **dandruff**. If the dandruff is linked to an inflammation of the scalp, this is called **seborrhoeic dermatitis**.

These conditions are considered in detail below.

## Dandruff (pityriasis)

Dandruff, or 'scurf', is a common scalp condition caused by the **flaking** of the cornified (or horny) layer of the skin epidermis. This flaking of the outermost skin layer occurs all over the body, all of the time and each person loses millions of these tiny flakes per day. The main reason for this general flaking is to remove skin bacteria, and thus keep the numbers of bacteria on the skin under control.

On the scalp, the hair tends to trap these flakes and they 'build up', or accumulate, into the large flakes which are characteristic of the condition. The damp, warm conditions under these flakes favour the multiplication of **bacteria** and **yeasts**.

At one time it was thought that dandruff was caused by bacteria. It is now known that it is not and that some people have a tendency to produce a large number of skin flakes on the scalp, while others do not. Whether bacteria are involved in the itching which often accompanies severe dandruff is not clear at the moment, but antiseptics are included in many medicated or anti-dandruff shampoos to keep the number of bacteria under control. These shampoos also contain substances like **selenium sulphide** and **zinc pyrithione**, which reduce the flaking by reducing the activities of the germinative (or basal) layer of the skin epidermis.

The most common form of dandruff is where the flakes fall freely from the hair when brushed or combed (this is called dry dandruff or **pityriases simplex**). If dandruff occurs in connection with seborrhea (an overproduction of sebum) then the oil tends to make the flakes stick to the scalp (this is sometimes called oily dandruff or **pityriasis stearoides**). This can lead to seborrhoeic dermatitits. In this case the client should be referred to their doctor.

## Sebaceous cysts

These appear as raised areas on the skin and are caused by a blockage in a sebaceous gland. The sebum normally released onto the hair and skin in that area accumulates and causes the swelling. This type of cyst is sometimes called a **wen** and they are harmless.

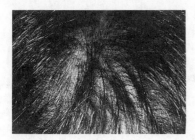

Fig 7.14

## Baldness (alopecia)

The most common type of baldness is **male pattern** baldness, which affects about 40 per cent of males by the age of 40. Figure 7.14 shows a developing alopecia. This condition is inherited and is not as common in females as it is in males. The necessary trigger for the hair loss is the presence of the male sex hormone and this is the reason that this type of hair loss is relatively rare in women. Older women may suffer a version of this balding as their levels of female hormones fall after the **menopause**.

How the male hormone triggers the condition is not known. For no apparent reason the hair follicles start to die when they reach the end of **telogen** in the hair growth cycle. Because of this, no new hair grows to replace the old when it falls out of the follicle. For this reason, this type of balding is a gradual process, with the hair 'thinning' and disappearing from around the crown and above the forehead. At the moment it is not possible to prevent the hair follicles from dying, and the only effective treatment is a hair transplant.

Male pattern baldness accounts for about 90 per cent of hair loss encountered by the salon. The other 10 per cent are made up of conditions where the balding tends to be patchy or scattered; these conditions include:

(a) alopecia areata
(b) diffuse alopecia (alopecia diffusa)
(c) traction alopecia
(d) cicatrical (scarring) alopecia

## Alopecia areata

This is the appearance of roughly circular bald patches on the scalp. The skin of the area is soft, smooth and has no hair. These features are important in distinguishing alopecia areata from ringworm. With ringworm, the bald patches have a stubble of broken off hairs running across them and the skin is often red and inflamed. There is no itching with alopecia areata and the condition also has 'exclamation mark' hairs around the borders of the bald patches. 'Exclamation mark' hairs are caused by the hair breaking and the hair root breaking down. Hairs are wider and darker near the broken end and about 0.5 cm (¼") long. They are easily pulled out and appear like an exclamation mark (!).

Alopecia areata usually disappears in two to three months, but may recur at intervals. The precise reasons for the development of the condition are not known.

## Diffuse alopecia (alopecia diffusa)

This describes a general 'thinning' of the scalp hair, often most noticeable at the crown and along the parting. It can occur in young women, who find it very distressing, due to hormone changes after childbirth and sometimes as a result of oral contraception. It can also occur after serious illness and drug treatments. The hair usually regrows.

Another type of 'thinning' is **alopecia senilis** which is associated with old age.

## Traction alopecia

This is a general term used to describe hair being pulled out of the scalp. This can result from the tension caused by tight rollers and due to the hair style adopted, e.g. tight plaits or hair rolled into a tight 'bun', etc. It can also be caused by a nervous twisting of the hair around the fingers. If the cause of the tension on the hair is removed, then the hair usually grows back.

## Cicatrical (scarring) alopecia

This results from skin damage and scarred areas in which hair will not grow.

**Table 7.2 – Summary: the main infections and infestations**

| Name of condition | Caused by | Major symptoms | Infectious or contagious? | Stop hairdressing operations? | Medical advice needed? |
|---|---|---|---|---|---|
| Impetigo | Bacteria | Blisters and yellow crusts. | Yes (very) | Yes | Yes |
| Boils (furuncles) | Bacteria | Red, raised area in skin. Very tender. Central pus. | Yes (if pus released) | Only if boil in scalp area | Yes, if persistent |
| Barber's itch (sycosis barbae) | Bacteria | Swelling and pus formation in beard hair follicles. | Yes | Yes, on beard area (*NB* avoid contact in this aea) | Yes, if persistent |
| Folliculitis | Bacteria | Yellow spot with hair in centre | Yes | Yes | Yes, if persistent |
| Ringworm (scalp) (tinea capitis) | Fungus | Round bald patches (stubble of hair), skin may be inflamed. | Yes (very) | Yes | Yes |
| Cold sores (herpes simplex) | Virus | Weeping scabs around mouth. | Yes | No, but care to prevent transmission | Not usually, but yes if persistent and extreme |
| Warts (verrucae) | Virus | Lump in skin (rough or smooth). | Yes | No (but avoid nicking with scissors | Not usually, unless removal wanted |

INFECTIONS BY PATHOGENIC MICRO-ORGANISMS

| Name of condition | Caused by | Major symptoms | Infectious or contagious? | Stop hairdressing operations? | Medical advice needed? |
|---|---|---|---|---|---|
| Conjunctivitis | Bacteria or virus | Inflamed eyes, possible weeping of fluid. | Yes | Yes | Yes |

INFESTATIONS BY ANIMAL PARASITES

| Name of condition | Caused by | Major symptoms | Infectious or contagious? | Stop hairdressing operations? | Medical advice needed? |
|---|---|---|---|---|---|
| Head lice (pediculus capitis) | Head louse | Itching, eggs (nits) glued to base of hair. Sometimes adults seen. | Yes | Yes | Yes (but advice can be given by hairdresser) |
| Flea (pulex) irritans) | Human flea | Red spots surrounded by pink patches. Itching. | Yes | Yes | Yes |
| Scabies | Itchmite (sarcopies scabiei) | Intense itching, especially in joints and at night (burrows sometimes visible). | Yes | Yes | Yes |

## Summary – Other problems

This part concentrates on the non-infectious and non-contagious conditions which a hairdresser may encounter. The major areas are outlined below.

**Table 7.3**

| Condition | Symptoms | Notes |
|---|---|---|
| Split ends (*Fragilitas crinium*) | Splitting of the hair at the points. | Often occurs at the points of long hair with a tendency to be dry. Breaks can occur along the length of the hair and there is no real 'cure'. Restructurant conditioners can be used but the only real answer is to cut the split ends off. |
| *Trichorrhexis nodosa* | Swellings occur along the hair. | These are weak points and the hair tends to break. It can be caused by rollers or by strong alkaline chemicals. |

| Condition | Symptoms | Notes |
|---|---|---|
| | | Conditioners which are absorbed into the hair shaft (restructurants) help to prevent breakage. |
| Monilethrix | Bead-like swellings along the hair shaft. | A very rare condition that is inherited and appears mostly in children. Tendency for hair loss as the hair tends to break off near the scalp. |
| Hypertrichosis | The growth of thick secondary (terminal) hair in an area which usually shows only the fine 'down' (vellus) hair. | Can occur on a facial 'mole' for example. |
| Hirsutism | Where male type secondary (terminal) hair growth patterns occur in females. | Includes 'bearded ladies' of which there is a number of medically certified cases. |
| Psoriasis | Silvered coloured scales. Reddened skin. No itching. | Inherited condition. Tends to clear up and recur. |
| Dermatitis and eczema | Swelling of skin. Sometimes cracking and weeping of fluid. | Terms are used inter-changeably. Contact dermatitis is the major occupational risk to hairdressers. |
| Seborrhea | Greasy hair and skin. | Caused by over-production of sebum. Implicated in acne. |
| Dandruff (pityriasis) | Flaking of scalp. | Can be dry or oily. Not caused by bacteria. Some people more prone than others. |
| Sebaceous cyst (wen) | Appearance of roughly circular 'lumps' on the skin. | Caused by a blockage which prevents release of sebum onto the skin. Sebum accumulates under skin. |
| Baldness (alopecia) | Hair loss. | Most common in 'male pattern' type. Inherited and triggered by male hormone. Other types, alopecia areata and alopecia diffusa have unknown causes. Traction alopecia is caused by physical pulling out of hair. |

## Self-assessment questions

1 What is meant by the term 'parasite?
2 What is the difference between an infection and an infestation?
3 What is meant by the transmission of a disease?
4 What is the main purpose of salon hygiene?
5 What is the key word for dealing with a client possibly suffering from an infectious or contagious scalp condition?
6 List the three main parts of the body defence system against disease.
7 List the four conditions which favour multplication of bacteria.
8 What are the major symptoms of head louse infestation (pediculosis)?
9 What precautions should be taken with a client suffering from 'barber's itch' (sycosis barbae)?
10 What are the major symptoms of scalp ringworm (tinea capitis)?
11 What are the major symptoms of psoriasis?
12 What is meant by 'sensitisation'?
13 What are the major precautions to protect:
    (a) the client
    (b) the hairdresser
    from developing contact dermatitis?
14 Why does eczema sometimes produce a secondary infection?
15 Which two factors cause male pattern baldness?
16 List the major differences in the symptoms of alopecia areata and ringworm of the scalp (tinea capitis).
17 What is traction alopecia?
18 Give two possible causes of diffuse alopecia in a female.
19 For which type of alopecia would the glass bulb be the most suitable electrode to use?
20 What is the technical name for dry dandruff?

## Practical assignment – Diagnostics

Of the various skin and scalp complaints listed in this section there are some which you may never see and others which are far more common. The infectious conditions you will almost certainly come across are clients with head lice while common non-infectious conditions will include male baldness and dandruff. These exercises are designed to give you extra information about hair and scalp conditions and to help you tell a client that he or she has head lice.

## Tasks

1  Go to a pharmacy, chemist, hospital out-patient or local health clinic and pick up leaflets and pamphlets on hair and skin conditions. Make a summary of the information given and actions to take.
2  Contact your local area health authority and find out what activities they are involved in concerning hair and skin condition. Do they, for example, screen school children for head lice? If so, how often, and what do they advise for the infestation? Do any other skin or scalp conditions arise?

3   Imagine you have just discovered that a client has head lice. What are the most likely signs? How can you be sure? How would you tell the client?

Explain your answers clearly.

# 8 CONSULTATION – designing a hairstyle

Advising a client on the type of hairstyle best suited to them is a common yet fundamental aspect of a hairdresser's work.

## What can influence a hairstyle?

The shape of the hair can alter the shape of the face by emphasising good features and minimising others. When designing a hairstyle for the client there are five main points to be taken into consideration:

1 facial structure (shape of face)
2 problem features
3 texture of hair
4 personality of client
5 lifestyle of client

### Facial structure

It is important that the professional stylist is able to recognise the various facial shapes. An oval face shape (*See* Fig 8.1(*a*)) is believed to be the perfect shape and the stylist must aim to achieve the illusion of an oval shape on their client. Other face shapes are shown in Fig. 8.1.

### Long face

To avoid a long face effect, create width at the sides using loose, soft waves or curls. Medium length hair is best with the fullness around the ears. Fringes can shorten the effect of an over-long face. This is shown in Fig. 8.2.

### Round face

Short hair is most suitable for a round face, with height on top of the head and the side hair flat, preferably covering the cheeks. An

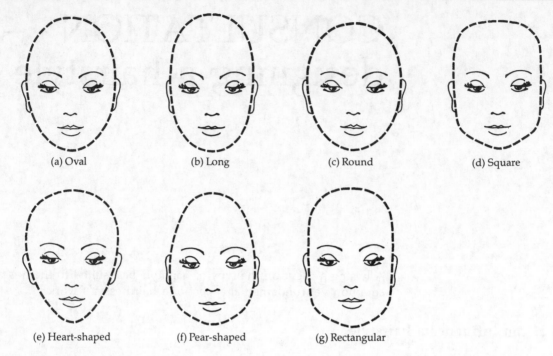

(a) Oval          (b) Long          (c) Round          (d) Square

(e) Heart-shaped     (f) Pear-shaped     (g) Rectangular

**Fig 8.1 Basic face shapes**

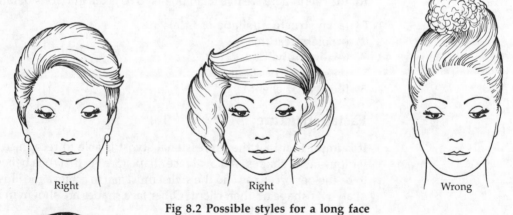

Right                    Right                    Wrong

**Fig 8.2 Possible styles for a long face**

Wrong

**Fig 8.3 Possible styles for a round face**

asymmetrical hairstyle or a parting will minimise the roundness but a full fringe across the forehead will emphasis the roundness of the lower face. This is shown in Fig 8.3.

## Square face

A soft design is needed to reduce the angular jawline. Fullness at the temples and cheekbones gives an illusion of roundness and the face shape can be softened by covering the jawline if possible. This is shown in Fig 8.4.

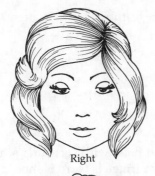

Right

## Heart-shaped face

Play down width at the temples and create fullness round the chin. An asymmetrical style or a side parting also looks effective on this face shape, as shown in Fig 8.5.

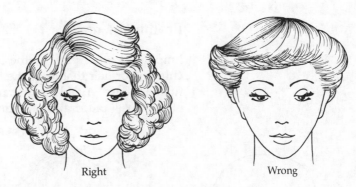

Right                                                Wrong

**Fig 8.5 Possible styles for a heart-shaped face**

## Pear-shaped face

Hair should be given width above the chin and left soft at the nape to soften the lower part of the face This is shown in Fig 8.6.

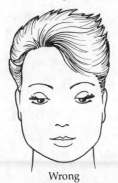

Wrong

**Fig 8.4 Possible styles for a square face**

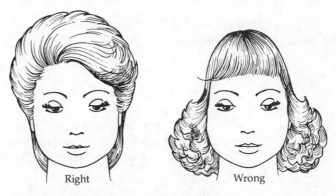

Right                                                Wrong

**Fig 8.6 Possible styles for a pear-shaped face**

## Rectangular face

Longer than a square-shaped face but with the same strong jawline that should be disguised with softness around this area. A fringe will help reduce the length of the face and a side parting offsets the angular features of this face shape. This is shown in Fig 8.7.

### Problem features

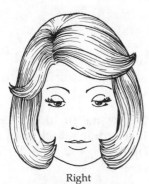

Right

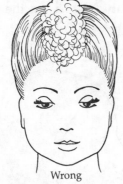

Wrong

**Fig 8.7 Possible styles for a rectangular face**

Where features are good, the hair may be pulled back to reveal them but problem features should be disguised so that the eye is drawn away from them and the more attractive features then gain attention. Less attractive features include:

- prominent nose
- heavy jawline or chin
- high or receding forehead.

## Prominent nose

Emphasise other parts of the face and head with soft curls at the chin line or hair that hugs the face. If a fringe is worn it should be full and loose. Avoid centre partings as this emphasises the length of the nose and draws attention to it. (*See* Fig 8.8)

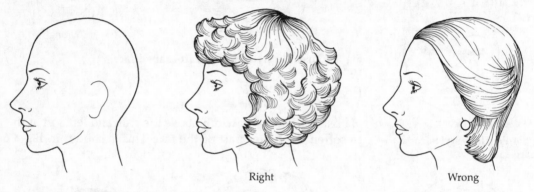

Right                    Wrong

**Fig 8.8 Styling for a prominent nose**

## Heavy jawline or chin

A smooth definite style that clings to the jawline should be used. Fringes help to balance the face. Hair that is drawn back from the face will accentuate the jawline. (*See* Fig 8.9)

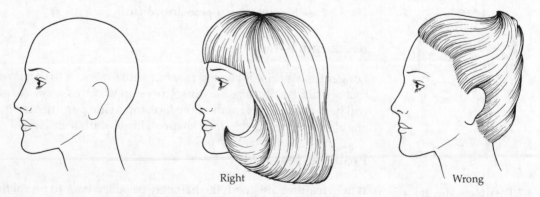

Right                    Wrong

**Fig 8.9 Styling for a heavy jawline**

## High or receding forehead

Full fringes minimise a high forehead and a medium length hairstyle, either smoothly curving or flicked back at the sides will emphasise the shape of the head rather than the forehead. Centre parting should be avoided but a side parting may be used if the hair is draped across the forehead. A side parting will make the forehead appear broader and so will only be effective on a narrow high forehead. This is shown in Fig 8.10.

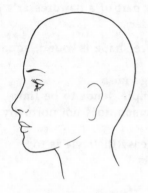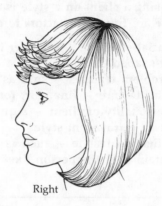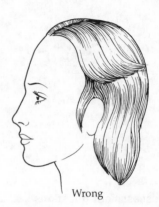

Right                                                                    Wrong

**Fig 8.10 Styling for a high forehead**

## Texture of hair

Fine hair is narrow in diameter and tends to be limp. It looks its fullest when it is club cut and allowed to grow no longer than chin length. Extremely fine, lank hair may also require a soft perm to give it extra body without a great deal of curl.

Coarse hair has a larger diameter and is usually strong and wiry. It can be allowed to grow longer unless it is also very curly in which case it will go very bushy. Coarse hair may have to be layered or thinned to make it more controllable.

Medium hair is the easiest type of hair to manage and combined with medium body it is suitable for most hairstyles and most hair lengths.

## Personality of client

The personality of the client is important when designing a hairstyle. A quiet subdued person will not thank the stylist for an extravagant hairstyle which will draw unwanted attention to themselves. Likewise a client with an outgoing and extroverted personality will require a style which is different and individual. A client who is neat and meticulous will need a hairstyle that is sleek and uncluttered.

## Lifestyle of client

A hairstyle should meet the client's needs and their lifestyle has a definite effect on the type of style they require.

Sporting hobbies create the need for a sleek, well cut, easy-to-manage hairstyle, whereas a client who entertains a great deal will probably require a more elaborate hairstyle.

## Summary

Advising a client on a style is a key part of a hairdresser's job. There are five main factors to consider:

1  Facial structure – whether the face shape is round, square, heart-shaped etc.
2  Problem features – such as a large nose
3  Hair texture – fine hair, for example, tends to be limp
4  Personality of client – a quiet person does not normally want an extravagant style
5  Client's lifestyle – such as how easy the style is to maintain or if the person likes sports.

## Self-assessment questions

1  List the five main factors which need to be considered in hair design.
2  What type of style favours a long face?
3  How can a style be designed to minimise a heavy jawline or chin?
4  What type of cut makes fine hair appear fullest?
5  What contrast could there be for a hair design for a person who regularly:
(a) plays sports?
(b) entertains guests?

## Practical assignment – Client consultation

## Task

Talking to clients can be a very daunting prospect for some trainees. To help you overcome any initial shyness fill in the following checklist for *each* client over a period of one week. At the end of this time you should then feel more comfortable when talking to the clients.

### Checklist for client consultation

1 Is the Client:    NEW.........................................................
                     BEEN ONCE BEFORE.............................
                     REGULAR...............................................

2 What is the Client's name?

.........................................................................................

3 Where does he/she live?

.................................................................................................................

4 What is his/her occupation?

.................................................................................................................

5 Does he/she have any hobbies? If yes, what?

.................................................................................................................

6 Does he/she have a family (including pets)? If yes, what?

.................................................................................................................

7 Is he/she going somewhere special? If yes, where?

.................................................................................................................

8 Is he/she going on holiday? If yes, where and when?

.................................................................................................................

9 What product/s does the client usually use on his/her hair? (e.g.
mousse, gel, lacquer etc)

.................................................................................................................

10 Does his/her hairstyle usually 'stay in' well? If no, what could be the
cause?

.................................................................................................................

11 Does his/her hair need a perm/conditioning treatment/colouration?

.................................................................................................................

12 If yes, what have you recommended?

.................................................................................................................

13 What after-care advice have you given to this client?

.................................................................................................................

14 Are there any retail sales suitable for this client's hair? If yes, what?

.................................................................................................................

15 Has the client made another appointment?

.................................................................................................................

# 9    HAIR AND SCALP TREATMENTS

## Hair condition

Hair looks its best when it is in good condition. Exactly what 'good condition' means is hard to define, but it does involve factors such as:

(a) the hair being **manageable** (i.e., easy to brush, comb and set)
(b) having a good **shine** (or **lustre**)
(c) being **pliable** and **elastic** (to produce a natural looking movement)
(d) to feel **soft** and to have **'body'**

The hair shaft is dead and cannot repair itself in the way that living parts of the body can. Yet the condition of the individual hair shafts determines the overall condition of the whole head of hair.

In the average life of a typical scalp hair, it may have been:

- brushed and combed nearly 10 000 times
- washed (using a shampoo) about 600 times
- blowdried (after the shampoo) about 600 times
- permanently waved about 16 times
- tinted (perhaps with a bleach included) 40 times.

It says much for the toughness of the hair structure that it can stand up to all this punishment without disintegrating. Hair does 'age', however, and the oldest hair is that at the hair points, which has usually suffered more damage than that near the scalp. This needs to be considered in terms of the processing time in bleaching, tinting and perming hair.

A key factor in hair condition is the degree of **cuticle damage**. This can result from a number of factors which will be classed here as 'internal' and 'external'.

## Internal factors influencing hair condition

### Age

General slowing down of hair growth and production of the natural sebum results in dry hair and scalp. Unpigmented hair may have a coarser texture than pigmented hair which can also create difficulties when styling hair.

### Diet

A well balanced diet is essential for healthy hair. It has been suggested that there is a link between high sugar and oil intake and greasy hair and skin. However, expert opinion tends to be divided on this.

### Drugs and illness

Both can have a profound effect on the hair, even an illness as simple as the common cold can alter hair condition. With more serious illnesses, the drugs and treatment used can cause rapid thinning and even baldness, e.g. chemotherapy. A hormone imbalance or fever illnesses, e.g. glandular fever, can also cause thinning of the hair.

Internal reasons for hair in poor condition are largely beyond the control of the hairdresser. However, even if the hairdresser is only able to improve the hair superficially, there are still psychological benefits to the client by improving the hair visually.

## External factors influencing hair condition

These can either be physical (or mechanical) damage – caused by brushing, combing and heat or chemical damage – caused by the chemical treatments and the ultraviolet rays in sunlight.

In reality both types will almost certainly be involved in determining the condition of a client's hair.

### Physical (or mechanical) damage

When the hair is in good condition the cuticle scales of the hair shaft are tight into the hair. This makes the hair smooth and shiny (or have a good lustre). When combing or brushing (and especially backcombing or backbrushing) hair, the mechanical scraping of the brush bristles or comb teeth across the cuticle roughens it. This leaves the hair dull and liable to further mechanical or chemical damage. The increased friction caused by roughened hair can lead to the production of static electricity in the hair and this can cause 'hair fly', thus making the hair less manageable.

Tight rollers, pins or clips on the hair can cause physical damage, especially on chemically treated hair. The hair normally contains some water, chemically bound to the cortex fibrils. Some of this water can be lost from the hair by blowdrying or by the drying effect of the atmosphere. Reduction in the water content of hair reduces its elasticity and this influences the movement of the hair.

## Chemical damage

This includes both the 'natural' damage caused by the ultraviolet rays in sunlight and that caused by the chemical treatments used in hairdressing.

1 *Damage by ultraviolet rays.* Ultraviolet radiation is invisible to the human eye but is present in sunlight. These rays produce the natural bleaching action of sunshine on hair by breaking some molecules of oxygen gas (symbol $O_2$) trapped in the air spaces of the hair cortex into the highly reactive nascent oxygen (symbol O:). That is:

$$O_2 \xrightarrow[\text{rays}]{\text{ultraviolet}} 2\ O:$$

*(oxygen gas)*           *(2 atoms of nascent oxygen)*

Nascent oxygen is produced chemically by the decomposition of the hydrogen peroxide used in chemical bleaching, oxidising perms and developing the oxidation ('para') tints. The nascent oxygen produced in the hair by ultraviolet rays splitting oxygen molecules, attacks the colouring pigments and decolourises (or bleaches) them in the same way as nascent oxygen released by peroxide. The damage caused by ultraviolet light is that it breaks some of the sulphur linkages (or disulphide bonds) between the polypeptide chains in the cortex and this weakens the hair.

2 *Damage by chemical treatment.* The chemical treatments routinely used in the salon may damage the hair cuticle and the cortex, but it is the outer cuticle which is the most vulnerable. The condition of the cuticle affects the hair porosity, which is a measure of the speed at which water and chemicals are absorbed. Even for hair in good condition the points of the hair will be more porous and therefore process more quickly. The damage to the cortex is sometimes called sensitivity; so 'sensitive' hair is more badly damaged than 'porous'.

Chemical treatments used in the salon include:

- shampooing
- perming

- tinting (or colouring)
- bleaching.

The damage caused by these operations will now be considered. Washing the hair using a **shampoo** may cause:

(*a*) Removal of too much natural oil, i.e. sebum. This leaves the hair dry and liable to crack and splinter.

(*b*) Bleaching and perming hair often causes some of the cortex keratin to become soluble in water. These water soluble materials can be washed out of the hair during a shampoo and thus weaken the hair.

(*c*) If the shampoo used contains soap, an alkaline deposit may be left on the hair. This causes the cuticle to swell and become rough and dull. If a soap-containing shampoo is used in a hard water area, the soap scum produced by a reaction between the soap and minerals in the water coat the hair shaft and also leave it rough and dull.

**Perming** hair involves breaking and then re-forming some of the sulphur linkages (or disulphide bonds) between the polypeptide chains of the hair keratin. Not all of these are rebuilt during the oxidation or normalisation process which fixes the style in the hair. This leaves the hair in a weakened state which is more likely than untreated hair to split and break.

In addition, the traditional perm lotions (those containing ammonium thioglycollate and having a pH of 9.5) leave the hair alkaline at the end of the perming process.

When the hair is alkaline at the end of perming, the cuticle scales are raised, so the hair is rough and dull.

A further point is that the chemical action of the perm lotion and the peroxide tends to remove much of the hair's coating of sebum (this is often described as 'stripping' the oil from the hair). Thus, at the end of the process the hair is very dry and therefore liable to crack and splinter.

When **tinting** the hair, permanent and semi-permanent hair dyes often contain a 'para' compound whose colour in the hair is developed by oxidation by hydrogen peroxide. The peroxide used is made alkaline in order to speed its decomposition and release of nascent oxygen, which then oxidises the small tint molecules into large coloured molecules trapped in the hair shaft. The alkali mixed with the peroxide leaves the hair with a roughened cuticle so it appears dull.

**Bleaching** is generally thought to cause the greatest amount of damage of any of these chemical treatments. This is especially true if the amount of lightening required is large, e.g. from dark hair to blond. The strength of the peroxide used is sufficient not only to destroy areas of the cuticle leaving the cortex unprotected and therefore liable to further chemical damage, but also very porous and likely to split and break. The hair is left alkaline at the end of the process, due to the alkalis used to speed the decomposition of the hydrogen peroxide which is used as the main bleaching agent. The alkaline hair has a swollen cuticle with the scales open, so the hair is rough and dull.

## The pH scale and hair condition

The pH scale is a 14-point scale which measures acidity or alkanity.

*pH7* is neutral, neither acid nor alkaline
*Below 7* is acid
*Above 7* is alkaline.

Hair is in its best condition if slightly acid (pH 5.5) but many hairdressing processes upset this pH 'balance' as can be seen in Fig 9.1 below:

Details on how conditioners are used to restore or balance hair pH are given in the section Acid type conditioners on p. 122.

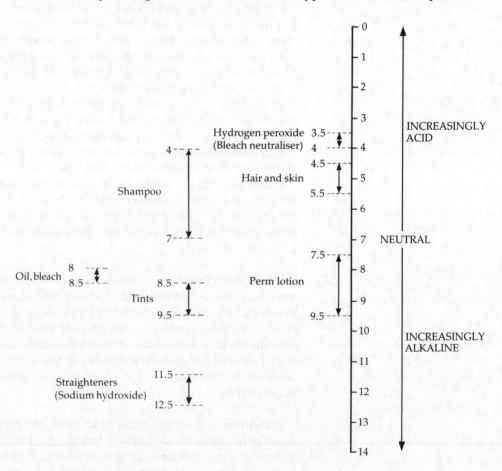

**Fig 9.1 Effects of chemicals on the pH balance**

# Types of conditioners

There are three general types of conditioners, based on their main ingredients and actions. These are:

(*a*) oil-based (or emollients) – which are the traditional conditioners

(*b*) substantive type – where material 'adds' to the hair

(*c*) acid type.

## Oil-based conditioners: external conditioners

Sometimes called **emollients** or **conditioning creams,** these are the simplest method of conditioning. The oil added to the hair, in a measured dose, is to replace the natural oils removed by shampooing, perming, tinting or bleaching. The oils used are often in the form of an **emulsion** in water, which makes spreading on to the hair easier, and are left coating the hair when the water evaporates. **Lanolin** (from sheep's wool) or slightly altered forms of lanolin are a good substitute for human sebum and are often used.

To ensure that the conditioning effect lasts beyond the next shampoo, moist heat, e.g. hot towels or a steamer, can be used to swell the cuticle allowing the conditioner to penetrate deeper into the hair shaft. As the hair cools, the cuticle scales close, trapping some of the conditioner between them, thus preventing complete removal at the next shampoo.

## Substantive-type conditioners: internal conditioners

These become fixed to, or absorbed into, the hair shaft, mainly due to the **electric charge** on the conditioner molecule and the hair shaft. This category includes some soapless detergents and **polyvinylpyrrolidone** (PVP) which acts as both a setting agent and a conditioner.

Other materials which appear to be absorbed by the hair include the protein conditioners (sometimes called **restructurants**). Because the hair is dead it cannot be 'fed', but does have the ability to absorb small polypeptide chains and single amino acids. These are produced by breaking down animal or plant proteins and the evidence is that some is deposited on the cuticle and some passes through the cuticle into the cortex. The amount absorbed by the hair seems to increase in the more damaged areas of the hair shaft, which is a very good property for a conditioner to have. The evidence does show, however, that this type of conditioner is most effective at protecting the hair from damage; so it is best applied before a perm, tint or bleach is carried out. Whether protein conditioners used after the treatment in any way increase the tensile strength or elasticity of the hair is not clear, although some evidence seems to indicate that they do.

## Acid type conditioners

These are based on the natural skin and hair secretions (e.g. sebum and sweat) having a pH of between 4 and 6. They produce an **acid mantle** over the hair and since pH does influence hair condition in that at acid pH the cuticle scales are flat, the hair is then smooth and shines. In alkaline pH the cuticle swells and the scales open slightly so the hair is rough and dull and more liable to both physical and chemical damage. Acids also help to hold the water soluble products produced by perm lotion and peroxide attacking the hair. Without an acid pH these can be washed from the hair during shampooing and weaken it.

There are two types of acid conditioners:

(a) *pH restorers* contain organic acids, e.g. **citric acid**, and have a pH of about 3. They are used to chemically neutralise the alkaline deposits left on the hair after perming, bleaching and tinting and are formulated to leave the hair with a pH of about 4.

(b) *pH balancers* are mildly acidic, e.g. pH6 compared to pH restorers. They are used, for example, in pH balance shampoos to ensure the final pH of the hair is acidic. Organic acids are used, e.g. **citric, tartaric** and **lactic acids**.

## Rehabilitating rinses

These are a general name given to mild conditioners which can be used after shampooing the hair. A wide variety of ingredients are used and although not used much in commercial salons they can be made at home. Some act as acid conditioners, e.g. vinegar (acetic acid) and lemon juice (citric acid) rinses. Others add 'body' by coating the hair, e.g. beer rinse. Others contain herbs which colour the hair slightly and bring out highlights, e.g. rosemary on dark hair camomile on blondes, henna on reddish/brown hair. Some contain egg (both yolk and white); these coat the hair producing body and shine. Many shampoos contain these types of ingredients to condition and shampoo in one operation.

## Conditioning treatments

The term conditioning treatments involves the practical methods used to improve the condition and a first step is to find the cause of a client's hair being in poor condition.

## How to find the cause of poor hair condition

Before starting any treatment, first make a visual analysis of the hair and scalp. A visual assessment will give a good indication as to the extent of the damage and will also indicate the depth of treatment that will be needed to restore the hair to a natural, healthy state.

Question the client as to the possible reason for the damage. Very often the client will have a good idea as to the cause of the hair's present condition, particularly if prompted with suggestions from the hairdresser. However, always remember to question the client tactfully and sympathetically – they obviously know that their hair is not at its best otherwise they would not want the treatment!

Consider the following areas when assessing the hair and scalp:

## Hair assessment

(*a*) *Hair types:* is the hair dry, brittle, greasy or wiry?

(*b*) *Hair texture:* is the hair fine, medium or thick?

(*c*) *Hair porosity:* is there a high degree of porosity? If so, has this been caused by chemical or physical factors such as bleach, tint, straighteners, permanent wave solution, sunlight or heat? Or is it because the client's hair has above average porosity?

(*d*) *Hair abnormalities/diseases:* are there any of the following present: fragilitis crinium (split ends), monilethrix (beading), alopecia (baldness)? If so, what has caused this?

## Scalp assessment

(*a*) *Skin type:* is the skin dry, greasy or normal?

(*b*) *Skin abnormalities/diseases:* are any of the following present: psoriasis, pityriasis capitis (dry dandruff), seborrhea (greasy dandruff)?

## Choosing the treatment

Before choosing any treatment the hairdresser must have a sound knowledge of the products available and must be aware of their limitations. Never promise the client instant, lustrous locks if the hair is badly damaged – instead, explain what the treatment will do, how many treatments will be needed and why. Hair can be so badly damaged as to be almost beyond repair and the only real remedy would be to remove it from the head by cutting until new, undamaged hair takes its place! However, even this type of hair can be made more supple and therefore easier to handle by careful and thorough use of restructurants, conditioners, oils etc. Knowing which product to use and how to make it more effective is essential if the client is to have confidence in the hairdresser's judgement.

The intended effect of any hair/scalp treatment is to make the hair more supple and to improve the circulation of the blood. An improved blood supply brings more food and oxygen to the hair and scalp which encourages hair growth and makes the sebaceous glands more active.

Heat and massage increase the blood supply to the scalp by causing the blood capillaries in the skin to dilate so that more blood flows into the skin; this can be clearly seen when the scalp turns pink in colour.

## Heat treatments

A heat treatment can be carried out in various ways depending on the source of heat.

### Sources of heat

(a) *Steamer:* produces warm, moist heat.

(b) *Hot towels:* produce warm, moist heat. Their temperature should be 60°C.

(c) *Accelerator or infra-red:* produces heat only, therefore has a more drying effect.

(d) *Hot oil:* used in conjuction with (a) or (b). The oil should be kept at a temperature of 55°C.

## Massage treatments

Massage is a form of manipulation which can be achieved either with the hands or mechanically with either the vibro or high frequency machine. The psychological value of massage has been very under-rated in the past and this is one area in hairdressing that the salons have not exploited to the full. Very few salons provide treatments which include the use of all the forms of massage, particularly when carrying out oil or conditioning treatments. A good massage, expertly carried out, not only benefits the hair and scalp but also gives the client a feeling of well-being.

### Uses of massage

1 To soothe and relax the client.
2 To stimulate the sebaceous glands of the scalp to produce the natural oil, sebum.
3 To increase blood circulation in the skin capillaries and therefore to aid nourishment of the hair and scalp. This condition is called **hyperaemia** (where the scalp appears pink).
4 To soften and improve skin texture by making it more pliable.
5 To ease contracted tissue, e.g. in the neck muscles.

### Types of massage available

There are three types of massage:

1 hand massage;
2 vibro massage;
3 high-frequency treatment.

## 1 Hand massage

Hand massage should be carried out with sure, firm movements – jerky, uncontrolled movements can be uncomfortable or even painful to the client. Nails should be kept to a reasonable length to prevent scratching the scalp and the hands and wrists should always remain flexible.

There are three main types of hand massage used in hairdressing:

(a) effleurage
(b) petrissage
(c) friction.

It must be stated that there are many other forms of hand massage but these are mainly used on other areas of the body and therefore do not come under the jurisdiction of the hairdresser.

**Effleurage** is a slow stroking movement applied to the scalp with the fingers and palms in a slow rhythmic manner. It is used at the beginning and end of each massage treatment to relax muscles and relieve tension.

Both hands are held at the centre, front of the head and then pulled firmly down the back of the head to the nape (*see* Fig. 9.2). The hands are then placed at either side of the head at the temples and again pulled firmly back round the contours at the sides of the head down to the neck and easing out to the shoulders; thus relieving any tension in the neck muscles.

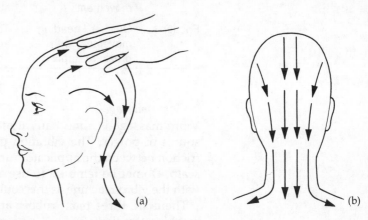

(a)      (b)

**Fig 9.2**

**Petrissage** is a slow, firm kneading movement in which the skin is gripped by the fingers and rotated over the skull. It increases the blood circulation and gives deeper stimulation of the glands and muscles.

Place both hands in a claw-like position on the scalp then rotate the skin over the skull without moving the fingers over the scalp.

The right hand moves in a clockwise direction while the left hand moves in the opposite, anti-clockwise direction.

The hands are lifted from their position one at a time and replaced elsewhere on the scalp until the whole scalp has been massaged. Always leave one hand in contact with the scalp when removing the other to ensure continuity of the massage. If both hands are removed together the massage becomes jerky and unpleasant.

**Friction** is the most well-known of all hand massage movements as this is the movement used when shampooing the hair. Friction is also a kneading movement and the fingers are still rotated in opposite directions for each hand. Unlike petrissage however, the movements are quite quick and vigorous with the fingers moving over the surface of the skin.

The hand is held in a claw-like position and the pads of the fingers are moved firmly over the scalp in circular movements away from the hair line up to the crown, then from the nape up to the front of the head and back down to the nape again.

Table 9.1 gives a summary of all hand massages.

**Table 9.1**

| Movement | Description | Use |
| --- | --- | --- |
| Effleurage | A gentle stroking movement. | To relax muscles and relieve tension. Used at the beginning and end of each treatment. |
| Petrissage | Slow, firm, kneading movement | To increase circulation and to stimulate glands and muscles. |
| Friction | Quicker kneading movement with pressure applied | To improve circulation and glandular activity, used when shampooing. |

2   *Vibro massage*

Vibro massage is a mechanical massage that uses electricity as its source of power. The vibration produced by the machine causes friction between the applicators and the scalp which stimulates the scalp. Do not be tempted to use added pressure when massaging with the vibro machine as this could be uncomfortable for the client.

There are three main rubber applicators for use with the vibro machine (*see* Fig 9.3):

(*a*) spiked applicator
(*b*) sponge applicator
(*c*) rubber-domed bell or flat vulcanite applicator.

**The spiked applicator (rubber pronged)** is the attachment most commonly used in hairdressing as the rubber prongs will move through the hair quite easily. It is used on the scalp in either circular or straight movements (*see* Fig 9.4).

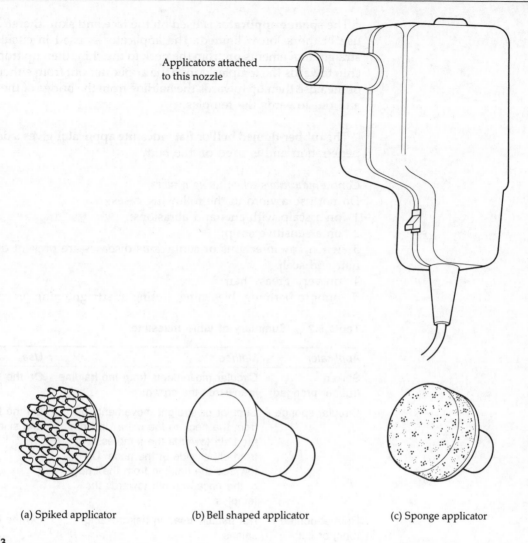

Applicators attached to this nozzle

(a) Spiked applicator

(b) Bell shaped applicator

(c) Sponge applicator

**Fig 9.3**

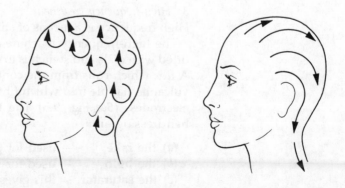

**Fig 9.4**

The **sponge applicator** is used on the face and skin; therefore its use in the salon is limited. The applicator is used in circular or straight movements up from the neck to the chin, then up from the chin towards the temples. Move the applicator out from either side of the nose then up towards the hairline from the bridge of the nose and out towards the temples.

The **rubber-domed bell** or **flat vulcanite applicator** gives a deeper penetration and is used on the body.

*Contra-indications when using a vibro*
Do not use a vibro in the following cases:
1  on a scalp with cuts and abrasions;
2  on a sensitive scalp;
3  when any infections or contagious diseases are present on the hair and scalp;
4  on very greasy hair;
5  prior to perming, bleaching, tinting or straightening processes.

**Table 9.2 – Summary of vibro massage**

| Applicator | Method | Use |
|---|---|---|
| Spiked (rubber pronged) | Circular movements from the hairline in towards the crown. | On the scalp. |
| Circular sponge | Circular or straight movements up from the neck to the chin. Up from the chin towards the temples. Out from either side of the nose. Up towards the hairline from the bridge of the nose and out towards the temples. | On the face and skin. |
| Rubber-domed (bell) or flat vulcanite | Not usually used in hairdressing salons. | On the body. |

*3  High-frequency treatment*
High frequency is a means of stimulation using an electric current.

The high-frequency machine consists of a control box which is fitted with dials and switches to control the strength of the current. A flex which runs from the control box is fitted with an insulated vulcanite handle into which fit three glass attachments known as electrodes. (*See* Fig. 9.5) The three main electrodes for use in hairdressing are:

(*a*) the **rake**  – used for general thinning;
(*b*) the **bulb**  – used for spot baldness (alopecia areata);
(*c*) the **saturator** – this gives deeper penetration.

'Mains' electricity is supplied to the salon at a voltage of 240 volts

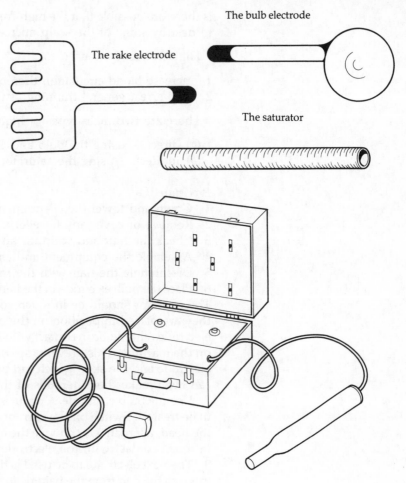

The bulb electrode

The rake electrode

The saturator

**Fig 9.5**

and a current of 13 amps. At these values electricity will pass through the body and cause an electric shock. The high-frequency machine converts (i.e. changes) the electrical supply to a high voltage (e.g. 2500 volts) but with a very small current. This type of electricity cannot pass through the body so does not cause electric shock. Mains electricity flows down cables in **surges** or **pulses** (100 of these happen per second). The high-frequency apparatus increases this to over 40 000 pulses per second.

The high voltage and the high frequency of the pulses produce the **sparking** in the electrodes which in turn produces small **ripples** of electricity in the skin (called **eddy** or **telsa** currents) to which the electrode is applied. The eddy currents produce heat in the skin which triggers increased blood flow to the scalp in a similar manner to hand massage. The sparking in the machine produces a 'sharp' smelling gas called **ozone** (chemical symbol: $O_3$). This rapidly breaks down into oxygen ($O_2$) releasing single atoms of oxygen called nascent oxygen (O:) which can destroy micro-organisms. It is therefore possible that the high-frequency machine has the ability to destroy some of the scalp micro-organisms.

High frequency is used to:

1 increase blood circulation thereby promoting hair growth;
2 help arrest general thinning of the hair and alopecia areata.

There are two main types of high-frequency treatments:

(a) direct – using the bulb and the rake;
(b) indirect – using the saturator.

*Procedure*
1 Gown and towel the client ensuring adequate protection.
2 Remove or cover any jewellery.
3 Check the hair and scalp for any contra-indications.
4 Assemble the equipment and check the machine.
5 Disentangle the hair with the rake end of a dressing comb.
6 Place the bulb electrode in the handle and switch on the machine. The operator should be in touch contact with the electrodes until they are placed in position on the client's scalp; alternatively, the electrodes should be in contact with the client's scalp before turning on the machine. This prevents sparking of the current between the electrode and the skin, which can be discomfiting to the client and can even make them nervous of the treatment.
7 Use the bulb electrode in circular movements on any bald areas to be treated. Switch off the current and remove the electrode from the head; alternatively, remove the electrode from the scalp keeping in touch contact with the electrode and switch off the current.
8 The next electrode to be used is the rake. This should be pushed through the hair from the hairline to the crown remembering to keep in touch contact with the electrode until it is placed on the scalp. Do not pull the rake electrode through the hair as it could become dislodged from the handle causing discomfort to the client.
9 Finally the saturator electrode is used. This is placed in the client's hand with one hand holding the electrode while the other hand holds the handle. Do not switch on the current until the operator's hand is firmly in position on the client's scalp. Switch on the current and gently massage the scalp with the fingers. Switch off the current before removing the hand from the scalp otherwise sparking may occur. When using the saturator the electric current passes through the electrode to the client in person and to the operator's point of contact which is the scalp.
10 Clean the electrodes and disinfect them to prevent the spread of infection.
11 Complete a record of the treatment giving details of the strength of the current used and the length of time for each electrode.

The first treatments should be of short duration, extending the length of each treatment as the tolerance of the client increases. It is usual to begin with two to three minutes for each electrode increasing the time by half a minute for each electrode at each subsequent treatment to a maximum of five minutes for each electrode.

The strength of the current is also increased for each treatment depending upon the tolerance of the client. Each client may have a different tolerance to the current so remember that the current should never be increased to the extent that it is uncomfortable for the client, as it could cause headaches or tenderness of the scalp.

No treatment should be extended beyond two months after which time there should be a lapse of at least one month when the treatment can then be restarted from scratch.

*Contra-indications*
You should not proceed with a high-frequency treatment in the following cases:

1   high blood pressure;
2   cuts, abrasions or inflammation present on the scalp;
3   client with heart complaint;
4   on excessively greasy hair – high frequency stimulates the sebaceous glands making them produce more sebum and thus aggravating the condition;
5   when there is spirit on the hair – a spark from the electrode could make it ignite;
6   never on wet hair;
7   when there are any diseases of the hair and scalp present.

*Precautions for high frequency*
1   High frequency should only be carried out on a clean, dry scalp.
2   The client should be kept away from wet floors, metal fittings, gas or water pipes. Remove or cover any jewellery as these are good conductors of electricity.
3   The electrodes should be pushed through the hair, never pulled or the electrodes may become dislodged.
4   If the client is nervous of a first-time treatment, show the strength of the current on the back of the client's hand to prove that the treatment will be quite painless. But remember to place it on the hand before switching on the current!
5   Always check that the scalp is free from cuts and abrasions and check all other contra-indications.
6   The treatment should not be used in conjunction with scalp lotions containing spirit or alcohol as the electrodes could spark and ignite the hair. Do not use on lacquered hair as lacquer is also highly inflammable.
7   Always have touch contact with the electrodes before placing them or removing them from the client's scalp or alternatively place the electrode on the scalp or in the client's hand (saturator) before switching on the machine.
8   The total treatment time should not exceed 15 minutes and no treatment should be extended beyond 2 months.

9   The electrodes should be sterilised after use by wiping them with ethanol and placing them in the sterilising cabinet.

10   The machine should always be thoroughly checked for frayed wires, faulty plugs, cracked electrodes etc., and corrected if faulty.

11   Always keep a very precise record of the treatment including the strength of the current and the duration of each electrode massage; this is very important when continuing the treatment over a period of time.

**Table 9.3 – High-frequency treatment**

| Electrode | Use |
|---|---|
| Bulb | Used on the skin and scalp in a circular movement to increase circulation, stimulate glands and muscles. Particularly useful for bald areas such as alopecia areata. Direct method of H/F. |
| Rake | Used on the scalp, it is pushed through the hair from hairline to crown. Direct method of H/F. |
| Saturation | Is held by the client so that the electric current passes through the client. Creates deeper stimulation of glands, muscles, etc. Indirect method of H/F. |

# Types of conditioning products

The hairdresser should not only know which conditioning products are available but also how they work before the client can be advised as to which is the most suitable for their particular hair type.

Hairdressing manufacturers spend a lot of money and research to produce whole ranges of hair care products for particular hair types and common hair or scalp disorders, the choice of which depends largely upon personal preference. However, before buying a whole new range of products, try them first to assess the results. Most manufacturers are only too willing to provide a sample of the product to prove its worth. It is very important that the hairdresser has every confidence in the product used and knows exactly the limitation of that product. Remember that the client will be disappointed if the results are not as good as they were led to expect. Do not be afraid to explain to the client how a course of treatments may be necessary to achieve a good result – if the hair or scalp has been mistreated or neglected it is unfair to expect it to be miraculously transformed overnight!

It would be virtually impossible to list every kind of hair/scalp disorder and give a full acount of each treatment. However, the two most popular types of treatment will be dealt with in detail as these can be adapted to meet a variety of needs.

# A basic conditioning treatment

A conditioning treatment will have a more lasting effect on the hair than a conditioning rinse which is merely rinsed through the hair after shampooing. Any types of conditioning agent may be used for the treatment, either a pH balance or the more traditional type depending upon the requirements of the hair.

## Uses of a conditioning treatment

1  To replace the natural oil of the hair and scalp.
2  To ensure that the hair has the correct pH.
3  To lubricate and moisten dry hair, thus making it more supple and easier to handle.
4  To soften and improve the texture of the skin by making it more pliable.
5  To relax the muscles and relieve tension.
6  To increase sebaceous activity if this is necessary.
7  To increase the blood circulation and stimulate the glands and muscles of the scalp allowing them to be more effective.

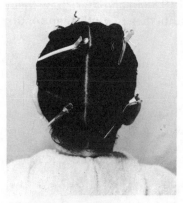

Fig 9.6 (a)

## Method of application

1  Check the hair and scalp thoroughly and question the client to ascertain the cause and extent of the damage.
2  Choose the correct conditioning agent for the extent of the damage.
3  Assemble the equipment.
4  Shampoo the hair. Towel dry then disentangle with the rake end of a dressing comb. Section the head into six sections (*see* Figs 9.6(a) and (b)).
5  Commence application at the nape and work up the section applying the conditioner where it is required. Sometimes it is only necessary to apply the conditioner to the ends of the hair. The conditioner may be applied with a brush (*see* Fig 9.7 (*a*)) or with a cotton wool swab made by wrapping a piece of cotton wool firmly

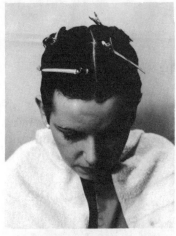

Fig 9.6 (b)

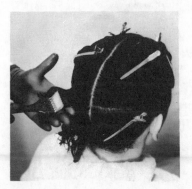

Fig 9.7 (a)

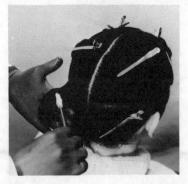

Fig 9.7 (b)

around an orange stick (*see* Fig 9.7 *(b)*) or around the tail end of a tail comb.

6  Continue working up the back of the head to the front sections. The meshes of hair at the front are taken back, away from the face to prevent any wet hair or conditioner falling onto the face.

7  When application is complete, check that all the necessary hair has been coated with conditioner, then begin the hand massage. The first massage movement to use is effleurage. Place both hands at the centre front of the head (*see* Fig 9.8 *(a)*) and then draw them firmly back in a stroking movement until they reach the nape of the neck (*see* Fig 9.8 *(b)*).

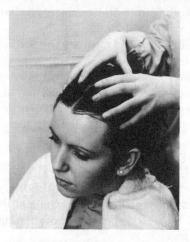

Fig 9.8 (a)

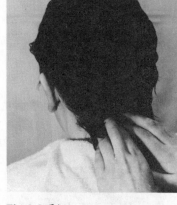

Fig 9.8 (b)

8  Replace the hands at the front sides of the head (*see* Fig 9.9 *(a)*) then draw them back following the contours at the sides of the head (*see* Fig 9.9 *(b)*). When the nape is reached, ease the hands out and follow through to the shoulders (*see* Fig 9.9 *(c)*). Make sure that the

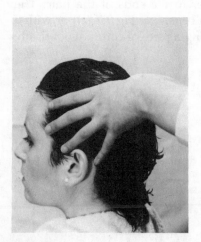

Fig 9.9 (a)

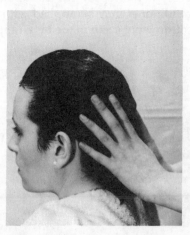

Fig 9.9 (b)

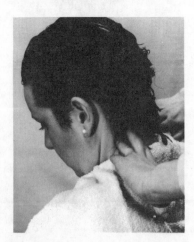

Fig 9.9 (c)

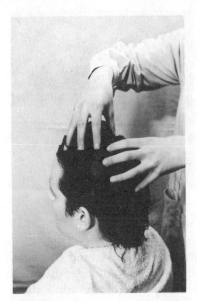

Fig 9.10

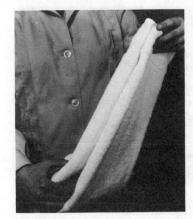

Fig 9.11

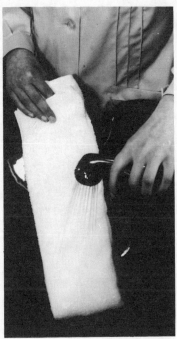

Fig 9.12

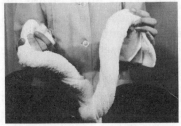

Fig 9.13

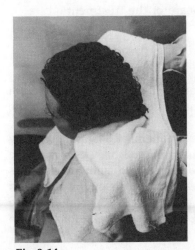

Fig 9.14

towel is tucked firmly down at the nape to prevent it from slipping from the shoulders.

9  Continue with a petrissage massage movement by placing the hands on the head in a claw-like position and slowly rotate the skin over the scalp (*see* Fig 9.10). When moving the position of the hands from one areas of the scalp to the next, do so one hand at a time. Removing both hands at the same time disrupts the continuity of the massage.

10  After completion of the massage use a steamer or hot towels to swell the hair and open the cuticle scales allowing deeper penetration of the conditioner.

11  To prepare the hot towel, first fold it in four lengthways, then place the two ends together forming a loop (*see* Fig 9.11).

12  Thoroughly wet the looped towel with very hot water without wetting the two ends held by the hand (*see* Fig 9.12).

13  Next, wring out the excess water by holding one end of the towel in each hand and then turn the ends in opposite directions. This twists the towel and wrings out the water without burning the hands (*see* Fig 9.13). Test the towel. It should only be damp, not wet and it should not be so hot that it will burn the client.

14  Unfold the towel so that it is double lengthways and place the folded edge at the nape of the neck (*see* Fig 9.14).

15  Then wrap each end of the towel firmly around the head, crossing the towel over at the front (*see* Fig 9.15).

16  The back section of the towel is then lifted up towards the front to make an envelope.

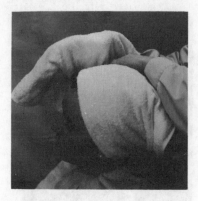

Fig 9.15

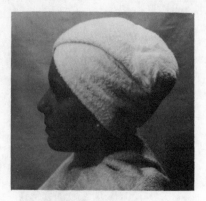

Fig 9.16

17  The hot towel should fit firmly and snugly round the head covering all of the hair. Any stray hairs can be eased under the towel with a tail comb. Figure 9.16 shows the completed towel application.
18  Seven hot towels should be used for a normal treatment and each towel should be replaced before it becomes too cool.
19  After removing the last hot towel, repeat the previous massage in reverse order. Do not allow the hair to cool down before this massage as the moist heat from the towels opens the cuticle scales allowing the conditioner to be massaged deeper into the hair shaft. After steaming, a vibro machine may be used instead of the petrissage hand movement but always end the treatment with an effleurage hand massage to make the client feel relaxed.
20  Rinse the hair thoroughly in warm water. If any conditioner is left on the surface of the hair after rinsing the finished result may be dull and lank.
21  Towel dry the hair and disentangle ready for setting or blowdrying.
22  Complete a detailed record of work carried out.
23  Advise the client on the after-care of the treatment.

## Hot oil treatment

Oil treatments are of maximum benefit to the client who suffers from a dry, tight scalp and dry brittle hair due to the inactivity of the sebaceous glands.

Vegetable oil is used in preference to mineral oil as it is more easily absorbed into the skin and hair than mineral oil. Deep massage movements with a combination of hand and vibro massage is recommended with this type of treatment to loosen the scalp and stimulate the sebaceous glands helping them to produce more sebum. The massage also helps to remove any flakes of dry skin that may adhere to the scalp.

## Purposes of hot oil treatment

1 To lubricate the scalp thus making it more supple and elastic.
2 To soften brittle hair caused by lack of sebum, giving it a healthier shine.
3 To loosen the scalp by relaxing the muscles and relieving any tension.
4 To increase sebaceous activity.
5 To increase the blood circulation and stimulate the glands and muscles of the scalp allowing them to be more effective.

## Method of application

1 Adequately protect the client with a gown and towel, making sure that the towel is tucked firmly down at the nape.
2 Assemble the equipment and heat the oil by pouring it into a small bowl then placing this in a larger bowl filled with hot water. This is known as a water bath. The oil should be heated to a temperature of 55°C.
3 Disentangle the hair and check the scalp for cuts and abrasions.
4 Divide the hair into six sections as for a conditioning treatment.
5 Wrap a hot moist towel around the head or steam the hair for five minutes under a steamer. This swells the hair and opens the cuticle scales thus aiding absorption of the oil.
6 Check the temperature of the oil and, while the hair and scalp are still warm, apply the warm oil to the scalp using a cotton wool swab or brush.
7 Application should commence at the nape and continue up towards the front, working from side to side as quickly as possible.
8 When application is complete, draw the oil through the lengths of the hair by massaging the scalp. First with the effleurage movements, to soothe and relax then with a petrissage hand massage to stimulate the sebaceous glands and loosen the scalp.
9 Apply the steamer for 10–15 minutes or use 7 hot moist towels.
10 Massage the scalp again while the hair and scalp are still warm. The vibro machine may be used at this point but the massage should be concluded with an effleurage hand massage.
11 To remove the oil, add soapless shampoo directly onto the hair before applying water. Massage the shampoo into the hair using friction movements until it emulsifies with the oil. This can be seen to happen when the oil becomes white and creamy and the hair no longer lathers.
12 Rinse the hair thoroughly in warm water and shampoo again with soapless shampoo. It is often necessary to shampoo the hair several times to completely remove all traces of the oil from the hair. Should any be left on the hair, the hair will become lank and greasy when it has been dried.

13  After the final rinsing, towel dry the hair then disentangle ready for setting or blowdrying.

14  Complete a detailed record of the work carried out.

15  Advise the client on the after-care of the treatment.

## Record keeping

A detailed record should be kept of all hairdressing treatments, particularly those that will be carried out over a period of weeks. This builds up a very clear picture as to how the hair is reacting and progressing with the treatment and any modifications to the

RECORD CARD

HAIR/SCALP TREATMENT

Name: .................................................... Tel No: .................

Address:  .............................................

.................................................................

| Hair assessment | Type | Porosity | Diseases/abnormalities | | |
|---|---|---|---|---|---|
| | | | | | |
| Scalp assessment | Skin type | | Diseases/abnormalities | | |
| | | | | | |
| Cause of damage | | | | | |

| Date | Conditioner/ lotion | Type massage | Time | Source of heat | Time | Result |
|---|---|---|---|---|---|---|
| | | | | | | |
| | | | | | | |
| | | | | | | |
| | | | | | | |
| | | | | | | |

**Fig 9.17**

treatment, e.g. increasing or decreasing the massage time or even changing the product can be done without getting in a muddle. Figure 9.17 shows an example of a record card.

## Summary

Because the hair shaft is dead, it cannot repair itself when damaged by factors such as:

(a) heat
(b) ultraviolet rays in sunlight
(c) chemical treatments like perming, bleaching and tinting
(d) brushing and combing, especially backbrushing and backcombing.

These chemical and physical factors tend to make hair rough and porous. This is mainly due to effects on the hair cuticle, although damage to the cortex can occur.

A wide variety of conditioners are marketed, often included in other products, e.g. shampoos. These can be grouped into thee basic types:

(a) oil-based conditioners (or emollients)
(b) substantive types
(c) acid types

Oil-based conditioners aim to replace the natural oil which has been removed from the hair. Lanolin is a common ingredient.

Substantive-type conditioners contain chemicals which may link on to or be absorbed into the hair. Examples include soapless detergents, polyvinylpyrrolidone and the more controversial protein conditioners, sometimes called restructurants.

Acid conditioners are designed to leave the hair with a pH value of between 4 and 6. In this pH range, the cuticle scales are tight to the hair shaft and this makes hair smooth and lustrous.

Rehabilitating rinses are mild conditioners, produced with a variety of ingredients which can be used after shampooing.

The first key step in deciding on which treatment to use is the assessment of the client's:

(a) hair, in terms of texture, porosity etc.;
(b) scalp.

Many conditioning treatments use heat and massage. Heat can be supplied by steamers, hot towels, accelerator and hot oil. Massage can be carried out by:

(a) hand, using techniques such as effleurage and petrissage;
(b) vibro machine, which has 'applicators' for various uses;

(c) the high-frequency machine which converts 'mains' electricity into a high voltage, high frequency with a low current. Tiny ripples of electricity (eddy currents) produced in the skin stimulate the blood flow and the ozone produced by sparking is an antiseptic. The high-frequency current can be applied direct (using electrodes) or indirect (using a saturator). There are a number of contra-indications and precautions involved in the use of high frequency.

A large number of conditioning products are available and there is a general method of application using hot towels or a steamer.

There are a number of practical remedies to hair in poor condition and it is important to keep record cards.

The check points, of a conditioning treatment are as follows:

1 know the products and treatments available, their use and their limitations.
2 assess the hair and scalp carefully;
3 determine the cause and extent of the damage;
4 keep a precise record of work carried out – remember, it may be necessary to adjust the treatment as the hair or scalp improves;
6 always advise the client on the after-care of the treatment and how any problems may be prevented.

## Self assessment questions

1 List four factors involved in hair condition.
2 What effect does heat have on hair condition?
3 Explain why backcombing or backbrushing hair may cause more damage than brushing or combing.
4 Why is hair that has been made alkaline by chemical treatments, rough and dull?
5 In what form are most oil-based conditioners applied to the hair?
6 Distinguish between 'pH restorers' and 'pH balancers'.
7 Why is a well balanced diet important to maintain healthy hair?
8 Why does age play an important part in the condition of the hair?
9 Which layer of the hair directly affects its porosity?
10 What is the purpose of a pH conditioner?
11 Name the layer of the hair which is most affected by restructurant conditioners.
12 What is the natural oil of the hair and scalp called?
13 Which type of vibratory application is most suitable for use on the head?
14 What effect does high-frequency massage have on the blood capillaries?

## Practical assignment – Conditioning

The condition of the hair has an important effect on all of our hairdressing services. This assignment aims to help you to identify the characteristics, both visual and tactile, which show whether the hair is in good or poor condition.

You will need:

- two sheets of A4 card
- scissors, pencils, ruler
- chosen materials for the collage
- glue or cow gum.

Now read the following two statements before beginning the task:

Hair in **poor** condition feels rough, dry and brittle. It looks dull, lifeless and without shine.

Hair in **good** condition feels supple, bouncy and pliable. It looks shiny, healthy and gleaming.

## Task

Using the above descriptions of the hair, create two collages: one to illustrate hair in poor condition and one to illustrate hair in good condition.

Each collage must be on an A4 size card with a 2.5-cm (1″) border. You may work with any medium to create the effect that you want, e.g. silver paper, foil, egg boxes, fabrics, dried pulses or pasta, empty cartons, tacks or nails and/or any other materials which you feel will give the visual and tactile (touch) illusion of the two hair conditions.

Assemble all your equipment and materials then work out your designs in rough before placing the materials on the card. Do not glue or stick your materials to the card until you are completely satisfied with the result. When the design is finished and firmly glued in place, either draw a 2.5-cm (1″) border around it or mount it on another larger piece of card which will give the same size border.

# SECTION 3
# ACTIONS AND REACTIONS

# SHAMPOOING

In hairdressing, to 'shampoo' hair has come to mean to 'clean' it. Shampooing is one of the most common operations in hairdressing salons and outside them most people wash their hair at least once a week. Washing the skin, using soap, is also an everyday event and both these cleaning operations involve:

- the use of water as the main cleaning agent
- the use of soap on the skin, or shampoo on the hair to help the water clean them more efficiently.

## Types of water

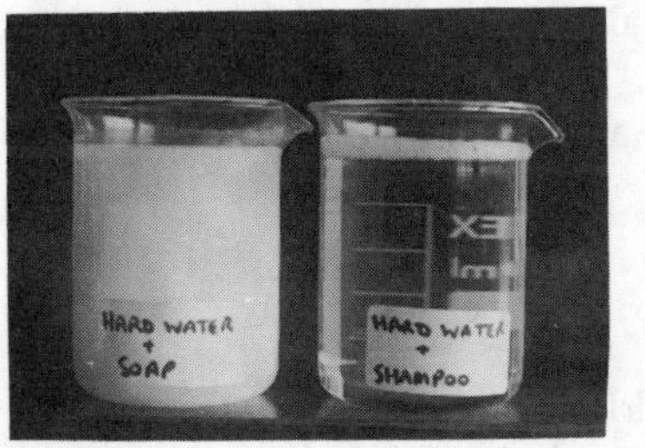

Tap water always contains some chemicals dissolved in it. These have mainly been dissolved from the soil and rocks with which the water has been in contact before treatment. Some calcium and magnesium salts for example, react with soap, producing an insoluble grey/white material called soap scum. It is also difficult to obtain a lather with the soap (see Fig 10.1). If these calcium and magnesium salts are present the water is described as hard, if they are not, then it is soft. Removing these salts from the water is called water softening, which can take place in a number of different ways.

Some types of hard water can be softened by boiling or heating to near the boiling point. This is temporary hardness. Other types will not soften when boiled and this is permanent hardness (this type of water has to be softened by other means). The effect of heating temporary hard water is to produce a deposit called **limescale**. This can be deposited on:

- the inside of hot water pipes, reducing the water pressure and eventually blocking them
- the heating elements of kettles, immersion heaters and steamers, so reducing their heating efficiency.

Both these are commercially important as they cost money to rectify.

Fig 10.1

## Softening hard water

This involves removing the calcium or magnesium salts which make the water hard. This is particularly important in hairdressing salons in areas where the water contains temporary hardness, as replacing hot water pipes because of blockage by limescale or heating elements from steamers, etc., is expensive. In any hard water area the **soap scum** produced in water can roughen the skin, or if soap is used on the hair the deposit of scum roughens and dulls the hair.

Water softening methods can be divided into two categories:

1   small scale softening, which includes boiling the water to remove the hardness and using chemicals which react with the soluble calcium or magnesium in hard water to produce insoluble forms, thus removing the hardness, e.g. softening water in a bath
2   large scale softening – where the supply is softened before use. The most common method of doing this is by **ion exchange** where the calcium and magnesium salt are absorbed by a material called **zeolite** leaving the water soft as it enters the salon.

## Cleaning process

Cleaning hair and skin involves removing the dirt which has become stuck or adheres to the surface. The process of cleaning requires the consideration of three factors:

1   the nature of the dirt and its solubility in water
2   the fact that on a microscopic scale the surface of hair and skin is rough
3   that at the end of cleaning, the hair and skin should be in good condition.

## The dirt on hair and skin

Hair (or skin) is made dirty by a wide range of materials like skin flakes, dust particles of many types, salt from dried sweat and so on. These in themselves may rapidly dissolve in water, but they are also mixed with the oily sebum which coats the hair and skin. This combination will not dissolve easily in water and therefore water alone is not able to clean the hair or skin efficiently.

## The surface of hair and skin

Skin, when viewed closely by the unaided eye, shows pits and small wrinkles. When seen through a microscope, the outer cornified layer of the skin appears as a rough, flaking surface. Similarly, the outer cuticle of the hair shaft, with its overlapping scales presents a rough surface, even when the hair is in good condition.

A rough surface, like those of skin and hair, presents a large number of places where dirt can lodge and means that the water must be able to penetrate into these microscopic hollows and cavities in order to remove the dirt.

## Conditioning

It is important that at the end of cleaning hair and skin their outer layers are left undamaged and that some natural oil remains. Sebum has an important function in preventing skin and hair from becoming dry and brittle. A cleaning action that is too efficient will 'strip' the hair and skin of all the sebum. With hair, the hair shaft is dead and the hair can be coated with a controlled amount of oil from a conditioner. With skin, the drying and cracking of the cornified layer is more important as it allows micro-organisms and chemicals to penetrate to the living cells of the germinative (basal) layer just underneath. The chemicals may cause dermatitis, and the micro-organisms, infections.

## Cleaning action of shampoo

Shampoos clean by their ability to:

- reduce surface tension of the water
- help the water to remove the oil and dirt from hair and skin and to prevent it being redeposited.

## Surface tension

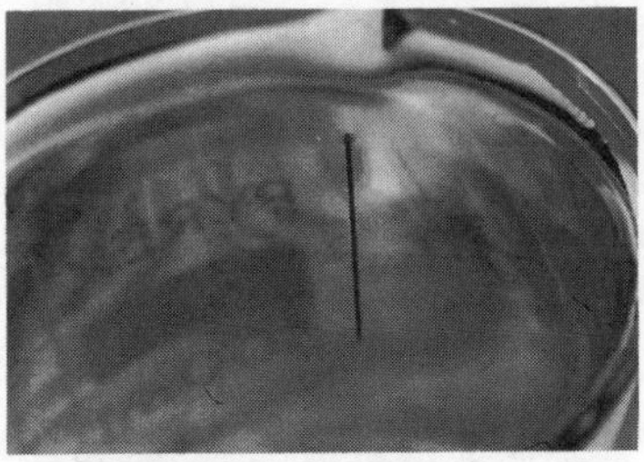

Fig 10.2

This results from the attraction of water molecules at the surfaces of the liquid, i.e. where it is in contact with other materials, towards the molecules in the rest of the liquid. This means that the water surface will tend to contract to cover the smallest possible area and form a surface 'film'. This can be seen at the air/water surface (a meniscus) on which it is possible to place an object (*see* Fig. 10.2), or in the way that droplets are spherical. This surface tension film occurs when the water surface is against the hair and skin and prevents the water from penetrating into the rough surface of the skin's cornified layer or the hair cuticle.

Shampoo reduces the surface tension of water, which allows it to penetrate into all parts of the surface of hair and skin. The process of bringing the water and surface to be cleaned into more intimate contact is described as **surface activity**. Because of this, soap and shampoo are sometime described as **surfactants**, (short for *surf*ace *active agents*).

## Removal of dirt

Water cannot properly dissolve oily materials, like sebum, but it can break them up into tiny droplets, i.e. emulsify them. Shampoos will attach to the oily dirt on hair and skin, remove them as tiny droplets, i.e. emulsify the oil (*see* Fig 10.3) and prevent the droplets from going back on to the hair in two ways:

(*a*) the shampoo molecules surround the oil droplets and keep them separate from one another, i.e. keep them emulsified

(*b*) the shampoo molecules coat the surface of the skin or hair and prevent the oil droplets from being redeposited.

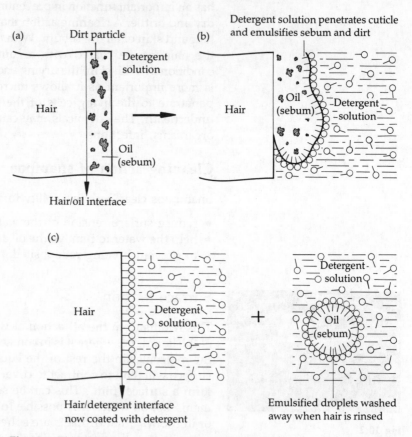

Fig 10.3 Cleaning action of detergents on hair

To summarise, shampoos help water clean hair and skin by:

- reducing surface tension in the water, allowing the water to wet or penetrate the surface of hair and skin more effectively
- act as emulsifying agents, causing the breaking off of the oily dirt into tiny droplets, which are then prevented from redepositing on the hair or skin.

## Agitation

This is the name given to the rubbing action involved in cleaning hair or skin. The rubbing or the massaging of shampoo on to the scalp causes:

(*a*) a good mixing of the water and shampoo or soap

(*b*) a good penetration by the soap or shampoo/water mixture on to the skin or hair surface.

(*c*) an emulsification of the oil and dirt as tiny droplets.

## Foaming

This is also called **lathering** and does not have much to do with the cleaning process. Because the cleaning action takes place on a microscopic scale the process is not visible to the unaided eye and therefore, it is important for the client's satisfaction to have some sign of the soap or shampoo's activity. Foam or lather provides this and helps to sell the product.

## Rinsing

After rubbing, or agitating, the water/soap or water/shampoo mixture on to the skin or hair, the oil and dirt will be suspended as the tiny droplets of an emulsion. This is then washed off the hair or skin by the water used to rinse.

## Other ingredients in shampoo

In addition to a soapless detergent, e.g. sodium lauryl ether sulphate, many shampoos contain:

1  an **auxiliary** detergent. These are weak detergents which alone are not very effective at removing oil from the hair, but they:

(*a*) thicken the shampoo

(*b*) help to maintain a rich lather

(*c*) condition the hair

(*d*) increase the solubility of the main soapless detergent.

2  common salt (sodium chloride) is often added to thicken the shampoo.

3  acids, e.g. **citric acid** (as lemon juice in lemon shampoo), which conditions the hair by leaving it slightly acid after shampooing. These are often called 'pH balance' or 'acid balance' shampoos.

4  antiseptics and chemicals which inhibit the early stages of dandruff. Zinc pyrithone has both properties and is found in medicated or anti-dandruff shampoos.

## Special shampoos for various types of hair

Various conditioners are used in the shampoos designed for various types of hair.

## Dry hair

This results from either insufficient sebum being produced by the scalp or too much sebum being removed during chemical processes like bleaching and perming.

The aim is to replace the natural oils in sebum with other oils which are:

(*a*) lanolin – used in cream shampoos

(*b*) plant oils, e.g. olive oil used in oil shampoos (designed for very dry hair).

*NB:* Shampoos designed for greasy hair have a higher proportion of soapless detergent to remove the surplus oil).

## Damaged hair

The aim is to coat the hair and, if possible, fill in the missing particles of cuticle. This group includes:

(*a*) *egg shampoo* – where a raw egg is added. The egg proteins coat the hair and the scalp and act as a barrier on the scalp to other chemicals in the shampoo. For this reason, it is recommended for sensitive scalps.

(*b*) *beer shampoo* – where beer is added. The coating slightly thickens each hair and so adds body to the whole head.

(*c*) protein shampoo – these contain proteins which have been broken down into a mixture of single and short chains of amino acids. There is some evidence that these will be absorbed by the porous regions of the hair, i.e. they are *substansive* to the hair, but this is not entirely accepted.

(*d*) herbal shampoo – may contain one or a variety of herbal extracts. Whether these substances condition the hair is far from clear, but they are usually used to add a sheen and gloss to the hair. Examples of herbal extracts include rosemary, sage, camomile, etc.

## Brightening shampoo

This is a mild bleach containing a soapless detergent with 10 vol (3 per cent) hydrogen peroxide.

## Colour shampoo

This contains a temporary dye in addition to the soapless detergent. The dye belongs to the azo group and coats the hair cuticle but is easily washed off after a few shampoos.

## Dry powder shampoo

This is used where it is difficult to carry out a wet shampoo; when a person is bed-bound for example. It contains a mild alkali mixed with an absorbant powder like starch. The alkali breaks down (or saponifies) a little of the sebum on the hair, so making a soap. This soap then cleans the hair during the thorough massage that follows. The powder absorbs the soap/oil mixture.

Table 10.1 gives a summary of the main types of shampoo and their uses.

**Table 10.1**

| Type | Use |
| --- | --- |
| Cream | Dry, brittle hair. Bleached, tinted, permed. |
| Oil | Extremely dry, bleached, tinted, permed. |
| Medicated | Mild dandruff. |
| Egg | Sensitive scalps, children's hair. |
| Beer | Lank, fine hair. |
| Lemon | To adjust pH to between 4–6 after hair has been bleached, tinted or permed. |
| Protein | Limp, chemically damaged hair. |
| Herbal | To add sheen. |
| pH balance | To adjust pH to 4–6, useful on chemically damaged hair. |
| Dry powder | Invalids, in between shampoos. |
| Brightening | Mild bleach, e.g. to highlight dull hair. |
| Colour | Temporary tints. |

# Comparisons of soap and soapless detergents

Soapless detergents have a number of advantages over soap and this explains the almost total use of soapless detergents in shampoos.

## Reaction with hard water

Soaps react with chemicals in hard water producing soap scum which can coat the hair, making it rough and dull. Soapless detergents do not produce any kind of scum. In addition, it is difficult to get a lather with soap in hard water, soapless detergents lather well. This is important because although the lathering is not directly related to the cleaning process, people do expect it.

## pH

Soap is produced with a surplus of alkali in the soap which gives a final alkaline pH of 8–9. This alkali causes the hair to swell and the cuticle scales to open slightly. This leaves the hair rough and dull. Soapless detergents have a pH of 7 (neutral) which leaves the hair in better condition.

# Precautions when shampooing

1  The client must be adequately protected, i.e. clothes should be completely covered by a gown and towels tucked well down at the nape. If a front wash is to be used, the client should be given a face cloth to protect their eyes (and possible make-up).

2  Hair must by thoroughly disentangled prior to shampooing.

3  The temperature of the water should be checked on the wrist or the back of the hand before allowing the water to run on to the scalp.

4  Correct shampoo should be used for the type of hair.

5  Liquid shampoo should be allowed to run over the back of the hand then on to the scalp to minimise coldness.

6  Cream shampoo should be applied to the palm of the hand before being evenly distributed over the whole head.

7  Friction hand massage should be used in circular movements from hairline to crown, throughout the whole head.

8  Hot water taps should be turned off during massage unless a mixer tap is used, in which case the whole tap is turned off. This is to conserve hot water.

9  Care must be taken to ensure that the hair is thoroughly rinsed after each massage.

10  After shampooing, hair should be towel dried and disentangled away from the face. Never allow the client to leave the shampoo area with hair dripping on to the face. Always wrap hair in a towel to keep the head warm if the client is required to move about in the salon.

# Greasy hair

Greasy hair is caused by the over-activity of the sebaceous glands which produce far more sebum than is necessary to coat the skin and hair. This excess sebum forms a sticky coating on the skin and hair enabling dirt and bacteria to adhere to it easily. Without regular attention the bacteria can cause dandruff, and if a fringe is worn, it can also be the cause of spots and blackheads on the forehead.

Young teenagers, particularly during puberty, are especially prone to this condition, and unfortunately, the over-activity of the sebaceous glands is not confined to the scalp area alone. The skin on the face is often affected and this can give rise to common acne (acne vulgaris). It is possible to give help and guidance for this on three important factors.

### Diet

Whether a high level of fats or sugars in the diet is linked to excessive sebum production is not clear. There is conflicting evidence for and against the view. As the majority of people take in far more fat and sugar than is necessary there is no harm in erring on the side of caution and suggesting their intake be reduced.

## Drying aids

There are many products which are now manufactured especially for greasy hair. These include: shampoos, setting lotions and special conditioners without the addition of oils or waxes. Common salt also has a drying effect on the hair. However, it is well worth remembering that bleaching, tinting and perming are all processes that dry the hair and can be used to combat oiliness. They also have the added advantages of making the hair look better and also increase trade in the salon.

## Shampooing

There is no evidence that frequent shampooing results in the excess production of sebum. Most oily hair requires washing every two or three days. A dry shampoo used between shampoos is often useful to absorb some of the unwanted sebum but vigorous brushing of the hair should be avoided at all times as this stimulates the sebaceous glands and distributes the excess sebum along the entire length of the hair shaft.

Shampoos containing oils or creams should be avoided. A soapless shampoo with no additives is the most effective, but it should not be used at too high a concentration, particularly if the hair has to be shampooed frequently.

## Summary

The water used in the salon may contain minerals dissolved in it which when mixed with soap forms soap scum. This can coat the hair and make it rough and dull. Water which reacts with soap to make scum is called 'hard' water and removing these minerals 'softens' it.

Shampoo helps water to clean dirt from the surface of the hair by reducing surface tension – this allows the water to penetrate between the hair cuticle scales and remove oil and dirt making the oil break up into tiny droplets – to emulsify it. The shampoo then prevents the oil going back on to the hair.

There are a range of ingredients in shampoos such as auxiliary detergents which help lathering, salt for thickening and other chemicals for pH balance. Anti-dandruff action shampoos can be formulated for various types of hair such as dry or damaged. There are also brightening, colouring and dry powder shampoos.

## Self-assessment questions

1  Name three sources of fresh water.
2  Which calcium and magnesium salts are present in temporary hard water?
3  What is the chemical name for limescale? What effect may this have on hot water pipes?
4  How can temporary hard water be softened without adding chemicals?
5  What produces 'soap scum'?
6  Give the effect of soap scum on hair.
7  What is meant by the term 'surface tension'?
8  Shampoos reduce surface tension. Explain why this is important in cleaning hair.
9  What is meant by the term 'emulsify'?
10  Why should the water used for a shampoo be run over the hairdresser's hand before spraying on to the client's head?
11  After shampooing, why should hair be dried and disentangled away from the client's face?
12  List three common additives in shampoo and explain what each does.
13  What is a 'pH balance' shampoo? How do such shampoos work?
14  Name the solvent commonly used to 'dry' clean hair before using for making postiche.
15  What types of shampoo should be avoided with a client with greasy hair?

## Practical assignment – Shampooing

The following three tasks have been devised to help you to recognise various hair types, to choose the correct shampoo and to be aware of necessary safety procedures when shampooing.

## Tasks

1  Collect hair cuttings of the following types of hair then attach them to a piece of paper. Select a suitable shampoo for each type giving reasons for your choice.
Set out your work in the format shown below.

| Hair type | Hair cutting | Suitable shampoo | Reasons for choice |
| --- | --- | --- | --- |
| Permed | | | |
| Fine textured | | | |
| Coarse textured | | | |
| Tinted | | | |
| Bleached | | | |

2   You have been asked by the senior stylist to write out safety procedures on shampooing for a new trainee who has just joined your company. Think carefully how the trainee can avoid accidents both to themself and the client while they are carrying out a shampoo, then make a list which can be pinned up in the staff room for future reference.

You can obtain information for this task from your own experience, your employer, your tutor and textbooks.

3   Read the following scenario carefully then answer the questions below.

'Jane is a 23-year-old model with shoulder length, tint-lightened hair. She has just returned from a modelling assignment in Africa and her hair is now extremely dry.'
(a)  What type of shampoo would you suggest and why?
(b)  What do you think has caused the dryness to Jane's hair?
(c)  What advice would you give to Jane to improve her hair?

4   By looking around retail outlets, carry out a survey of the information given on the packaging of shampoos and their prices.
Draw up a table including your findings on:

● Types of ingredients
● What particular function these ingredients have (where given)
● Special purposes of the shampoo (frequent use, medicated, anti-dandruff, pH balance etc)
● Prices – convert these to 'per 100 cc' so that you are comparing the price for the same volume of shampoo.

As a result of your survey try to answer the following questions:

(a)  Is the emphasis in the information given on the ingredients or on what the shampoo is **claimed to do**?
(b)  Why is there a range in price?

5   Take samples of five (or more) different shampoos. Try to make these a range of types and prices. You may also find it interesting to include your own favourite type.
On small sections of your own or someone else's hair, try out shampooing with equal amounts of each shampoo.
Compare them in terms of:

● thickness
● colour
● scent
● lathering
● cleaning action
● hair condition after shampooing.

Put your findings into table form.

You can set the shampoos a more difficult task by moisturising the fingers with a little mineral or vegetable oil and putting this on to the hair first. This will produce hair which is very greasy. Wash the small sections as before.

In each case which shampoo is best? Which one seems the best value for money (consider its action against its cost). Explain your answers.

# 11 CUTTING HAIR

The cutting of hair is one of the most important of all the hairdressing skills. A good haircut, skillfully executed, can transform the most mediocre head of hair into something special. To cut hair proficiently the hairdresser must be aware of where and how the length and bulk (thickness) need to be removed from the hair in order to create a desirable shape with good line and balance. Each head of hair differs in some way and each haircut should be carefully cut to emphasise any good points and minimise any defects.

Remember that a good haircut is the basis for all good hairdressing. When a blowdry or set has 'dropped' from the hair, all that remains is the shape of the haircut!

## Basic haircutting techniques

There are three main haircutting methods that can be employed to produce particular effects on the various types of hair. Blowdrying and the movement towards natural looking hair has helped to encourage a greater responsibility on the part of the hairdresser to produce better haircutting. To this end, it is necessary to become proficient in the various methods of cutting to enable the hairdresser to adapt these methods to any fashion changes.

The basic techniques are:

- tapering
- thinning
- clubbing.

### Tapering

This method removes bulk and length from the hair, in other words, it will thin the hair at the same time as removing the length. By thinning the hair, a lot of the hair bulk (or weight) is also removed, thus it will allow the hair to curl more easily. Obviously, this type of cutting will not make straight hair curly, but it can encourage any natural curl or wave movement already present in the hair.

Hair can be tapered either wet or dry. The scissors are used in a slithering movement to taper dry hair. Taper cutting wet hair with the scissors can tear the hair and may also cause 'steps' because of the hair's tendency to stick together when wet.

When taper cutting wet hair the razor is used. Using a razor to cut dry hair is undesirable because the blades of the razor tends to pull the hair, making it a painful experience for the client!

## Taper cutting dry hair

Hold the mesh of hair to be cut firmly between the first and second fingers. Then, using a backcombing or slithering action with the open blades of the scissors near to the crutch, direct the scissors from the points of the hair to the middle lengths. The blades should be closed very slightly during the stroke towards the scalp, then opened again drawing the scissors away from the scalp. Never completely close the scissors during the stroke towards the scalp as this could remove too much hair and create 'steps' in the haircut.

Alternatively, the mesh of hair may be backcombed slightly before cutting. This will produce less taper than without using backcombing. The more the hair is backcombed, the less taper is produced.

## Taper cutting wet hair

Take the mesh of hair to be cut and with the razor blade held at a slight angle to the mesh, make a light slicing movement from the midlengths to the points of the hair, either on top or underneath the mesh of hair. The pressure on the blade will determine how much of the hair is cut away and the length of the stroke will determine the amount of taper. (*See* Fig 11.1(*a*), (*b*).)

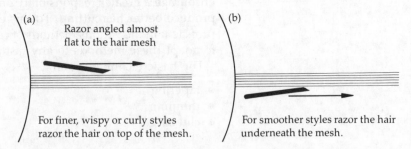

(a) Razor angled almost flat to the hair mesh

For finer, wispy or curly styles razor the hair on top of the mesh.

(b)

For smoother styles razor the hair underneath the mesh.

**Fig 11.1**

## Uses of tapering

- To remove excess length and bulk (thickness) from thick hair.

- To encourage natural curl and wave movement by removing the weight from the points of the hair.
- To re-introduce natural taper into over-clubbed hair.
- Before a basic permanent wave, to aid winding – hair which had finer, tapered points will bend much more easily around a perm rod than thicker, clubbed hair.
- To produce a lighter, feathered effect to the hairstyle.

## Thinning (or bulk reducing)

This method removes unwanted bulk, but not length from the hair. It may be done with the scissors, razor or aesculap scissors but it must be remembered that the scissors and aesculap scissors should only be used to thin out dry hair and the razor used to thin out wet hair.

Check the hair carefully to decide where on the head the bulk needs to be reduced, as it is not always necessary to thin out the whole head.

The following areas on the scalp should never be thinned because of their growth direction patterns and the possibility of unwanted spiky effects or odd hairs sticking out from the scalp if the hair is cut too short:

- the hairline, particularly at the front
- along a parting
- the crown area.

## Thinning dry hair using scissors

Divide off the areas that should not be thinned, then taking approximately 10 mm (½") width meshes, hold the hair out from the scalp at right angles. Using the points of the scissors, remove a few hairs from the root area and along the hairshaft. Continue in this manner until the whole head, or the parts that require thinning, have been completed. Take care not to remove too much hair at the root area as these hairs will tend to 'spike out' when they grow if too many have been removed.

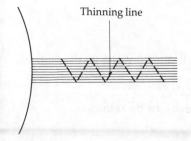

Thinning line

Fig 11.2

## Thinning dry hair using aesculap scissors

Divide off the areas that should not be thinned, then taking larger width meshes than thinning with the scissors, approximately 2 cm (1") in depth, hold the hair out from the scalp at right angles. The aesculap scissors are then inserted into the mesh at an angle. The hair is cut in a zig-zag pattern along the length of the mesh (see Fig. 11.2). Continue in this manner until the whole head, or the parts that require thinning, have been completed.

## Thinning wet hair using a razor

Divide off the areas which should not be thinned, then taking approximately 1 cm (½") meshes, hold the hair out from the scalp at right angles. With the tip of the razor, remove a few hairs at the root and along the hair shaft. Alternatively, the hair may be thinned out by using shorter and extra slicing movements on each hair mesh while actually razor cutting the hair (removing length at the same time); in this case, the slicing movements are commenced closer to the scalp.

## Uses of thinning

- to remove excess bulk from the hair
- to give a finer, feathered effect to certain areas of a hairstyle
- to remove the weight from over-clubbed hair.

## Club cutting

Club cutting is a method of cutting the hair bluntly straight across, thereby removing the length from the hair but retaining the bulk. Because the weight is left on the points of the hair it tends to discourage any natural tendency of the hair to curl. Hair can be club cut wet or dry, either using the scissors or a razor. However, club cutting with a razor requires a lot of practice and should only be attempted when the operator is fully proficient in razor cutting.

Club cutting allows the hair to be cut very precisely, but it must always be remembered that the head is a curved object, and although the hair may be cut in a straight line, the angle at which the hair is held away from the scalp is very important to produce the correct shape for the finished haircut.

## Club cutting wet or dry hair

Vertical or horizontal meshes of hair are held from the scalp at an angle and the points of the hair are cut straight across either between fingers or, if the hair is to be cut very close to the scalp, over the comb, with the scissors. (*See* Fig 11.3.)

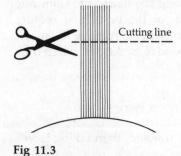
Cutting line

**Fig 11.3**

## Uses of club cutting

- on fine hair, to retain as much bulk and weight in the hair as possible
- to discourage curl on over-curly hair
- for fashion cutting, where bulk needs to be retained.

# Haircutting terms and effects

There are many terms used to describe varying effects produced by either taper cutting or club cutting. The most common of which are given below:

- graduation
- reverse graduation
- texturising
- bevel cutting
- scissors over comb
- precision cutting.

## Graduation

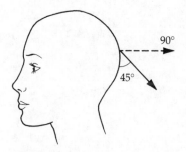

Fig 11.4 (a)

Graduation can be achieved by either club cutting or taper cutting, whichever is the most suitable for the hair type and the finished dressing. It is attained when the top layers of the hair lie above the lower layers. The top layers may lie well above the lower layers, in which case there would be a high degree of graduation, but if all the top layers lie just above the lower layers then there is less graduation.

### Increasing graduation

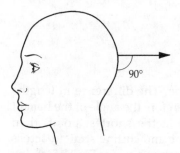

Fig 11.4 (b)

By increasing the graduation the amount of layering in the hair is also increased. The more the hair sections are lifted, the greater the graduation. When the hair is held down close to the head, at a 0° angle, a bob effect is the result, which contains no graduation. At each degree of lift of hair away from the head the more graduation is achieved. To help with the understanding of the degrees of lift, it is useful to remember tht a 90° lift means that the hair is held straight out from the head at right angles. Thus, a 45° lift is half this amount and a 180° lift is twice the lift of 90°.

1 *45° lift.* (*See* Fig 11.4(*a*).) This will create slight graduation, usually used for wedges, etc.

2 *90° lift.* (*See* Fig 11.4(*b*).) This will create twice as much graduation, usually used for short, high layered styles.

3 *90°–180° lift.* (*See* Fig 11.4(*c*).) This will create a great deal of graduation, usually used for long, high layered styles.

### Examples of graduation

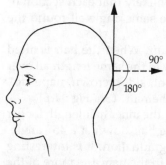

Fig 11.4 (c)

Graduation is sometimes referred to as **layering.** Increased layering is when the hair is steeply graduated and low layering is when there is little graduation.

1 *Increased layering graduation on long hair.* Increased layering is a good example of extreme angles, where the hair is cut from short

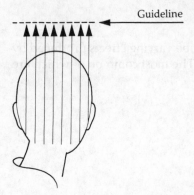

Guideline

**Fig 11.5 (a)**

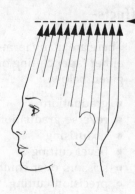

Guideline

The further the front hair is dragged back towards the crown before being cut then the longer it will become.

**Fig 11.5 (b)**

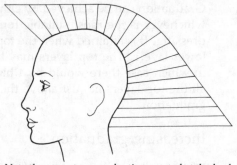

Note the very steep graduation created at the back.

**Fig 11.5 (c)**

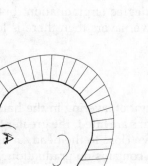

**Fig 11.6**

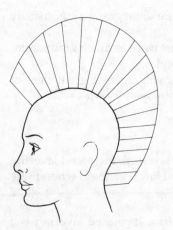

**Fig 11.7**

on the top or front, to long at the nape. The difference in lengths at these two points is very great and therefore the angle of the haircut is very steep. By cutting a guideline at the shortest point, then combing all the hair up to this guideline and cutting straight across at this point, very steep graduation is achieved. (*See* Fig 11.5(*a*), (*b*), (*c*).) To cut the hair vertically and to hold the fingers at this steep angle would be very difficult and it is unlikely that each section or mesh of hair could be cut at exactly the same angle all round the head.

2   *Uniform layering graduation on short hair.* When the hair is lifted out from the head at a 90° angle and cut to the same length all over the head, i.e. the same length at the front, sides, crown, nape etc., the result is a basic, short, graduated haircut. (*See* Fig 11.6)

3   *Low layering graduation.* A haircut with the inner hair length longer than the outline hair length. Pulling the hair down at a 45° angle, as opposed to lifting it up, creates less graduation. It is interesting to note that the less graduation there is in the hair, the more of the hair bulk remains. (*See* Fig 11.7.) Thus, finer hair can have as much thickness as possible retained by club cutting the hair into a style with very little graduation, while thicker hair can have some of the

weight or thickness removed by thinning and cutting the hair into a style which requires layering.

### Reverse graduation

This technique is used when the top layers of the hair are longer than the underneath layers of the hair, e.g. a bob or pageboy style. (*See* Fig. 11.8.)

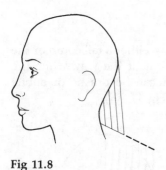

**Fig 11.8**

### Texturising

This has a more drastic effect than thinning the hair. Certain hair lengths are cut shorter than others without blending. The shorter hair lengths are used to support the longer lengths giving increased root lift. Alternatively, it can be used to soften the outline either within the haircut or around the hairline. There are many methods of texturising the hair the most popular of which are:

- chipping in
- channel cutting (scaffolding)
- weave cutting
- under cutting

## Chipping in

This technique can also be employed around the front hairline and fringe to soften or even spike, the front hair onto the face by combing the hair forward and on to the face, then snipping away the hair as it lies flat on the skin (*see* Fig. 11.9). Remember to be very careful when using the points of the scissors near the eyes and ears.

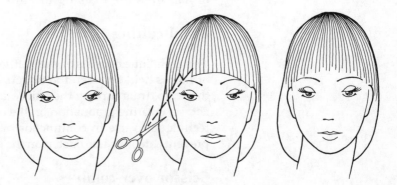

**Fig 11.9 Chipping in on front hair line**

## Channel cutting

This is the drastic removal of hair to produce a 'spikey' effect. A 'grid' of shorter hair is cut to support the longer hair lengths. The hair is cut first one way and then across the other to create the grid effect.

## Weave cutting

The hair to be left long is woven out using either a tail comb or the closed scissors. This hair is then held out of the way while the remaining hair in the section is cut. It can be drastic or subtle depending on the required effect. (*See* Fig 11.10.)

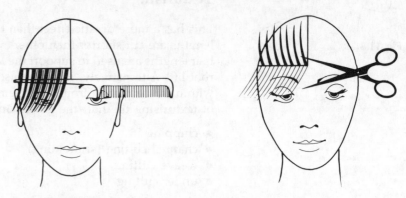

**Fig 11.10 Weave cutting**

## Under cutting

The underneath sections of a mesh of hair are cut shorter to support the longer hair lengths. This technique can be done using either the scissors or a razor. If a razor is used, hold the blade at a slight angle to the mesh and make light, slicing movements underneath the mesh of hair from the roots up towards the points.

## Bevel cutting

This technique consists of club cutting the hair on a curve. The mesh of hair is held between the fingers and then bent up and towards the scalp, thus curving the hair round. The hair is then cut straight across, creating graduation on the ends of the hair. This is a useful technique to use in conjunction with low layering to soften and prevent a definite line or step on the edges of wedged or bobbed hair.

## Scissor over comb

This technique can cut the hair extremely short and was originally used in men's haircutting and the ladies' shingle of the 1920s.

A fine, pliable comb is used to allow the hair to be cut as close to the scalp as possible. The hair is combed upwards from the nape and the hair which protrudes through the teeth of the comb is cut off. The scissors should rest along the length of the comb and should open and close quickly whilst the comb is moving up the head. If the scissor movement is too slow then steps will occur in the haircut.

The angle at which the comb is held will determine the length of the hair, if it is held next to the scalp then the hair will be very short, the further away from the scalp that it is held then the longer the hair.

Electric or hand clippers can be used in place of the scissor and comb. The clipper heads have attachments which are numbered according to their depth, thus the lower the number the shorter it will cut the hair.

A special comb known as a *Brian Drummer Flat Topper* can also be used with the clippers in place of the attachments. It has a spirit level incorporated into it so that the stylist can make sure that the hair is completely level when cutting. However, no matter what type of haircut is being carried out it is very important to keep the client's head in the correct position. If it is inadvertently held to one side during cutting then the finished haircut will be lopsided!

## Precision cutting

This technique consists of cutting the hair very precisely to give a very clean line. Although there are many ways of precision cutting, it is often easier and more precise to cut the hair in a straight line, either vertically or horizontally. By considering carefully the shape of the finished style, then taking into account where the hair needs to be short and where the length has to be kept, it is often possible to use the shape of the head to create the angles needed for the amount of graduation required.

The geometric lines of the 1960s era are a very good example of precision cutting, where the angles and lines of the hair are precisely cut to form a distinctive shape, be it soft or angular (*see* Fig 11.11).

The hair needs to be kept thoroughly wet when precision cutting to ensure that cutting meshes are smooth and straight from root to point.

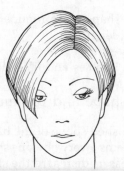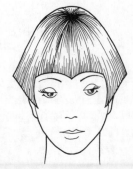

**Fig 11.11**

# Assessing the head for cutting

It cannot be stressed too often that before placing a pair of scissors near to a head of hair, the hairdresser must know exactly what the client requires and how best to achieve that result. It is too late when the hair has been cut to realise that the client's requirements have been misunderstood, or even ignored!

Clients are often nervous when they visit a salon for the first time, particularly when they require a haircut. Talking to the client and discussing the requirements enables the hairdresser to find out exactly what the client needs and expects from the haircut. It also helps to build up a relationship of trust and confidence between the client and the hairdresser. Remember that the client is a very important person and if displeased with the finished result the client will not return to the salon, nor will they recommend the salon to their friends.

To prevent unnecessary mishaps, and to gain enough information to allow the hairdresser to proceed with confidence, two main areas must be explored:

- assessment of the client
- assessment of the hair.

## Assessment of the client

This is meant to determine the client's requirements and enables the hairdresser to advise the client on any modifications of the chosen haircut that may be necessary.

It is important to question the client closely; they may know exactly what they have in mind but have great difficulty in describing the exact haircut. If this is the case, it is often useful to keep a book of fashionable hairstyles available in the salon to show the client. Thus, the hairdresser will have a visual description of the style or 'look' that the client is aiming for.

The following factors must also be taken into consideration as they will influence the suitability of the chosen haircut:

- face shape and prominent features
- neck length
- body size
- age, hobbies and lifestyle.

## Face shape and prominent features

The finished shape of the haircut should suit and flatter the client. This seems a very obvious statement, but it is surprising how many hairdressers disregard the shape of the client's face when restyling the hair. Take a good look at the client's face by drawing the hair away from the face to determine whether it is round, square, long, oval, etc.; this can affect the amount of hair that needs to be removed and will also help to determine the shape of the finished haircut. Next, check whether there are any prominent features or blemishes that need to be camouflaged, e.g. a receding chin. Some prominent features can be attractive and therefore need to be emphasised, e.g. the eyes can be emphasised by a fringe.

## Neck length

If the client has a very long neck the hair needs to be left longer in the nape. Alternatively, a very short neck looks less obvious if the hair is kept shorter in the nape or is swept up towards the top of the head to make the neck appear longer.

## Body size

The finished haircut should be part of a total look, not just a separate item that happens to be attached to the client's head! For example, a very tall, slim client with a small head would look ridiculous with a short, scalp-hugging haircut.

## Age, hobbies and lifestyle

The age of the client is a very important consideration. A middle-aged person does not always suit the same style as a teenager, although a current fashion trend can often be adapted to meet the needs of both, as long as it is not too extreme.

The general lifestyle and hobbies of the client also need to be considered. When assessing a client's personality, clothes etc., it is important not to gown up until starting the procedure. Also find out if the client will have enough spare time to spend on an elaborate hairstyle or whether they will need a style that requires the minimum amount of time spent on it between salon visits. These and many other questions need to be asked to find out exactly what the client expects and requires of the haircut.

### Assessment of the hair

This is to determine the type and method of cutting to use. Remember that it is sometimes necessary to combine a variety of haircutting techniques on one head to achieve the required shape.

Whenever possible, use the type of hair to its best advantage – it is very difficult, if not impossible, to create a long, smooth bob style on very thick, wiry, naturally curly hair. it is far better to utilise the curl and thickness of the hair to create a style that requires these features. Consider the following:

- hair texture
- hair volume
- hair length

- amount of natural curl or movement present in the hair
- growth direction of the hair.

## Hair texture

The texture of the hair refers to the diameter of the hair and can either be fine, thick or medium. Fine hair will need all the bulk retained, heavy clubbing helps to do this. Thick or coarse hair may need to have some of the bulk removed, in which case it may be necessary to thin, taper or high layer the hair, depending upon the finished style. Medium textured hair is usually no problem and adapts to most cutting techniques, again depending upon the finished style.

## Hair volume

This is the amount of hair on the scalp, or how densely the hair grows. A client may have fine textured hair, but with plenty of hairs on the scalp making it quite abundant or thick, coarse hair which is very sparse. The density of hair can vary throughout the head, e.g. hair may be denser at the nape than the crown. Therefore there are many combinations making each head slightly different.

## Hair length

Clients often do not realise that some haircuts require a lot of length in certain areas and often do not appreciate how long it takes for the hair to grow to the length they require. Often it is necessary to compromise with a hairstyle, and it may take a few months and quite a few haircuts to achieve the final effect. A good example of this is when a client has had a layered or steeply graduated haircut and wishes to 'grow out' the top layers until the hair is all one length. This can take up to 12 months, depending upon how short the hair was originally. Advice should be given to the client on the type of styles and haircuts they can have during this period, in order to keep the hair well shaped without loss of length from the areas which need to grow longer.

## Amount of natural curl or movement present in the hair

Always try to utilise any natural curl or movement in the hair. Ignoring or fighting against the curl can often ruin a haircut. By using and incorporating any natural curl or movement the haircut will stay in shape longer and will be easier for the client to manage.

## Growth direction of the hair

Strong growth direction patterns can cause some difficulties when cutting the hair, e.g. a double crown, strong napeline, etc. Cutting the hair when wet without tension allows extra length in these areas and prevents an uneven line when the haircut is finished.

## Sections for cutting

Sections are necessary when cutting hair to allow the hairdresser to proceed with the haircut in a neat and methodical manner. When cutting a basic haircut it is often more efficient to commence cutting at the nape. Sectioning is necessary therefore to hold the remaining hair firmly out of the way for greater ease when working.

## Cutting angles around the hairline

The hair may be cut at many angles around the hairline to create different shapes and styles. But always remember to take into consideration any strong hair growth direction patterns, e.g. strong napeline, cow's lick, etc.

The areas to consider when cutting angles around the hairline are:

- the forehead or fringe (*see* Fig 11.12)
- the sides of the head (*see* Fig 11.13)
- the nape of the neck (*see* Fig 11.14)

*NB* When using the features of the face or ears etc., as a guide to form the cutting angles, always check that they are even on either side.

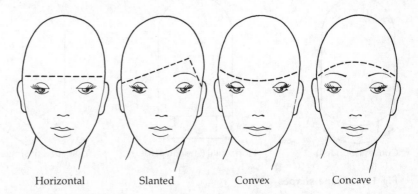

Horizontal          Slanted          Convex          Concave

**Fig 11.12 Fringe outline shapes**

## Cross-checking the hair

After cutting any head of hair the haircut should be checked very thoroughly across the sections to ensure that the haircut is level and even from all angles. This is known as **cross-checking.** However, remember when cross-checking a fashion cut not to get too

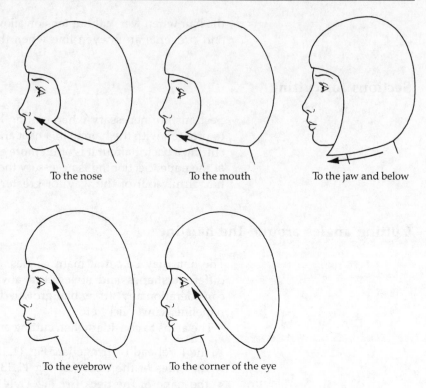

To the nose      To the mouth      To the jaw and below

To the eyebrow      To the corner of the eye

**Fig 11.13 Cutting shapes around the face**

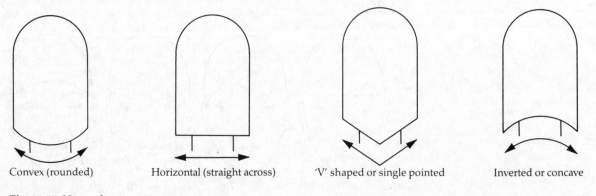

Convex (rounded)      Horizontal (straight across)      'V' shaped or single pointed      Inverted or concave

**Fig 11.14 Nape shapes**

enthusiastic and alter the line or shape of the style, particularly if the angles already cut are very steep.

Check carefully around the hairline at the sides, front and nape. If the hair has been held and cut away from the head, the underneath hair will be slightly longer, leaving wisps of hair which can make the finished line untidy. Unless this was intended to be part of the finished style they should be removed.

## Basic rules when cutting hair

1  Decide the exact shape of the finished haircut before starting to cut the hair.
2  Choose the correct type of cutting necessary for the type of hair.
3  Always cut a guideline from which to work.
4  Cut the guideline at the shortest point of the haircut.
5  Comb each mesh of hair to be cut cleanly and thoroughly from the root to the point.
6  Do not take cutting meshes that are too large. The guideline must be clearly visible through the mesh.
7  Try to cut the hair on a straight line as this gives a more precise result. Use the fact that the head is a round object to create the angles, rather than holding the hair, scissors or fingers at an awkward angle.
8  Cut with the hair growth direction and utilise any natural curl or movement to enhance the style.
9  Never cut the hair too short. It is easy to remove more hair but impossible to put it back on again.
10  When cutting wet hair, allow for the fact that hair will lift 5 mm (¼") when dry.
11  When precision cutting, do not allow the hair to dry out – always keep it wet.
12  When cutting around the ear, allow for ear protrusion and do not cut the hair too short.
13  Always cross-check a basic haircut by lifting the hair away from the head in the opposite direction from which it has been cut.
14  Give a final check to the haircut when the hair is dry and dressed.
15  Always advise the client on the care and maintenance of their haircut, especially if they have had a new style.
16  For beginners – if the guideline at the nape is cut with the client's head bent forward it will help to avoid the risk of cutting the hairline too short when the head is lifted upright.

## Example: cutting a short graduated haircut

Commence the haircut at the shortest point which in this particular case is at the side of the head. Section off a small mesh of hair and if the hair is to be cut very short at the sides, comb the mesh smoothly from root to point then rest the fingers against the scalp. The hair is then cut to the width of the fingers. This will be the guideline. (*See* Fig 11.15.)

Work up the side of the head to the temple, bringing the hair down in fine meshes and cut to the guideline. The more the hair is lifted away from the head the greater will be the graduation. (*See* Fig 11.16.)

Create a guideline from the sides through to the nape by taking a mesh of hair parallel to the hairline, above and just behind the

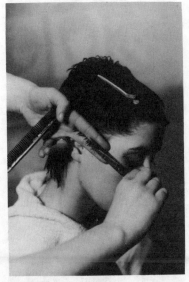

**Fig 11.15 Guideline for a short graduated haircut**

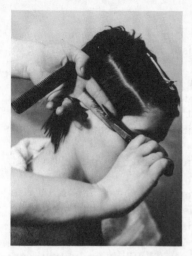

Fig 11.16

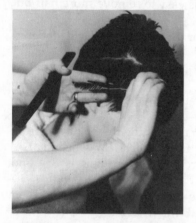

Fig 11.17

ear and combing it towards the sides. Use a small section of the previously cut hair to give the required length then cut the hair down towards the nape with the scissors parallel to the hairline. Continue down the side back to the nape in the same manner. All the hair is then brought to this perimeter guideline until the centre of the head is reached. (*See* Fig 11.17.)

Cut the other side of the head in the same manner (*see* Fig 11.18) working up the sides to the centre of the head. (*See* Fig 11.19.)

Create graduation in the hairstyle by lifting the hair out from the head at right angles and cutting straight across to the desired length. (*See* Fig 11.20.)

A guideline is cut to the length required down the centre back (*see* Fig 11.21 and Fig 11.22) and through to the front but omitting the fringe (*See* Fig 11.23).

To cut a slanted fringe, take a diagonal section across the front of the head and comb the hair in the opposite direction to the longest point of the fringe (*See* Fig 11.24). Cut the hair parallel to the section parting. When the hair is combed back the opposite way it will graduate from short to longer. To check where to commence cutting, comb the fringe area down on to the face. Decide which is the longest

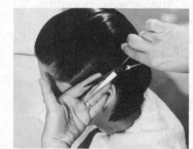

Fig 11.18

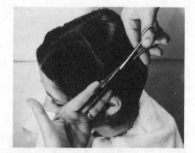

Fig 11.19

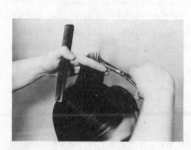

Fig 11.20 Creating graduation

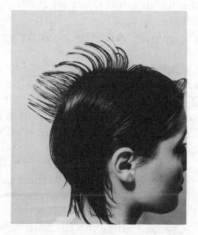

Fig 11.21

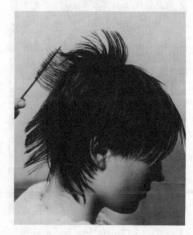

Fig 11.22

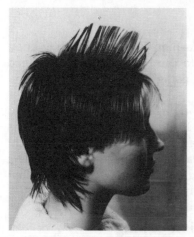

**Fig 11.23**

point of the fringe and cut a small piece of hair at this point, then take the cut piece of hair across the forehead to the opposite side. this will show where the hair has to be cut.

Cut in the shape at the nape, taking off any stray neck hairs. (*See* Fig 11.25 and Fig 11.26.)

Check all of the hairline, removing any stray hairs that may spoil the line of the haircut. Take particular care if the hair is cut short around the ears to protect the ears with the fingers (*See* Fig 11.27). Cross-check the entire haircut.

The finished haircut is illustrated in Fig 11.28.

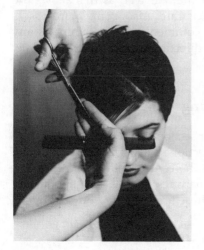

**Fig 11.24**

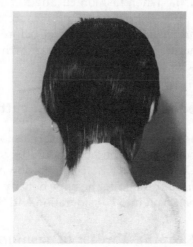

**Fig 11.25**

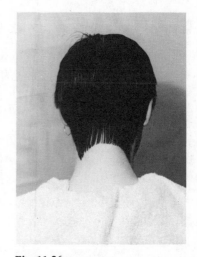

**Fig 11.26**

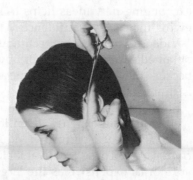

**Fig 11.27**

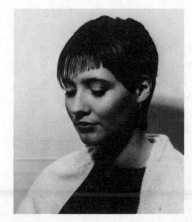

**Fig 11.28**

# Fashion cutting

Techniques vary considerably for fashion cutting depending upon individual preference. Two separate hairdressers could cut a head of hair into exactly the same style using different techniques and finish with the same result.

Hair fashions are continually changing and it is very difficult to lay down any hard and fast rules. If the technique used produces a good result and the client is satisfied then that technique is right in that particular case and for that particular hairdresser. By utilising basic techniques and working imaginatively it is possible to adapt basic cutting skills to produce high fashion work.

## Preparing the head for fashion cutting

Assess the client and the hair as for a basic haircut, however, it is usual when fashion cutting to cut the hair wet, as this allows the hair to fall naturally and is more accurate. Also, some hairdressers prefer to see the hair wet before commencing the haircut as any natural movement, curl or growth direction patterns are more easily seen and identified.

## Sectioning for fashion cutting

There are no hard and fast rules for sectioning the hair when fashion cutting and the hair should be sectioned as and where required. Often the hair is sectioned down the centre of the head from the front through to the nape but any partings, fringes, etc., should also be taken into consideration and these are sectioned off separately.

## Keeping abreast of fashion trends

It is sometimes difficult to keep ahead of current fashion trends, but there are many different ways to overcome this problem.

Attending demonstrations and seminars gives an insight into new methods. Actually seeing enthusiastic stylists at work and exchanging new ideas helps to motivate and stimulate staff often giving them fresh confidence to try out any new ideas in the salon.

Videos of new cutting techniques are readily available and can be obtained either by renting or buying outright. They are very useful because they can be shown time after time until the cutting technique is thoroughly understood.

Short courses at leading schools are also beneficial and are often well worth the expense, even if only attended for one day.

Local colleges of further education often run short refresher courses too. These are invaluable to the small salon owner as they are not as expensive as the large hairdressing schools.

As can be seen, there are many ways in which to learn and

improve new cutting skills, each of which promotes an awareness of new ideas, and benefits not only the hairdresser but also the client and therefore the salon itself.

## Summary

**Table 11.1**

| Method/ technique | Description | Effect |
|---|---|---|
| Tapering | Slithering movement with scissors on dry hair. Slicing movement with razor on wet hair. | Removes length and bulk. Encourages curl. |
| Thinning | Aesculap scissors or scissors on dry hair. Razor on wet hair. | Removes bulk only. |
| Clubbing | Cutting straight across the hair mesh. | Removes length only. Retains bulk and discourages curl. |
| Graduation | Cutting the hair so that the top layers lie above the underneath layers. Increased layering – steep graduation. Low layering – very little graduation. | Can give a layered effect or a full effect depending upon the degree of graduation. |
| Reverse graduation | Cutting the hair so that the top layers are longer or lie below the underneath hair. | Gives hair maximum volume where the ends turn under, e.g. pageboy, bob. |
| Texturising | A technique used to give root lift and remove weight from the hair. | Can soften the outline of a haircut or give a spiky effect depending on the method used. |
| Bevel | Cutting the hair on a curve over the fingers. | Creates slight graduation on the ends of the hair. |
| Scissor over comb | Cutting the hair through the teeth of the comb or with the clippers. | Can create very short haircuts on both men and women. |
| Precision | Cutting the hair precisely to give a very clean line and shape. | Hair falls into a very definite shape which can be either soft or angular. |

## Self-assessment questions

1 Which method of cutting reduces length and bulk?
2 Which method of cutting reduces bulk only?
3 Which method of cutting retains the bulk?
4 Which method of cutting encourages any natural wave movement or curl present in the hair?
5 What is the correct name for thinning scissors?
6 What is meant by graduation?
7 What is meant by reverse graduation?
8 Which method of cutting facilitates ease of winding when permanently waving the hair?
9 How does sectioning the hair prior to cutting aid the hairdresser?
10 How is the basic haircut cross-checked?

## Practical assignment – Cutting

# Hair growth patterns

This assignment should help you to get used to diagnosing the hair growth patterns of your clients and give you practice in selecting suitable haircuts.

## Tasks

1 Look carefully at the hairgrowth of *two* of your friends or family members then draw the position of the hair growth pattern at the front, nape, sides and crown area.
2 Compare the different growth patterns for each person and write a brief summary of each.
3 Describe a suitable haircut for each and give reasons for your choice.
4 Draw or cut out from magazines haircuts which would be suitable for someone with a:
   (a) double crown
   (b) strong upward-growing napeline
   (c) cow's lick at the front of the head.
Give reasons for your choice of haircuts.

# 12  BLOWDRYING AND SETTING HAIR

When a client comes into a hairdressing salon to have their hair styled, one of the basic ways a style is produced is to wave or curl the hair; or sometimes to straighten naturally waved or curly hair. Setting is carried out using either dry methods or a wet technique. This will be covered in two sections:

1  what happens to the hair during setting
2  basic techniques for producing hairstyles using these methods.

## What happens to the hair during setting

The most important aspect of hair structure (how hair is held together) to do with setting is the way the minute chains of molecules making up hair are held on to some of their neighbouring chains, or to explain it technically, the way the amino acids making up the **polypeptide chains** of hair **keratin** are able to make **cross-linkages** between the chains. This is shown in Fig 12.1.

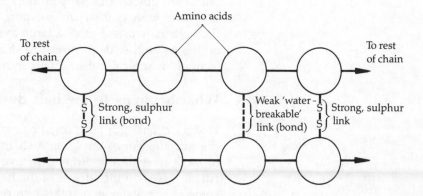

Amino acids

To rest of chain

To rest of chain

S⎫
S⎬ Strong, sulphur link (bond)

Weak 'water-breakable' link (bond)

S⎫
S⎬ Strong, sulphur link

**Fig 12.1**

There are two types of cross-linkage:

1 types that can be broken by water (these are the weaker of the two sorts and we will call them **water breakable** cross-linkages).
2 a stronger type of linkage that cannot be broken by water (these are the ones involving atoms of sulphur, called **sulphur bonds**).

At a first stage dry and wet sets involve breaking some of the weaker water breakable cross-linkages. At a second stage setting involves making the polypeptide chains change their position (which is possible when the cross-linkages are broken) and at a third stage the chains are fixed in their new position by reforming the cross-linkages so that at the end the hair is styled.

## Why sets are not permanent

The air around us usually contains some water molecules that make up an invisible gas, called water vapour, and the measuring scale, called relative humidity (or just humidity for short), indicates the amount of water vapour in the air in a particular place. If the air does not have much water vapour in it (that is, it is 'dry'), it is described as having a low relative humidity. If, on the other hand, it has a high water vapour content (which is most often the case in hairdressing salons), it is described as humid or moist, and can be said to have a high relative humidity. The humidity influences how much water enters the hair since hair is able to take in (or absorb) some of this water vapour. Hair is therefore described as hygroscopic. How much it takes in depends on two main factors:

1 the quantity of water already in the hair
2 the air's relative humidity – the higher this is, usually the more water vapour the hair takes in.

This water taken in from the air breaks some of the water breakable cross-linkages which have been fixed in their positions during the setting process. When these are broken, the polypeptide chains slip back into their original positions and the style disappears or 'drops out'. How quickly this happens depends on air humidity, so set hair drops out more quickly when exposed to damp (humid) air. When the style is 'washed out', a large amount of water is put directly on the hair either deliberately, in shampooing, or accidentally, for example when caught in a rain shower.

## What happens to the hair during wet setting

When a client's (or your own) hair is wet, most of the water is on the outside. For example, in a shampoo, the hair is wet in order to wash away oil and dirt which have collected on and between the cuticle scales on the surface of the hair shaft. As the cuticle is wet, some of the water penetrates into the hair which breaks some of the water breakable cross-linkages between the polypeptide chains of the hair (*see* Fig. 12.1). When some of the cross-linkages are broken, the polypeptide chains can be moved past each other very slightly, which over the length of the whole hair adds up to waving or curling the hair. The hair is then fixed in position when removing the water by drying it. This **wet, move and fix by drying** sequence is the basis of wet or cohesive sets.

## What happens to the hair during dry setting

Here the hair is not wet. In other words, no extra water is added but some of the moisture naturally in the hair is driven out by heat. Much heat is supplied by the techniques used in dry setting, for example heated rollers. The heat is in direct contact with the hair, which means it is carried into the hair with less being lost.

Some of the water is turned into hot water vapour (technically, steam), some is lost through the cuticle and the rest breaks some of the water breakable cross-linkages, which allows the polypeptide chains to be moved, for example, by stretching the hair around a heated roller. Next the cross-linkages re-form, fixing the chains in their new positions as the hair cools. Because some of the water vapour usually present in the hair has been lost during dry setting, the hair ends up with less moisture inside after dry setting, compared to wet setting. The hair will therefore quickly absorb any water vapour from the air around it as soon as any is available (and that is as soon as the set is finished). The equipment used when dry setting includes heated curling tongs, crimping irons, straightening irons, hot brushes, Marcel waving irons and heated rollers etc., all of which involve the use of heat very close to the skin of the face and scalp. Extreme care must therefore be taken to prevent skin burns.

With a wet set, it is mostly the water added during 'wetting' that is driven off, so the hair at the end of this process contains only a little less, or the same amount, of water than at the beginning. Thus, it does not usually absorb water as quickly as a dry set and, therefore, lasts longer. To make both types of set last longer, **setting aids** are used. How they work and what is in them are covered in the next section.

## Setting aids

Setting aids are applied to the hair before waving. The main types are:

- setting 'lotions'
- gels
- mousses.

Which one is used depends on the type of finished style. Gels, for example, have the greatest moulding facility.

All setting aids contain weak glues which 'hold' the hair in place.

Glues (or adhesives) are not necessarily 'sticky'; some work by 'bonding' together and these can be used in setting aids.

Setting lotions are the most 'runny' of the setting aids (they are about as viscous as water). This may cause problems with application due to dripping and running.

Gels contain chemicals which 'stiffen' the material but which do become much less viscous when rubbed on the hairdresser's hands and then the client's hair. Materials which are viscous until brushed or rubbed and then become more liquid are called **thixotropic.** They have the advantage of giving a 'non-drip' application of a relatively large amount of setting agent and give a good moulding ability to the stylist.

Mousses are foams which contain very small bubbles. The smaller the bubbles the 'denser' the foam. The bubbles are produced by the **propellent** in the pressurised container when it is released. Mousses are often used for 'scrunch' and 'natural' drying.

The active ingredients of setting aids depend on the type being used. Some use natural gums, for example, **tragacanth** and **karaya.** Many use an artificial gum or plastic called **polyvinylacetate** (PVA for short) which coats the hair. In practice, PVA is often mixed with polyvinyl pyrrolidone (PVP) to make it stick to the hair better. The mixture is often 60 per cent PVP and 40 per cent PVA.

As well as gluing the set hair to some extent, some setting lotions also contain a dye used to temporarily colour the hair (these are called **rinses**).

In either wet or dry setting, whether a setting lotion is used or not, putting lots of water on the hair during shampooing immediately breaks enough cross-linkages in set hair to allow the polypeptide chains to slip back into their original position, so both types of set can be easily washed out.

Having covered the basics of what happens to hair during setting, the practical aspects of setting hair in the salon will now be considered.

## Practical methods of setting hair

The main methods used are:

1 rollers
2 pincurls
3 finger waving
4 blow waving and blowdrying.

### Rollers (roller setting)

Rollers are used in setting to give lift, height and volume to a hairstyle. To produce a successful style that is durable and lasts well, careful planning is needed. The planning can be divided into two areas:

(*a*) pli (set direction)
(*b*) the size of rollers.

## Pli direction

The rollers should be placed in the hair in the direction of the finished style; therefore, it is very important to decide beforehand the direction and movements of the finished style. Before placing any rollers in the hair, always comb the hair thoroughly to see which way the hair falls naturally. The growth direction of the hair is known as the hair growth pattern. This growth direction of the hair is 'built into' the hair due to the distribution and angle of the hair follicles in the skin.

Setting the hair against the hair growth pattern may produce a good result when it is combed out initially, but the style will not last very long and will tend to 'stick out' at odd angles to the scalp the following day. As most clients expect their sets to last from one shampoo to the next, it is important to make full use of any natural features like hair growth patterns and incorporate them into the style.

Different results can be achieved depending on how the roller mesh and roller are angled from the scalp. Remember that the hair will dry where it is placed and it is therefore important to angle the roller and roller mesh correctly to achieve the desired result.

Figure 12.2 shows how:

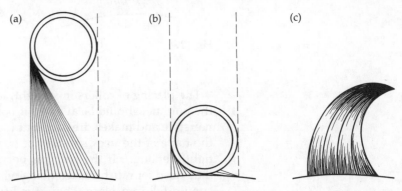

**Fig 12.2**

(*a*) hair is wound at right angles to the scalp
(*b*) the roller should be placed exactly in the centre of its own mesh
(*c*) the setting gives a normal root lift.

Figure 12.3 shows how:

(*a*) the hair is dragged forward at an obtuse angle from the scalp
(*b*) the setting gives more lift and volume.

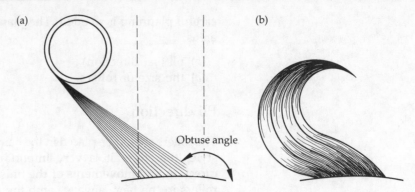

**Fig 12.3**

Figure 12.4 shows how:

(*a*) the hair is dragged back at an acute angle from the scalp
(*b*) the setting produces dragged roots and less lift and volume.

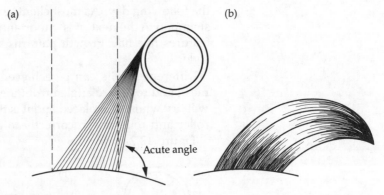

**Fig 12.4**

The placing of rollers in straight, ladder-like rows, particularly at the hairline, should be avoided if possible as it causes breaks in the hairstyle and makes dressing out more difficult. Any wispy hair at the nape of the neck should not be dragged as this will not curl it tightly enough. If the hair has been correctly set there should be little need for much backcombing when dressing out as the hairstyle should fall into place when it is brushed.

## The size of rollers

After planning the direction of the pli, the next step is to choose the size of the roller to use in order to achieve the required result. Various factors will influence the size of curler to use:

- the texture and density of the hair
- the length of the hair

- the amount of curl already present
- the required result.

### 1  *The texture and density of the hair*

It is important to check carefully, not only the texture of the hair, but also the density, before selecting the roller size to use.

The texture of the hair refers to its diameter; a large diameter applies to thick hair and a small diameter to fine hair.

The density refers to the amount of hair on the head. It is possible to have fine textured hair that it very abundant (i.e. a lot of hairs per square inch on the scalp); likewise, it is possible to have thick textured hair that is very sparse (i.e. few hairs per square inch on the scalp).

Fine textured hair usually requires a smaller roller than thick textured hair to produce the same amount of curl because there are fewer water breakable cross-linkages in fine hair, although if the hair is very abundant (or dense) this can create too much curl because of the amount of hair present.

Thick textured hair usually requires a larger roller, but again the density of the hair must also be taken into consideration because if the hair is very sparse this does not always apply.

### 2  *The length of the hair*

The longer the hair, the heavier it becomes, therefore very long hair may require a smaller roller than is usually necessary to counteract the 'dragging effect' of this length of hair, particularly if a curly style is required. However, the size of roller is very dependent upon the amount of curl that is required in the finished style.

Long hair styles that are very smooth require extremely large diameter rollers and in this case the use of too small a roller would result in too much wave and curl movement which would be difficult to eliminate when dressing the hair.

### 3  *The amount of curl already present*

Naturally curly hair and permanently waved (permed) hair may require a larger roller than straight hair because of the amount of curl and body already present in the hair.

### 4  *The required result*

The final decision depends on the type of style the client requires, i.e. whether the finished dressing is to be smooth, curly, wavy or a combination of any of these.

The main rule to remember is that a small roller will produce a small curl with a lot of bounce, while a large roller will produce a large curl with less bounce. The reason for this is that the more times the hair is wound round the roller, the more polypeptide chains are moved when the cross-linkages are broken, so when they are fixed in their new positions by drying, a tighter curl is produced.

## Method of placing a roller in the hair

1  Divide off a mesh of hair the same size as the roller. This should

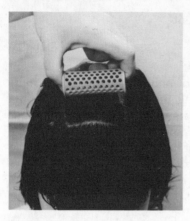

**Fig 12.5**

be the same length and the same width as the roller. (*See* Fig 12.5.)

2 Comb the hair thoroughly from the roots through to the points at a right or obtuse angle from the scalp. (*See* Fig 12.6.)

3 Place the points of the hair in the centre of the roller, making sure that the tension is even on either side of the mesh. Then turn the roller, using the thumbs to hold the points in position until they are locked round the roller. (*See* Fig 12.7.)

4 Wind the hair and roller evenly down to the scalp. The wound roller should be in the centre of the mesh when wound. (*See* Fig 12.8.)

Note the position of the securing pin. It should hold the roller firmly in position without marking the hair and it should never be secured in such a way as to mark the client's scalp or cause discomfort.

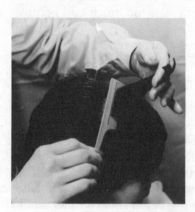

**Fig 12.6**

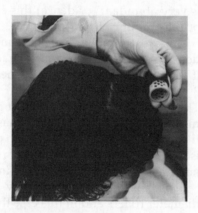

**Fig 12.7 Start winding on to the roller**

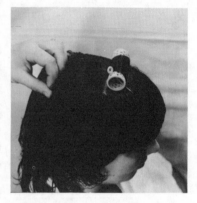

**Fig 12.8 Wound roller in centre of mesh**

Once the skill of correctly placing a roller in the hair has been mastered, it is possible to experiment with different roller positions to create different effects. Combing the wet hair into the direction of the finished style before setting, then placing the rollers in the required direction leads to more interesting styling and also produces a more durable hairstyle for the client. Figs 12.9(a) and (b) show how to set the hair directionally.

## Mistakes and precautions when roller setting

1 Hair mesh too wide – this causes drag at the roots, either in front of the roller or behind the roller. (*See* Fig 12.10(*a*), (*b*).)

2 Hair mesh too narrow – the roller will overlap onto the next hair mesh so that the root hair of this mesh will be dried completely flat to the head (*see* Fig 12.11). If all the hair meshes are too narrow,

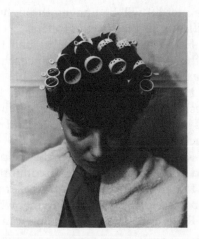

Fig 12.9 (a) Front directional
winding

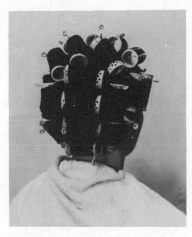

Fig 12.9 (b) Back directional
winding

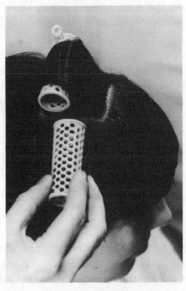

Fig 12.10 (a) roller setting drag
caused on roots behind roller

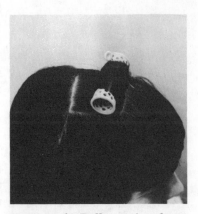

Fig 12.10 (b) Roller setting drag
caused on roots in front of roller

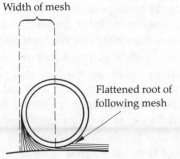

Width of mesh

Flattened root of
following mesh

Fig 12.11

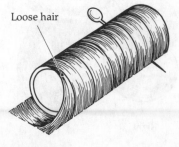

Loose hair

Fig 12.12

the root lift will be uneven throughout the head and there will be difficulty in placing the rollers.

3   Hair mesh too long – the hair has to be dragged at the sides of the mesh causing loose hair at each end of the roller when winding (*see* Fig 12.12).

4   Hair mesh too short – creates the same problem as the hair meshes which are too narrow, i.e. the roller will overlap and flatten the hair at the sides of the roller and can also cause difficulties when placing the other rollers.

5   Roller pin pressing on to the scalp – will leave marks on the skin and will cause the client discomfort.

6   Roller pin not securing the roller properly – the roller will drop or become displaced while drying, which will spoil the finished style.

7   Roller pin marking the hair – can create 'kinks' in the hair when dry.

8   Hair points bent back or not wound completely round the roller when winding will create 'fish-hook' ends, which when dressed makes the hair appear frizzy on the ends.

9   Uneven tension or winding – leads to uneven movements in the hair.

10   Avoid placing the rollers in straight, ladder-like rows as this can cause breaks in the style and create difficulties when dressing the hair.

11   Wispy nape hairs should be wound correctly. If they are dragged the napeline of the finished style will be uneven.

12   Never underestimate the importance of a good pli. A well placed set, skillfully carried out not only helps the dressing of hair but is also the basis of a long-lasting style.

## Pincurls

To style the hair with pincurls the hair should be thoroughly wet to enable the operator to mould the hair correctly. It is important to use and incorporate any natural hair growth patterns and movements that may be present in the hair to give durability to the style. As with roller setting, the hair should be combed in the direction of the finished style and the pincurls placed in that direction. A pincurl is usually taken from a square mesh and the curl must be kept as round at the points of the hair as it is at the roots. The durability of the pincurl depends on the perfect roundness and how smoothly it is wound from the roots. Twisting or buckling the hair either at the roots or along its length will not give a stisfactory result as the hair will dry where it is placed.

Pincurls may be secured with either one-pronged or two-pronged clips, depending upon personal preference, but these should be inserted in such a way that the ends of the clip secure the points of the hair firmly in position while the head of the clip rests on the stem of the curl so that the clip does not hinder the formation of the next pincurl. (*See* Fig 12.13.)

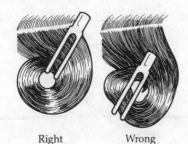

Right          Wrong

**Fig 12.13**

Special care should be taken when securing hair that is either fine, bleached or highly porous as this type of hair marks easily.

Pincurls are best suited to medium textured hair with a slight natural movement. Very thick or extremely curly hair is difficult to pincurl and buckles easily while very fine, straight hair usually requires extra lift and body.

The size of the pincurl is determined by the hair texture and the required result. Thick hair usually requires a larger pincurl than fine hair to achieve the same result. The diameter of the pincurl will determine the amount of curl in the finished movement, but the set will loosen and drop slightly when it is dressed, so allowance should be made for this by making the diameter of the pincurl slightly smaller than the required result.

## Types of pincurl

**Fig 12.14**

There are several types of pincurls to produce various results:

- clockspring
- flat barrel spring
- barrel spring or stand-up
- stem curls
- sculptured curls
- reverse pincurls.

**Fig 12.15**

### 1  Clockspring (See Fig 12.14)

This type of pincurl is small and tight with a closed centre which produces a tight curl on the ends and a looser wave at the root. A clockspring pincurl is usually used at the nape of the neck when a curly effect is required.

### 2  Flat barrel spring (See Fig 12.15)

An open-centred curl which is formed flat to the head. This is the most common type of pincurl and is also used when reverse pincurling to form wave movements.

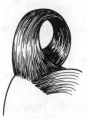

**Fig 12.16**

### 3  Barrel spring or stand-up (See Fig 12.16)

This type of pincurl also has an open centre and is formed so as to stand up from the head. it is secured by passing a clip through the curl at the base. The stem direction of a stand-up pincurl is directed up and away from the direction of the finished dressing, thus creating lift and volume in the same manner as a roller. If it is used in conjunction with rollers, the pincurl must be the same diameter as the rollers used.

### 4  Stem curls (See Fig 12.17)

Stem curls are open-centred pincurls with a long stem. A mesh of hair is taken from a square base and wound either from root or point. The curl is then placed above, below or to either side of the base, depending on the direction of the finished style; this produces a long stem to the pincurl and can be used to accentuate hair growth direction at the nape or sides of the head.

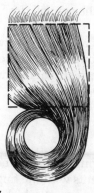

**Fig 12.17**

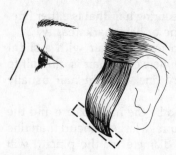

**Fig 12.18**

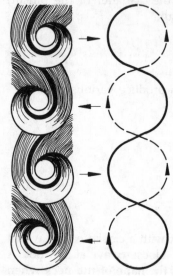

**Fig 12.19**

5 *Sculptured curls* (*See* Fig 12.18)
The hair is combed thoroughly and moulded in the exact position in which it is going to be dressed and is then secured by either tape or clips. Tape is usually used in preference to clips as it does not mark the hair and it holds the moulded hair more securely in position. A sculptured curl produces a soft effect at the nape, sides or fringe area, especially on very short hair.

6 *Reverse pincurls* (*See* Fig 12.19)
Reverse pincurls are, as the name suggests, curls that are formed in one direction and then reversed back around the head in the opposite direction. On looking closely at a wave movement, it can be seen that it is an 'S' shape, which bends in one direction and then bends back in the opposite direction. By reversing the pincurls one way and then another it is, therefore, possible to achieve wave movements in the hair.

## Precautions and considerations when pincurling

1 Hair should always be thoroughly wet when pincurling.
2 Consider the hair and hair growth patterns carefully before starting to pincurl the hair.
3 Use and incorporate any natural wave movements into the style.
4 Always work to the shape of the hed, i.e. in curved movements, not straight lines.
5 The durability of the curl is maintained by its perfect roundness, therefore a pincurl should be as round at the points as it is at the roots.
6 Do not twist or buckle the hair, either when forming the pincurl or when securing it.
7 Special consideration should be given to permed, tinted, bleached or highly porous hair, as these hair types are often more difficult to pincurl and can mark or buckle more easily.
8 The hair should be kept flat when forming the pincurl unless it is a stand-up pincurl.
9 The diameter of the pincurl determines the size of the final curl, therefore, care must be taken to wind the correct size of pincurl for the desired effect − bearing in mind that the set will drop slightly when dry.
10 When reverse pincurling, the pincurls along each row should be wound in the same direction but in the opposite direction to the previous row. The curls should be a uniform size and arranged in a brickwork pattern to eliminate unwanted partings.

## Finger waving

Also known as 'flat waving' or 'water waving', this is a method of moulding the hair into 'S' shaped movements with the fingers and comb, producing a wave movement. The point at which the hair changes direction is known as the **crest** (*see* Fig 12.20(a)) and the height of the crest and, therefore, the depth of the wave depends on the amount of moulding with the fingers. Finger waving (*see* Fig 12.20(b)) can be achieved on straight or wavy hair but naturally tight curls, coarse or permanently waved hair will not usually wave successfully.

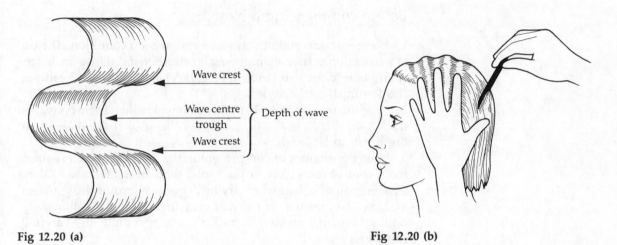

Fig 12.20 (a)                                    Fig 12.20 (b)

## Precautions and considerations when finger waving

1   The hair should be clean and thoroughly wet. A thick gel setting lotion will help to keep waves in position.
2   The hair should be well tapered and of reasonable length, particularly on the crown.
3   Utilise any natural wave movement in the hair – do not fight against the natural growth. To find the natural wave, comb all hair back from the client's face, then push forward. The hair will fall in its natural line.
4   Do not use clips, grips or wave claws unless absolutely necessary as they mark the hair and flatten the wave centres.
5   Use the coarse end of the comb and avoid scratching the scalp by leaning the comb slightly towards the operator.
6   All waves should be the same width and slightly smaller than the required result to allow for slight loosening.
7   Always wave towards the parting and never wave in straight lines.
8   Ensure that the underneath hair is waved. 'Lifting' the hair into place when finger waving can distort the roots.

### Blowdrying

Blowdrying is used to create a natural, soft effect and the finished result should be smooth and 'bouncy'. The success of the finished blowdry is very dependent on the shape of the haircut and the expertise of the operator when blowdrying.

There are many methods of blowdrying the hair and each operator may use slight variations to achieve the same result. However, there are certain precautions to take regardless of the method used, to ensure a successful result.

## Before commencing a blowdry

1  Hair must be scrupulously clean and in good condition. The use of a conditioner after shampooing is often beneficial (use an oil-free conditioner if the hair tends to be greasy) and will give a healthier, shinier finish to the style.

2  Note the texture of the hair. Fine hair will require more body than thick hair, therefore the finer the hair the smaller the diameter of the brush to be used.

3  Note the amount of curl present in the hair. Curly hair requires more control (especially at the roots) than straighter hair. Taking smaller meshes of hair when drying helps to overcome this problem.

4  Note the direction of the hair growth. Any imperfections, e.g. double crown, awkward hairline etc., should be carefully camouflaged.

5  A conditioning blowstyling lotion ensures a more durable style and helps reduce static electricity.

6  The sectioning of longer hair helps the operator to work more quickly, methodically and efficiently.

7  Combing hair in the direction of the desired style, particularly short hair, helps the operator to dry the hair in the correct direction.

## While blowdrying

1  The jet of air should follow the direction of the brush and hair. Never blow against the cuticle of the hair as this can be damaging and give a rough finish to the style.

2  Never allow the jet of air to flow on to the client's scalp as it can cause burns to the skin.

3  Maintain plenty of lift at the roots, particularly at the crown area.

4  Ensure that each mesh of hair is completely dry before proceeding to the next. If the hair is not sufficiently dried then a capillary action takes place between this damp hair and any dry hair and the shape of the style will not last.

5  The size of the meshes depend on the size of the brush. The smaller the brush, the smaller the section. Taking too large a mesh and dragging the hair can make the style flat.

6  Greater curl and body can be achieved by winding the hair round the brush, drying with a hot jet of air and then allowing the hair to cool still wrapped around the brush. For speed, the brush is left in the hair while cooling takes place and another brush of the same size is used on the next mesh of hair.

7  Ensure that the points of the hair are dried evenly round the brush. Rotating the brush while drying helps to prevent 'kinking' of the hair. Remember that hair will dry where it is placed and if the points or roots of the hair are buckled while drying, the finished result will be buckled.

8  In the case of very short hair, finger drying (i.e. drying the hair with the fingers instead of a brush) is sometimes more effective. Short hair at the nape, on the sides or on the fringe are often better dried by this method as a brush imparts too much lift to this length of hair.

9  Blowdrying long hair can be tedious and time consuming. To save time it is often easier to dry off the roots of the hair by brushing it in the opposite direction than the finished style and allowing the jet of air to dry the root section only in this position. When the hair is combed back into its original position there is then a good degree of lift at the roots. The points of the hair are then dried in the direction of the style.

## After blowdrying

1  When blowdrying is completed, allow the hair to cool thoroughly then check that the hair is completely dry. Warm hair often gives the illusion of dryness while it is still damp.

2  Comb or brush the hair into the finished style ensuring that the sides are blended into the back and that all partings are straight and clean. Pay particular attention to the nape area to ensure that the shape is pleasing and check the balance of the finished dressing from the front, sides and back of the head, making full use of the mirror.

3  Apply a fine spray of lacquer or shine and smooth down any fly-away hairs with the back of the comb or palm of the hand.

## Blow waving

Blow waving the hair is a method of waving the hair producing soft natural movements with the aid of a comb or brush and heated air from a hand hair dryer. The hair is held in a wave position and a flattened nozzle dryer attachment directs and concentrates the flow of heated air. The control required to form wave shapes is determined by movements of the comb or brush and dryer, in relation to the hair position. It is mainly used in men's hairdressing.

## Method

1  Commence at front hairline and follow any natural movement.

2  Insert the comb in the hair, using the coarse end of the comb, and with a backward combing movement, grip and hold the hair in a wave crest.

3  Direct the hot air on to the centre of the wave in the opposite direction to which the comb is held.

4 The comb movement is similar to a finger waving movement and half strength air flow should be used or the force will blow the hair out of the comb.

5 Continually move the dryer along the hair; in this way the heat is evenly directed and does not burn the head.

## Summary – Blowdrying and setting hair

**Setting hair involves the breaking and re-forming of water breakable linkages between the polypeptide chains of hair keratin. Setting can be divided into:**

**1 wet sets – where the hair is wet before processing and thus water breaks some bonds in the hair. Examples are roller setting, pincurls, finger waving, blow waving and blowdrying.**
**2 dry sets – where the hair is processed dry by directly applying heat and the moisture already in the hair breaks the cross-linkages. Examples are heated rollers, heated brushes, etc.**

**Setting lotions make the set last longer by glueing the hair in place. Some contain natural gums, but most modern setting lotions contain a mixture of polyvinylpyrrolidone (PVP) and polyvinyl acetate (PVA).**

## Self-assessment questions

1 What holds the polypeptide chains of hair keratin together?
2 Define the term 'hygroscopic'.
3 Give four examples of both dry and wet sets.
4 What is meant by 'pli direction'?
5 Why should placing rollers in straight, ladder-like rows be avoided?
6 What effect does using a hair mesh too wide for the roller produce?
7 List the main types of pincurls.
8 How does a setting aid produce a longer lasting set?
9 What type of accident is particularly associated with dry setting techniques?
10 In wet sets, what causes the cross-linkages to re-form?

## Practical assignment – Roller setting

This assignment has been devised to help you to understand the effects of different roller sizes on the hair.

## Task

Divide your tuition head into six sections. Wind a different size roller onto each section. Dry the hair and remove the rollers. Examine the result then write your findings in the form of a table as shown opposite.

|  | *Size of roller* | *Result* |
|---|---|---|
| Section 1 |  |  |
| Section 2 |  |  |
| Section 3 |  |  |
| Section 4 |  |  |
| Section 5 |  |  |
| Section 6 |  |  |

# 13 DRESSING HAIR

Dressing the hair is of equal importance to either setting or blowdrying for, although good setting or blowdrying will make the style durable and easier to dress, the actual dressing of the hair will give the final image, and it is this final image which will either please or displease the client and will also serve as advertisement for the salon.

Dressing the hair requires plenty of practice to gain the confidence to work quickly and efficiently and to know when enough work has been carried out on the head. It is almost like putting the finishing touches to a painting. A good artist will know almost instinctively when the picture looks 'right' and therefore stop working on it. By dabbling about too much after this stage the image can be completely ruined!

## Considerations when dressing hair

- Use of tools.
- Use of dressing creams.
- Amount of volume required.
- Line and balance.
- Final image.

### Use of tools

Dressing the hair can be made much easier and simpler by using the correct tools for the effect required.

### Use of dressing creams

Dressing creams are used to reduce static electricity and to replace any natural oil that may have been removed when shampooing. They will also add a shine or gloss to dull, dry hair.

Most dressing creams are made from mineral oil as an emulsion with perfume added. Mineral oil is used in preference to vegetable oil because it does not go rancid and does not penetrate the hair shaft but remains on the surface only, so giving a better shine than vegetable oil. This also helps to protect the hair from dampness.

Dressing creams do not need to be used on every head of hair but only if the hair is dry or very 'fly-away'. Do not use them on hair which tends to be greasy as they will encourage this condition.

*Method of applying dressing creams*
After brushing the hair thoroughly apply a small amount of the cream to the palm of the hand (about the size of a pea). Rub the hands together then gently stroke the hair with the hands making sure that the cream is also applied to the underneath layers. Care must be taken to avoid applying too much cream as this will make the hair too greasy and lank. When the cream has been applied, rebrush the hair thoroughly to distribute the cream evenly throughout the whole head.

Dressing oils as opposed to creams can be obtained in aerosol can form and are known as conditioning sprays or hair gloss. They can be sprayed onto the hair after brushing, as with dressing creams, or they may be applied after completion of the dressing to add shine and lustre to the hair. Hold the can about 30 cm (12") away from the scalp and direct the spray just above the head to prevent the oil being concentrated in one area. The oil will then drop on to the hair and will coat it more evenly if applied in this manner. It is very important to use this type of dressing oil sparingly – if used liberally the excess oil will make the hair appear greasy and lank.

## Amount of volume required

Some hairstyles require very little volume while others need more than can be created by either the amount of hair itself or by the way that it is set/blowdried. There are two methods of creating extra volume when dressing the hair:

- backcombing
- backbrushing.

## Backcombing

This is pushing the hair back on itself at the root to give a lifted full effect using a comb. Tapered hair is easier to backcomb than clubbed hair as the finer ends are more easily pushed back on themselves. Backcombing is also sometimes used to temporarily straighten over-curly hair.

Backcombing the hair at the roots underneath the hair mesh will give volume, while backcombing on top of the mesh will help to blend the hair together and will give an even spread of hair; this is often called **teasing.**

**When backcombing hair:**
1 Brush the hair into the shape and direction of the style then decide which area of the head requires extra volume; usually this is on top of the head and crown area but sometimes the whole head will require extra volume.
2 Start at the top or front of the head and take a narrow section of hair in the direction of the style.
3 Lift out from the scalp at right angles.
   Holding the hair mesh firmly in one hand and the comb in the other, insert the comb into the hair mesh approximately 2–3 cm (¾–1⅛") away from the scalp.
4 Push back the hair to the root repeatedly until enough hair has been pushed back to form a padding at the root. The more the hair is pushed back the greater will be the lift.
5 Continue in this manner until the areas which require extra volume are completed.
6 Always remember to hold the hair firmly while backcombing. Allowing the hair mesh to sag while the comb is pushing back the hair to the roots prevents the hair from being pushed back correctly and will make the style flop.
7 The side of the section depends upon the density and thickness of the hair and the amount of volume required, but the finished backcombing should not be visible at the front of the mesh as this creates difficulties when smoothing the hair over the backcombing.
8 If the backcombing does penetrate through to the front of the mesh then the section or hair mesh is too fine.

   It is usually only necessary to backcomb the hair at the root area as this is where the lift is needed. Only if extreme height is required by the hairstyle is it usually necessary to backcomb the hair past the mid-lengths towards the points.
   A common fault when backcombing is not pushing the hair right back to the scalp thus creating a padded effect at the mid-lengths instead of the roots. When the hair is smoothed over, the root area remains 'floppy' resulting in no lift whatsoever!

**The teasing method:**
Teasing does not give the same lift to the hair but is used to blend the hair meshes together, thus giving an even spread of hair and a smoother finish to the dressing. It can be used in conjunction with backcombing or on its own.
   Larger sections of hair are taken where required and held between the fingers and thumb. The hair is then pushed back on itself on top of the hair mesh while the hair between the fingers is pulled in the direction of the style. When smoothing the hair after teasing,

care must be taken to smooth the hair gently so as not to remove all the backcombing.

## Backbrushing

This is pushing the hair back on itself either under or on top of the hair mesh to give a lifted effect using the brush.

Backbrushing gives a softer effect than backcombing and is useful for longer hair; backcombing long hair tends to create too much lift and there is the danger of the hair becoming too tangled.

## Removal of all backcombing and backbrushing

Clients should always be advised as to how to remove backcombing or backbrushing from their hair correctly. Incorrect removal can be very painful for the client and damaging to the hair.

Commence removal at the nape of the neck, with the wide spaced teeth of a dressing comb. Always start at the points of the hair and work down towards the roots.

### Line and balance

Balance refers to the shape of the dressing in relation to the client's face, head and neck. The lines of the hairstyle should compliment the wearer and each movement should flow naturally into or complement the next. Judging when the finished style is 'balanced' requires practice and that undefinable something – instinct or flair perhaps – that tells the stylist that the dressing looks right on the client.

The use of the mirror while dressing the hair helps to keep a check on the balance of the hairstyle by putting the style in perspective. Dressing the hair at close quarters limits the vision of the stylist to one area only; so by frequently checking the outline and shape of the dressing in the mirror the stylist can see at a glance where and if the shape needs to be altered.

When the dressing is complete, stand away from the head and check the line and balance of the style at the front, sides and back of the head. First look at the silhouette of the hairstyle; this will help to show up any defects in the balance of the dressing, then check that the movements and/or smoothness within the silhouette are correct. Next check that the edges along the hairline are even and that the lines blend into each other and compliment the face and neck.

### Final image

The final image is the culmination of the stylist's skills and no matter how good or bad the setting/blowdrying is, it is this final image on which the client, to a great extent, will judge the salon. It is worth a few extra seconds therefore to check that nothing mars the line of the hairstyle.

Remove any stray, wispy neck hairs with the scissors, and when completely satisfied with the result show the client the finished style from all angles in a hand mirror.

Do not apply any lacquer before seeking the client's assurance that they are pleased with the result – the style may have to be changed slightly and this is difficult after the lacquer has been applied.

## How to apply the lacquer

1 Protect the client's eyes and face with a face shield or with the free hand.
2 Aim the spray just above the dressing to allow the lacquer to drop on to the hair. While lacquering the hair, the spray should be moved in the direction of the hairstyle so that any movement of air does not disturb the dressing.
3 Spray the lacquer from a distance of 30 cm (12″) so that a fine even spray coats the hair. Spraying the hair too near to the head will saturate only one area and this could wet the hair too much causing it to drop. Alternatively, the lacquer may form 'blobs' on the hair which, when dry, will look like white nodules sticking to the hair.
4 When enough lacquer has been applied to the hair, re-check the dressing carefully and smooth any fly-away hairs with the flat of the hands or the back of the comb.

## Manufacture and design of hair fixing sprays

Hair fixing sprays are developed from synthetic **plastic polymers** dissolved in alcohol which coat the hair with a clear plastic film. A mixture of two plastic film-formers is often used. For example: polyvinylpyrrolidone (PVP) and polyvinyl acetate (PVA) in the ratios of PVP–PVA:

60–40 per cent for general use
70–30 per cent for hard holding.

When lacquer is sprayed on to the hair the alcohol evaporates leaving the resin or plastic coating on the hair. This tends to stick or mildly glue the hair in place when the alcohol solvent evaporates. Hair lacquers can be sprayed on to the hair using either a hand-pumped spray or a pressurised aerosol spray can. Public concern for the environment has made manufacturers more aware of the need to produce aerosol spray cans which are 'ozone friendly', i.e. they do not contain ozone destructive gases – **chlorofluorocarbons.** Aerosol lacquer contains:

(a) the **propellent** which produces the pressure inside the container
(b) the **nozzle** which when pressed releases the pressure and the can contents are sprayed out as the fine droplets of an **aerosol**

(*c*) the **film-former** which is the material which coats the hair.

## Safe use and storage of pressurised spray cans

Because the contents are often **flammable** do not allow a client to smoke when lacquering their hair. As the contents are under pressure, heat will increase the pressure and may cause the can to burst. Do not store on heaters or in direct sunlight. Do not puncture or burn (or incinerate), even when empty.

# Procedure for dressing a basic set

1  Gown the client to ensure that any loose hairs or flakes of skin do not fall on to the clothing.
2  Check that the hair is completely dry by removing one of the rollers (usually where the hair is thickest or longest) and test the ends of the hair. If the hair is damp it will lose its springiness and will not comb out into shape.
3  Remove the rollers and clips from the hair gently without tugging, then allow the hair to cool for a few minutes.
4  Loosen the set and help eradicate any roller partings by double brushing or using the brush and comb to brush the hair thoroughly from root to point in all directions over the head.
5  Apply a small amount of dressing cream if the hair appears dry or fly-away. If an aerosol type is used this may be applied at this stage or when the dressing is complete.
6  Brush the hair into shape using one brush and following each stroke with the other hand to smooth and shape the hair. Stroke the brush in the planned direction of the set taking into consideration any wave or curl movements.
7  Backcomb or backbrush any areas of the hairstyle that require extra volume or lift – but remember, not all styles require backcombing.
8  Lightly comb the surface of the hair to shape and smooth into position, the free hand can also be used to follow the comb to help to smooth the hair. It may be necessary to tease certain areas at this stage so that the lines and movements blend into the shape.
9  Check the line and balance of the hairstyle from all angles to ensure that it is the correct shape and suits the client. Remove any wispy neck hairs.
10  Show the client the finished result in the hand mirror and if they are satisfied with the style apply a light spray of lacquer, remembering to use a face shield or the hand to protect the face and eyes.

## Precautions and considerations when dressing hair

1  Ensure that the hair is completely dry before combing or dressing the hair. Straighter hair will drop if it is damp, while permed or

naturally curly hair will frizz and in either case the correct shape will not be achieved.

2  Use the correct tools for the effect required. For example do not use a tail comb for disentangling or smoothing the hair, the teeth are too fine and it can be painful for the client.

3  Fine hair should not be brushed as vigorously as normal or thick hair as it loses its springiness more easily.

4  Always work in the direction of the set when brushing, backcombing or smoothing the hair.

5  Use dressing creams and oils sparingly. Using too much may result in the hair having to be shampooed again to remove the excess grease.

6  Only backcomb or backbrush the hair where necessary. Putting too much backcombing into the hair is time wasting and not particularly beneficial to the hair as it can damage the cuticle scales.

7  Take hair meshes of the correct size when backcombing: too fine and the backcombing will be visible at the front of the mesh; too thick and the backcombing will not penetrate into the mesh far enough and it will be 'floppy'.

8  Do not backcomb right to the points of the hair, it will destroy any curl at the ends of the hair.

9  Make sure that the backcombing is at the root of the hair to give the necessary lift – if it is only present at the mid-lengths the hair will flop.

10  Do not let the comb penetrate too deeply through the meshes when smoothing backcombed hair as this can remove too much backcombing.

11  Any areas that still require lifting even after backcombing can be done so by inserting the tail end of a tail comb at the roots and gently lifting the hair.

12  Check regularly in the mirror when dressing the hair – it helps the stylist create the correct shape and balance.

13  Make sure that the movements within the style complement each other and that the hair is sufficiently blended.

14  The final dressing should be balanced from all angles, so check the style at the front, sides and back.

15  It is sometimes a good idea to check the finished dressing in relation to the client's body proportions by asking the client to stand.

16  When the dressing is complete remove any fallen hairs, etc. from the client's neck and shoulders with a neck brush.

17  Only use the lacquer after the client has been shown the finished style, then if the style needs to be altered slightly it can be done with the minimum of fuss.

18  Do not spray the lacquer too close to the head as this concentrates the lacquer into one area of the head and can wet the hair causing it to drop.

19  Use only a fine spray of lacquer. Using too much can cause 'beading' of the lacquer and when dry it will look like white nodules on the hair.

20  Finally, do not 'over-work' the hair. When the balance, shape and smoothness are correct – leave it!

## Summary

Dressing the hair produces the final image of the style and the task is made far easier by using the correct tools. Dressing creams containing mineral oils which coat the hair can be used after brushing to reduce static electricity and replace any oils lost during the shampooing, setting or blowdrying process.

Backcombing and backbrushing are techniques used to produce extra volume and can also help to straighten over-curly hair to some extent. Backcombing/backbrushing at the roots will give lift to the style while backcombing/backbrushing on top of the hair mesh (teasing) is used to 'blend' the hair and eliminate roller marks. Both types of backcombing/backbrushing should be removed from the hair carefully to avoid client discomfort or unnecessary damage to the hair. Any tangling should be removed using the wide teeth of a dressing comb starting at the hair points and working down towards the roots.

Care must be taken to check that the line, balance and shape of the finished style is in proportion to the client's head shape and body size. Remember that the final image is most important and should compliment the client.

The hair may be 'fixed' in place by 'fixing sprays' made from synthetic plastic polymers dissolved in alcohol which leave a plastic coating on the hair, thus protecting it from the effects of atmospheric moisture. However, care must be taken when using these sprays as they are usually flammable and additional precautions are necessary when using the aerosol sprays as the pressurised can will explode if exposed to excessive heat or sunlight, or if disposed of incorrectly.

## Self-assessment questions

1  Which type of oil is used in most dressing creams?
2  Why is it necessary to store aerosols out of direct sunlight?
3  What is the name given to backcombing on top of the hair mesh?
4  Why should a client not smoke when a lacquer is being applied?
5  Why is it necessary to use dressing creams sparingly?
6  Which teeth of the comb are used to smooth out backcombing?
7  Where should the hair be backcombed to create lift?
8  What is the effect of backcombing the points of the hair?
9  What is meant by 'balance' in relation to hairstyling?
10  Why is it necessary to show the client the finished style before applying lacquer?

**Practical assignment – Dressing**

Dressing hair is an important hairdressing skill as it is the final illustration and showcase of your work. Knowing how to dress the same head of hair in a variety of styles will enable you to give the client the flexibility to change their 'Look' to suit their mood, the occasion and the clothes that they are wearing.

The following task will give you practice and, as a result, confidence in the designing and dressing of the same head of hair into a variety of styles.

You will need:
- tuition head or live model
- tools and equipment for wet (cohesive) and dry (temporary) setting
- a variety of brushes and combs
- hair ornamentation
- dressing aids such as lacquer, wax, dressing cream, gels etc
- camera
- folder, glue, scissors, pen and plain paper or card.

## Tasks

1 Take a photograph of the tuition head or live model before you start.
2 Set, blowdry, scrunch dry, tong, crimp, straighten or use any other drying technique on the model to create **five** *different* hairstyles from the one head. Include the following:

(a) a smooth style
(b) a curly style
(c) a hairstyle which has backcombing/backbrushing
(d) a hairstyle with ornamentation
(e) a hairstyle which incorporates some form of temporary setting e.g. tonging, crimping, straightening etc.

3 Carefully dress the hair into each required shape and style, making sure that the completed dressing is checked from every angle to show off your work to its best effect.
4 Take a photograph of each hairstyle from the **front, side** and **back**.
5 Write a short report of how you achieved each hairstyle and the dressing aids that you used on each.
6 Mount the photographs together with the written summaries on a plain piece of card or paper showing the 'before' photograph and the effects which you achieved by the various methods.

# 14 PERMING, NEUTRALISING AND STRAIGHTENING

Perming and setting both involve the breaking of some of the cross-linkages between the polypeptide chains of hair keratin.

The type of cross-linkage broken in setting is different from that broken in perming, in that:

- in setting, some of the weak water breakable cross-linkages between the polypeptide chains are broken and re-formed
- in perming, some of the stronger linkages are broken and re-formed.

Perming is most often used to wave or curl the hair. The style is permanent in that it can only be removed by 'growing out' (new hair with the person's natural style replacing the permed hair), or by perming the hair again (which can be called a **reverse perm** or **straightening**). There are several methods of perming hair, the most common being **cold permanent waving** (or just **cold perm** for short) as it is cold in comparison to other methods that use heat to perm the hair.

## Cold perming – the chemical process

Much practical expertise is needed in perming but the basic operation can be thought of as three stages:

1 *Softening* – by using the **perm reagent** ('reagent' simply means 'something that reacts', in this case, with the hair).

2 *Moulding* – in practice this consists of rolling or combing the hair to give the required amount of curling or straightening.

3 *Fixing* – this permanently 'fixes' the hair in the styled position. This last stage is often called **neutralisation** and the chemical used, a **neutraliser**, but technically it is not really a chemical neutralisation at all. These three stages will now be considered in more detail.

## Stage 1 – Softening

Traditional cold perm reagent has a pH value of 9 to 9.5 (i.e. is alkaline on the pH scale) and this dissolves some of the cement-like keratin which usually holds down the hair cuticle scales. This alkaline factor in turn allows the reagent to get into the hair cortex and then the reagent works on the cross-linkages between the polypeptide chains in the cortex. First, the water in the perm lotion breaks some of the water breakable cross-linkages (in the same way as wet setting) and second (and more importantly in perming) a chemical called **ammonium thioglycollate** attacks and breaks the water unbreakable cross-linkages made up of sulphur bonds (about 60–70 per cent of them).

In the newer 'acid' perms, another chemical is used, called **glycerol thioglycollate**, which has a pH value of about 4, but the hair is made alkaline first to cause the outside scales to open and the reagent to penetrate the hair cortex. Another point about 'acid' perms is that only about 10 per cent of the sulphur bonds are broken, because these bonds are stronger in acid conditions.

In both cases, the sulphur bonds are broken by the reagent forcing some of the sulphur atoms making up the cross-linkages to take hydrogen atoms instead of linking together between the polypeptide chains.

Sulphur atoms can only form two links or bonds with other chemicals, i.e. one is used up holding the sulphur atom on to the polypeptide chain and the other is used to link to a sulphur atom of a neighbouring chain (i.e. from a cross-linkage). Accepting the hydrogen from the perm reagent means the bond that is used to form the cross-linkage is taken up by the hydrogen atom and the cross-linkage is broken. This is shown in Figs 14.1(a) and (b).

In chemistry, the adding of hydrogen atoms like this is called a **reduction**, with the chemical giving the hydrogen called a **reducing agent** (in this case the perm reagent) and the substance accepting the hydrogen being said to be reduced (in this case the hair keratin).

## Perm reagents and pH

The pH scale ranges from 0 to 14, a pH value of 7 being **neutral**, values below 7 being **acid** and values above 7 being **alkaline**. The main point is that the 9 to 9.5 pH values of traditional cold perm reagents do considerable damage to hair, although the amount of damage can be reduced by selecting a perm reagent marketed for a particular hair type. In fact, if a pH value is raised much above 9.5 to, say, 11, so many sulphur bonds are broken in the hair that is breaks up (or disintegrates). This is done deliberately in products which remove unwanted hair, called **depilatories**.

Traditional perm reagents (and the much stronger depilatories) also attack and weaken the keratin of the outer, protective layer of the skin called the cornified layer which is why great care must be

Small part of polypeptide chain

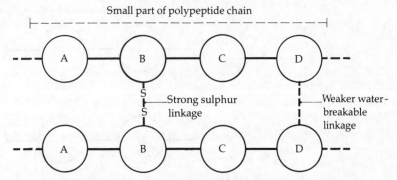

Fig 14.1 (a) **Hair before shampooing and applying perm lotion**

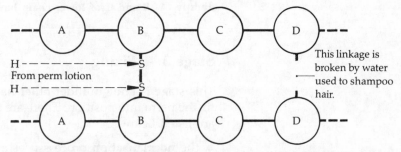

Fig 14.1 (b) **Hydrogen (H) released by perm lotion links to sulphur atoms (S) of sulphur linkage**

taken not to get perm solution on the scalp, and why over-use of depilatories can cause inflammation of the skin.

The newer 'acid' perms cause far less damage, although care is needed in their use, just as for any strong, reactive chemical.

Finally, the alkaline pH values of traditional cold perm reagents make them good at removing the hair's natural outer coating of oil (making the hair dry), so many perm reagents also contain **conditioners** which coat the hair cuticle and act like the natural oils.

## Stage 2 – Moulding

Most often, this involves winding hair around rollers (or it can be done by combing the hair in order to straighten it), in either case, the hair is stretched slightly (or putting it more technically, some **tension** is applied). Since some of the water breakable and non-water breakable sulphur cross-linkages are broken in Stage 1, the stretching causes the polypeptide chains to slip past each other very slightly. This very tiny movement on the minute scale of polypeptide chains adds up, by slightly moving millions of chains, and allows the individual hairs, and therefore the hair in general, to be styled. How much the chains are slid determines just how much curl will be in the hair when the perm is finished. This sliding of the polypeptide chains is shown in Fig 14.2.

The hair is then rinsed thoroughly to remove the perm reagent.

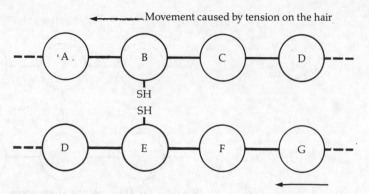

Fig 14.2 Winding hair causes the polypeptide chains to change positions slightly (A, B and C of lower chain have moved off to the left)

## Stage 3 – Fixing

This stage is known under other names as is the reagent used to fix the perm into position. There are three main alternatives, which are listed below:

- the **normalisation** process uses a **normaliser**
- the **neutralisation** process uses a **neutraliser**
- the **oxidation** process uses an **oxidiser** – this is the best term to use.

Normalisation does not give much indication about events inside the hair at this stage.

The term 'neutralisation' commonly used in hairdressing salons is technically incorrect. In chemistry, neutralisation has a strict and definite meaning which does not apply to the reaction which 'fixes' hair in perming. The term neutralisation is reserved for the following chemical reaction:

*Acid + Base → Salt + Water*

i.e. an acid and a base (an alkali is a base which dissolves easily in water) react chemically together to produce a 'salt' and water. Note that the word 'salt' also has a technical meaning in chemistry, that is, something produced by this type of reaction.

The best description for what happens in the hair is oxidation. In order to fix the perm, the polypeptide chains must be locked into the positions they are in after Stage 2. To do this, the hydrogen atoms added by the perm reagent in Stage 1 have to be removed and this allows the sulphur atoms to re-form cross-linkages between the polypeptide chains. As keratin, being a protein, contains a high proportion of sulphur-containing amino acids, there is a good chance that even after moving the polypeptide chains, the sulphur atoms of one chain will still be near other sulphur atoms of other chains.

The hydrogen atoms are removed by using a chemical which can pull hydrogen atoms away from the sulphur atoms. In practice this is done by one or other of two reagents, which are:

(*a*) hydrogen peroxide (often 6 per cent)
(*b*) sodium perborate (often 5 per cent).

Both these chemicals when applied to hair release highly reactive single atoms of oxygen (called nascent oxygen) which pull the hydrogen off the sulphur, allowing the cross-linkages to re-form. In fact, each atom of nascent oxygen pulls two hydrogen atoms off and combines with them to form water. All this is shown in Fig 14.3.

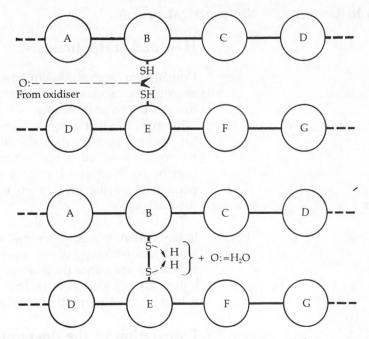

**Fig 14.3 Nascent oxygen removes hydrogen from the sulphur atoms and joins with them to form H$_2$O (water)**

In chemistry, the removal of hydrogen atoms in this way is called oxidation, with the chemical doing the removal called an oxidising agent, and the substance the hydrogen removed from being described as oxidised.

## Perming and hair condition

As mentioned before, alkaline perm reagents may remove the natural oils from the hair and these can be replaced by using a suitable conditioner.

Another measure used to improve hair condition after perming is that the reagent used to 'fix' the perm in Stage 3 of cold perming often contains a mild acid (citric acid for example) which reacts with any alkali left in the hair by the perm reagent and removes it.

This is technically a neutralisation as:

$$Ammonium\ thioglycollate\ +\ Citric\ acid\ =$$
$$(alkali\ or\ base)\qquad\qquad (acid)$$
$$Ammonium\ thiocitrate\ +\ Water$$
$$(salt)\qquad\qquad (water)$$

Having considered the chemical events in perming, the practical techniques and precautions involved in cold perming will now be considered.

## Cold perming – the practical process

### Hair and scalp analysis

Consultation with the client *before* starting the perming process is essential to allow the client's requirements to be thoroughly discussed and understood.

Examine the hair carefully to make sure that it is really suitable for perming and question the client on any previous treatments, referring to record cards if the client has attended the salon previously. If in any doubt as to the suitability of the hair for permanent waving always carry out a pre-processing test to support the analysis.

The client's scalp must also be checked for the presence of any inflammation, excessive dryness, cuts or abrasions (this can be done when disentangling the hair prior to shampooing). If these conditions are minor they can be protected with barrier cream but if they are major then the treatment must be postponed. Remember, if in doubt postpone the treatment.

### Preparation of the operator

Rubber gloves should be worn by the operator while applying the permanent wave reagent to prevent contact dermatitis of the hands. However, if the rods are wound with water and the reagent applied after the rods have been wound (i.e. post damping technique) it is not always necessary to wear the rubber gloves when winding the hair. In this case it is often a good idea to apply barrier cream to the hands as it will protect them if they should come into contact with the reagent at any stage of the perming process.

A tinting apron worn over the overall helps to prevent the reagent from splashing and drying on the overall. Although it does not stain in the same way as tint, the reagent can leave an unpleasant odour if allowed to dry on any clothing.

### Preparation of the client

The client's clothing should be protected at all times during the perming process. A gown should be placed around the client in such a way as to cover all the clothing and a towel should be securely tucked in at the nape to prevent it from slipping on to the floor. A neck strip or strip of cotton wool may be placed at the nape as a precautionary measure to prevent any reagent or water from seeping down the neck.

Barrier cream applied to the skin around the hairline protects it from any reagent that may accidentally run on to this area and prevents burning or sensitising of the skin by the reagent. This is particularly important if the client already happens to have a sensitive skin. But remember that the barrier cream must be applied to the skin only. Any cream that accidentally coats the hair will prevent reagent penetration of that hair and will therefore affect the curl.

## Preparation of the hair

The client usually, but not always, requires the hair to be cut when having a perm. It is the decision of the operator whether the hair is cut before or after the permanent wave (*see* Fashion permanent waves, p. 221). However, for a basic perm it is usual to shape the hair before winding the perm. Taper cut hair is easier to wind than hair that has been club cut because the points of the hair are finer and have had some of the weight removed, thus allowing them to be curled more easily around the rod.

Most cold permanent waves are wound on wet hair but the hair should not be over-saturated with water as this could dilute the reagent and makes it less effective. Towel drying the hair after shampooing removes the excess water but leaves the hair damp enough to give better absorption of the reagent.

The hair should be shampooed with a soapless shampoo as this not only cleans the hair and scalp but also removes any natural sebum that may be coating the hair. If the sebum remained, it could create a barrier between the reagent and the hair which would prevent the reagent from entering the cortex and the perm would not produce a satisfactory curl.

If the hair is structurally damaged or porous it may be necessary to apply a restructurant or special pre-perm treatment after shampooing to even out the porosity of the hair and to strengthen the cortex. Always take a test rod if the hair is very porous or damaged to make sure that it can withstand the perming process. If in any doubt at all, do not perm until the hair is strong enough.

## Preparation of the tools and equipment

All the equipment and tools that you will need should be assembled before beginning the permanent wave. A lot of time and energy can be saved if everything is to hand when it is needed.

## Sectioning for cold permanent waving

### Reasons for sectioning

- ease of working
- minimum of wasted time
- cuts down the risk of overprocessing
- divides the hair into neat, controllable divisions
- helps rod selection
- keeps the size of the rods balanced by dividing the head into smaller areas.

### Method of sectioning

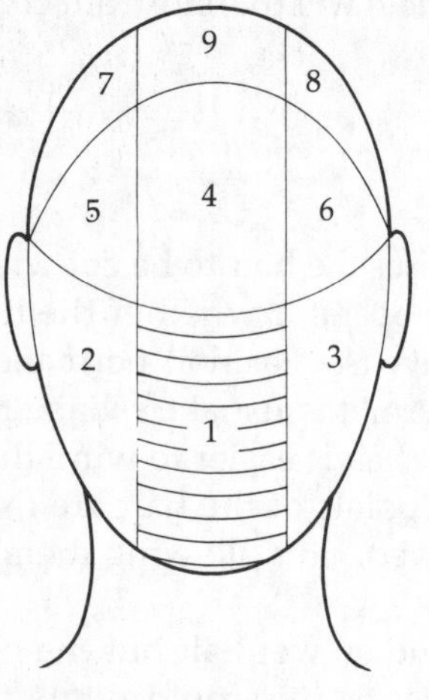

1 After shampooing with soapless shampoo, towel dry and disentangle the hair.

2 Divide the hair into nine sections as shown in Figure 14.4. The numbers refer to the order in which the sections are wound, Section 1 being divided into sub-sections. Note how the sections curve to the shape of the head. Start at the centre front.

Each section should be the same width and slightly longer than the perm rod. (*See* Figs 14.5 and 14.6.)

Figure 14.7 shows a completed section with the correct width and length.

Next, move on to the front, side section, checking for width with the perm rod at the top and the bottom of the section to ensure that the width is even along the length of the section. Allowance should be made for any problem hairlines.

When the side section has been completed, the other side can be sectioned in the same way, remembering to check the width at the top and bottom of the section (*see* Figs 14.8(*a*), (*b*)).

When the front sections have been completed, commence sectioning the crown area by extending the top front section down

Fig 14.4

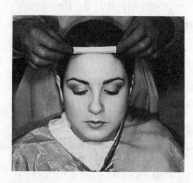

Fig 14.5

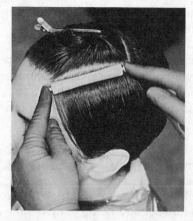

Fig 14.6

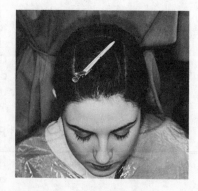

Fig 14.7 Completed section

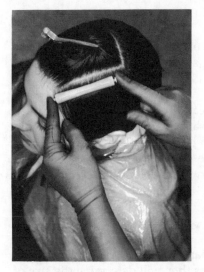

Fig 14.8 (a)

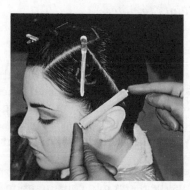

Fig 14.8 (b)

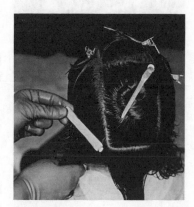

Fig 14.9

the back of the head. The length of this section is determined by an imaginary line from the top of both ears which curves round the back of the head. Secure the section. Next check that the side sections are the correct width for the rods.

Figure 14.9 shows how to measure the width of the side section.

Join both side sections to the centre back section, from the top of both ears. Make sure that all partings are straight and neat and that the hair is securely held with the sectioning clips (*See* Fig 14.10).

Commence sectioning the nape hair (*see* Fig 14.11), by extending the centre crown section down to the nape. Check the width of the centre nape section. The front, crown and nape sections should be the same width from the front of the head down to the nape.

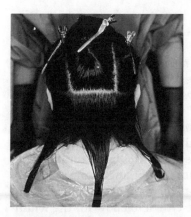

Fig 14.10 Hair securely held by sectioning clips

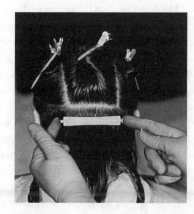

Fig 14.11

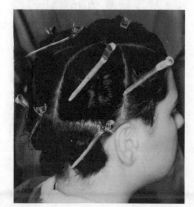

Fig 14.12

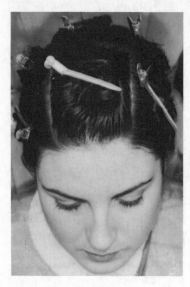

**Fig 14.13**

Next, secure firmly the sections that are left at either side of the nape.

Figure 14.12 shows a side view of completed sections; Fig 14.13 shows a front view of completed sections.

*Points to note:*
Always work to the shape of the head. If the hair is extremely short, thick or abundant it may be necessary to add extra sections to hold the hair securely. The sections can be altered slightly as sectioning progresses but remember that the sections should always be the same width as the rods used otherwise problems are created when placing the rods during winding.

## Winding a cold permanent wave

Before starting to wind a cold permanent wave, the following points must be taken into consideration as they will determine the size of rod to be used and the amount of curl to be achieved.
1 *Texture of hair:* thick hair will require a larger rod than fine hair to achieve the same effect.
2 *Type of curl required:* a tight curl requires small rods, a loose curl requires large rods.
3 *Type of hair:* i.e. bleached, tinted, porous, resistant, or normal. Bleached, tinted and porous hair will require a special weaker reagent while resistant hair will require a stronger reagent. If in doubt, take a test curl of the hair. Remember that the condition of the hair after perming is very important – using too strong a reagent for the type of hair will leave the hair in poor condition and could even cause hair breakage.
4 *Finished result:* this will also determine the amount of curl required.

## Method of winding a basic cold permanent wave

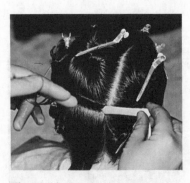

**Fig 14.14**

1 The hair is ready for winding when it has been cut into the desired shape (if necessary), shampooed with soapless shampoo, towel dried and sectioned into nine sections.
2 Commence winding at the centre nape. Using a tail comb divide the hair to produce a sub-section (mesh) which is exactly the same depth as the rod. Figure 14.14 shows how to produce the correct size of sub-section (mesh).
3 Apply the reagent, either with a perming brush or piece of cotton wool, approximately 1 cm (½″) from the scalp to prevent the reagent from running on to the skin. This is known as **presaturation.**
4 Comb the mesh out from the head at right angles making sure that the hair is thoroughly combed from the roots to the points. Then comb the mesh upwards towards the crown to allow for the width of the rod when wound.
5 Make sure that the tension is even on both sides of the mesh,

otherwise the hair will 'loop' at one end when it is wound, producing an uneven finished curl.

(*a*) When looking down the mesh from the ends (*see* Fig. 14.15), the points of the hair should be directly in the centre of the mesh at the roots, giving even tension to the hair on both sides of the mesh.

(*b*) If the hair is pulled slightly to one side the tension becomes uneven.

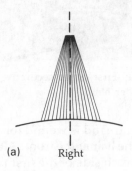

(a)  Right          (b)  Wrong

Fig 14.15

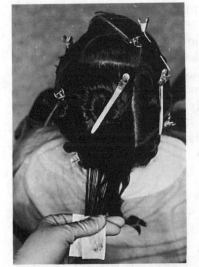

Fig 14.16 Applying end paper

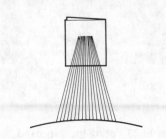

Fig 14.17

6   Place the end paper over the points of the hair and fold, keeping the tension of the hair even at all times. (*See* Fig. 14.16.) Note that the end paper is positioned past the end of the hair points (*see* Fig. 14.17) which helps to avoid the points being bent back when wound (this is known as '**fish-hook**' ends).

7   Carefully wind the end paper and points of hair around the rod and wind down to the root. Winding the hair from the points down to the root is known as **croquignole** winding. Do not pull the hair too tightly when winding as this creates undue tension on the hair and could cause hair breakage, or 'pull-burns' on the skin. Figure 14.18 shows hair and rod wound down to the root.

The hair should be evenly distributed along the length of the rod. 'Bunching' all the hair in the centre of the rod will give an uneven curl.

8   Secure with the rubber band across the top of the rod making sure that it is not twisted or cutting into the hair, otherwise breakage may occur (*see* Fig 14.19).

9   Proceed down the first major section in the same manner. Keep each mesh the same size as the rod. If the mesh is the correct size each rod will touch the one above, ensuring that there is no root drag on the hair. Figure 14.20 shows the first major section wound.

10   Continue winding each major section in the order specified in Fig 14.4 on p. 209, checking for development at frequent intervals during the wind.

Figure 14.21 shows the front view of head completely wound. The

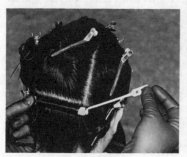

Fig 14.18

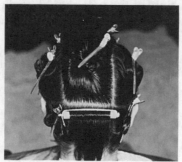

Fig 14.19 First curler secured
by rubber band

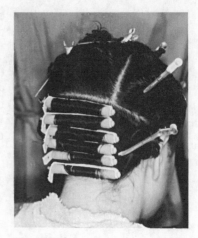

Fig 14.20

first centre rod is wound forward so that the rubber band does not
mark the hair at the front. Alternatively, plastic pins can be inserted
one at each side of the first two rods to lift the rubber band off the
hair and to hold the rod securely in place. Remember to ensure that
the pins to not mark the hair.

A side view of the completed wind is shown in Fig 14.22.

11  When the whole head is completed, post damp with reagent,
taking care that the reagent does not run onto the skin.

12  Check the first and last rod wound for development.

13  To contain and utilise the body heat from the scalp, place a
disposable polythene cap over the head and await development.
Check every three to five minutes. Figure 14.23 shows a polythene
cap used while the perm develops.

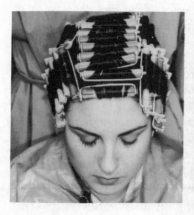

Fig 14.21

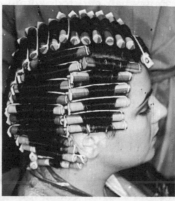

Fig 14.22

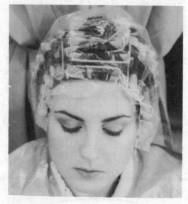

Fig 14.23 Polythene cap used
while perm develops

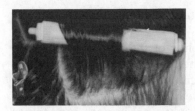

Fig 14.24

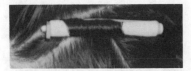

Fig 14.25

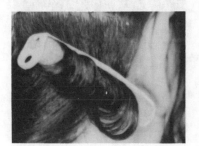

Fig 14.26

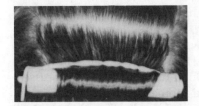

Fig 14.27

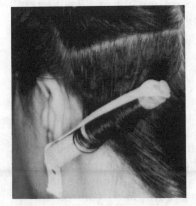

Fig 14.28

As a check on this section about winding, look at the photographs below to see what is wrong.

- Hair mesh too deep for the rod causes root drag (Fig. 14.24).
- Rod pulled back from front hairline, incorrect tension and positioning of rod. This will make the hair at the hairline straight and without root lift (Fig 14.25).
- No root lift and uneven tension on the hair causes 'looping' of the hair at the side and drags the root. The finished curl would be flat and uneven (Fig 14.26).
- Rubber band twisted and cutting into the hair, could cause hair damage (Fig. 14.27).
- Hair wound too loosely and without lift at the root would result in uneven curl on the ends of the hair only (Fig. 14.28).

## Neutralising a cold permanent wave

1  Before fixing the curl, make sure that enough disulphide bonds have been broken to obtain the amount of curl required. This is done by gently unwinding a rod (but not removing it completely) then pushing the hair gently back towards the roots. If the perm is ready the hair will form an 'S' shape movement, the size of which depends upon the amount of curl required. A large 'S' movement gives a loose curl while a small 's' shaped movement will give a tight curl. Check different rods at various parts of the head to ensure that there is even development throughout the whole head (*see* Fig. 14.29). Keep the hair points round the rod by holding with the thumbs while pushing the hair towards the roots.

2  Rinse the hair thoroughly for five minutes in warm water. If a front wash is used, take particular care to rinse the front rods thoroughly. If a back wash is used, particular attention should be paid to the rods at the nape.

3  Remove excess water by blotting thoroughly with cotton wool. Leaving the hair too wet will dilute the oxidiser and make it less effective. To check that enough moisture has been removed from the hair, press the palm of the hand onto the rods – if the palm is wet when it is pulled away from the head, the hair requires re-blotting.

4  Apply a strip of cotton wool around the hairline to protect the face and neck.

5  Apply the oxidiser to the wound rods, ensuring that each one is completely covered. It is important not to mix the oxidiser or pour out ready-mixed oxidiser until it is required otherwise much of the oxygen will be lost into the atmosphere.

6  Leave for five minutes.

Figure 14.30 shows wound hair covered with oxidiser. Cotton wool around the hairline prevents the oxidiser from dripping on the face and neck.

7  Carefully remove the cotton wool and the rods. The hair should

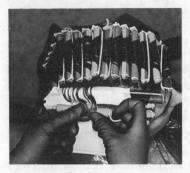

Fig 14.29 Checking perm development

not be pulled or stretched at this stage as the curl is not yet fully 'fixed'.

8 Apply oxidiser gently to the points of the hair as each rod is removed (Fig 14.31). Do not drag the hair or massage the oxidiser into the hair as this could alter the curl. Check that all the hair has been treated with the oxidiser then leave for a further five minutes.

9 Rinse the hair thoroughly and apply a pH balance conditioner if necessary to remove any traces of alkali that may be left in the hair.

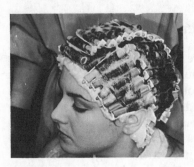

Fig 14.30

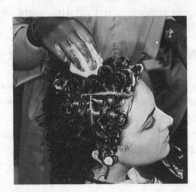

Fig 14.31

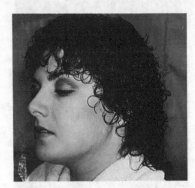

Fig 14.32

Figure 14.32 shows the permed hair before it is dried.

10 Always advise the client on the after-care needed for a permanent wave. Clients do not always realise that a perm will dry the hair and make it more porous, therefore the hair will usually need to be conditioned regularly. Other further chemical processes, e.g. bleaching, tinting, etc. should be approached with caution, again because the hair will be more porous and also because the scalp will be more sensitive for a few days after the perm. The hair should be protected from dampness after a perm, e.g. the rain, bathing etc., as it will revert back to its new alpha state when wet – therefore instead of a set or blowdry 'dropping' or loosening when it is damp it will become curly!

## Points to note

The sulphur bonds are not completely fixed until the hair is dry. This means that care should be taken when setting or blowdrying after the permanent wave. Stretching and pulling the hair at this point can loosen the curl so if the hair is to be blowdried after the perm (which does involve stretching and moulding the hair) it is often better to allow slightly more curl than required during development to counteract the loosening effect of the blowdry.

Alternatively, ask the client if the hair may be dried naturally without tension, although this is often not possible if the client does not wish to have a curly effect.

## Record cards

Always complete a client record card when the process is completed. This should contain the following information:

1  date
2  hair condition
3  product used, including the strength of the reagent
4  size of rod used
5  development time
6  any precautions necessary
7  finished result and any comments necessary
8  recommended after-care treatment.

## Precautions and considerations when permanent waving

1  Always test curl bleached hair. Bleached hair is in a very porous condition; therefore too strong a reagent can cause irreparable damage.
2  Always use a special or weaker reagent on tinted hair. Tinted hair is also in a porous condition.
3  Test unknown hair for any incompatible chemicals on the hair shaft, e.g. hair colour restorers, with an incompatibility test.
4  Before commencing a permanent wave, check the scalp for cuts and abrasions. If these are minor, cover and protect with petroleum jelly or barrier cream; if major, postpone the treatment.
5  The porosity of the hair must be taken into consideration when selecting the correct strength of reagent. The porosity can, in some instances vary along the shaft of the hair, in which case a pre-perm treatment may be needed to even out the porosity.
6  Use the correct size rods for the desired result. Hair meshes should be the same size as the rod, as too large a mesh will result in too great a difference between the root and point curl.
7  Partings should be clean and straight, unless 'weave winding' the hair to prevent rod partings on some types of hair.
8  Each mesh should be combed thoroughly from root to point.
9  The points of the hair should be wound completely round the rod to prevent fish-hook ends.
10  The tension on the wound hair must be even and the hair evenly distributed along the length of the rod. Do not 'bunch' the hair in the middle of the rod.
11  The rubber of the rod should lie flat and untwisted along the top of the wound hair.
12  The reagent should not be allowed to come into contact with the skin as it could cause dermatitis.

13   Barrier cream may be used round the hairline to prevent burning of sensitive skin.

14   Hair should be checked for development during winding, immediately after post damping and every three to five minutes thereafter unless otherwise stated by the manufacturer.

15   Reagent should not be allowed to come into contact with anything metallic as this could discolour the hair.

16   The hair should be thoroughly rinsed in warm water before the oxidiser is applied.

17   All excess moisture must be removed after rinsing and before the oxidiser is applied to prevent dilution of the oxidiser.

18   The oxidiser must be left in contact with the hair for the correct length of time to ensure adequate fixing of the curl.

19   When permanent waving above a graduated neckline, the curl should be large enough to blend into the straight hair at the neckline.

20   Always follow the manufacturer's instructions.

**Table 7.1   Permanent waving faults, causes and remedies**

| Fault | Possible cause | Action required |
| --- | --- | --- |
| Development time excessively long | Rods too large<br>Use of too few rods<br>Hair meshes too large<br>Wrong strength of reagent<br>Cold salon | Change rods if necessary<br>   Redamp with correct strength of lotion and leave until fully developed |
| Hairline and scalp irritation | Cuts and abrasions on the scalp<br>Reagent running on to scalp<br>Too much reagent applied<br>Cotton wool placed around hairline or between rods when processing | Apply a soothing lotion to the affected areas<br>   Use cool water for rinsing and do not massage the scalp |
| Pull-burn | Rods wound too tightly allowing reagent to penetrate hair follicle | Apply soothing lotion to affected area<br>   Refer client to doctor if serious |
| Hair breakage (within a week or two) | Rods wound too tightly<br>Rubbers too tight or twisted<br>Overprocessing<br>Reagent too strong<br>Incompatible reaction | Condition the hair using restructurants and deep penetrating conditioner |

| Fault | Possible cause | Action required |
|---|---|---|
| Straight finished result (no curl) | Rods too large<br>Insufficient processing<br>Reagent too weak<br>Insufficient oxidation<br>Too few rods used<br>Poor shampooing | Take test curls, if hair is in good condition, re-perm<br>If hair is in poor condition, treat with conditioning treatments and re-perm with weaker lotion |
| Discolouration of the hair | Use of metal tools<br>Use of containers used for other purposes<br>Presence of incompatible chemicals on the hair | If incompatible chemicals are present on the hair, rinse off reagent immediately<br>If the hair remains discoloured after rinsing, apply toning or semi-permanent or temporary rinse |
| Curl weakening | Use of wrong or too weak oxidiser<br>Incorrect timing or oxidiser<br>Insufficient blotting of hair after rinsing<br>Faulty oxidiser<br>Hair pulled excessively when not completely 'fixed' | Take test curls; hair in good condition can be re-permed; hair in poor condition should be treated with deep penetrating conditioners before re-perming. |
| Frizz (curl may appear straight when dry, excessively curly when wet) | Reagent too strong<br>Rod size too small<br>Overprocessing<br>Overheating during development | Condition the hair thoroughly using penetrating conditioner restructurant<br>Cut the hair if possible. |
| Fish hooks on hair points | Points of the hair doubled back while winding | Remove by cutting |
| Hair too curly | Rod size too small | Hair in good condition can be relaxed by combing through reagent then oxidising<br>Hair in poor condition should be treated with deep penetrating conditioners and restructurants and not subjected to further chemical treatments |

| Fault | Possible cause | Action required |
|---|---|---|
| Good curl result when wet, poor result when dry | Hair over-stretched when drying<br>Overprocessing | Condition the hair thoroughly and cut if possible |
| Uneven curl along the hair length | Mesh too large for rod size<br>Uneven tension along length of the rod<br>Incorrect use of end papers<br>Hair not combed smoothly from roots to points<br>Hair 'drag'<br>Uneven application of reagent/oxidiser | When hair is in good condition, relax with perm lotion if curl strength is too great; re-perm if curl strength is too weak<br>If hair is in poor condition treat with conditioning agents first. |
| Uneven curl throughout the head | *See* section above<br>Insufficient mesh for rod length, causing drag at the sides of the section<br>Wind commenced at the more porous area instead of most resistant<br>Reagent insufficient or unevenly applied<br>Lack of control when winding causing 'looping' | When hair is in good condition, relax with perm lotion if curl strength is too great; re-perm if curl strength is too weak<br>If hair is in poor condition treat with conditioning agents first |
| Straight hair at sides and nape | Incorrect angling or placing of rods<br>Rods too large for length of hair<br>Mesh too large for rod size<br>Wispy hair around the head left out of the rod | If hair is in good condition re-perm the straight hair, making sure that the perm lotion does not come into contact with the curled areas |

## Contra-indications for permanent waving

The hairdresser should not go ahead with permanent waving in the following cases:

1  incompatible chemicals are present on the hair shaft
2  hair is excessively porous or weakened, e.g. over-bleached
3  the tensile strength or elasticity of the hair has been impaired

4 if previous permanent wave is present – remember that a permanent wave will remain in the hair until it is cut off. However, specialised techniques like 'blocking-out' with conditioner or specially designed restructurants may be used over the old curl in some cases.

5 hair or scalp suffers from contagious or infectious disease, e.g. tinea, pediculosis capitis, etc.

6 after childbirth. The nutriments in the blood which are usually given to the hair to feed it are required to return the body to normal, leaving the hair in poor condition. It is usually more successful to perm the client's hair before the birth of the baby, during pregnancy.

7 after/during illness or when the client is taking drugs. Perming hair during this time is often unsuccessful. If in doubt, always take a test curl.

# Other types of permanent waves

## Acid perms

These are believed to be less damaging to the hair than alkaline perms. They are usually supplied with an activator and their own oxidising agent. When the hair has been wound, the reagent (lotion) is mixed with the activator and applied to the hair making sure, as with all post damping, that each rod is thoroughly dampened with the lotion.

Most acid perms require heat to speed up their development and even then they tend to be slow-acting. When checking the development of an acid perm look at the 'stranding' of the hair mesh as well as the 'S' shape formed. The hair mesh should separate into about seven strands when it has developed.

## Foam perm

This requires a special machine which is powered by electricity and has two separate guns, one to pump air into the perm lotion and the other for the neutraliser making a foam of each. Because of its aerated nature, this perm is applied after the rods are wound and is very comfortable for the client as the lotions do not drip.

## Uni perm

This perm is processed by heat from a machine similar to the old heat perm machine. The machine has heated bars which then heat up the clamps attached to it. The hair is wound taking large sections to accommodate the size of the clamps which are placed over the wound rods and then left to cool. The hair must be pushed to the centre of the rod and the rubber band placed along its top to allow the hair to be properly heated and prevent the rubber band from melting.

## Exothermic perming

This type of permanent wave is wound in exactly the same manner as a cold permanent wave except that the reagent is applied after waving instead of during the wind. It is therefore important not to allow the hair to dry out during winding – if it does, redamp with water. When the wind has been completed, mix the two chemicals together according to the manufacturer's instructions. The mixture will become warm. Apply this warm mixture evenly over the wound rods and await development. When the required amount of curl is achieved, rinse and oxidise according to the manufacturer's instructions and complete a client record card.

## Fashion permanent waves

There are many types of fashion permanent waves and many techniques are employed to achieve the desired effect. However, the main objective of each is to give curl and/or body to the style wherever it is required.

It is often more desirable when fashion perming to wind the hair with water and then post damp with the reagent when the wind is completed. This enables winding to be commenced anywhere on the head as the reagent is only in contact with the hair when the whole head has been wound. It also ensures a more even curl throughout the head as the processing time is the same for each strand of hair. However, the resistance of certain areas of the head, e.g. the nape, must be taken into consideration and the size of the perm rods in these areas must be adjusted accordingly, otherwise the finished curl will be too loose in comparison with the rest of the head.

The cutting of the hair for fashion perming is of the utmost importance. Tapering before a basic permanent wave gives the best results, but to achieve a particular fashion style or shape the hair very often requires club cutting. Winding hair that has been club cut is more difficult than winding tapered hair because of the thickness or bulk left on the points. Very often it is preferable and gives a better result to perm the hair first and then cut the style into the curl.

Sectioning for a fashion permanent wave depends largely on the direction of the wind and the finished hairstyle. Any sectioning of the hair is used to help not hinder the operator by keeping the hair out of the way and under control while winding. However, when perm winding directionally, i.e. in the direction of the finished style, any sections should be placed where they are required, to make the actual winding easier. It is impossible to give any hard and fast rules as to how and where to section the hair for fashion perming and it is up to the individual to decide exactly where the sections are necessary for each particular head according to the technique used and the direction of the finished style.

Particular care must be taken when the hair is permed and left to dry naturally, without setting or blowdrying. Mistakes in this case cannot be hidden so they must not be made! Avoid some of the perming pitfalls by taking the following precautions:

1  Communicate fully with the client to ensure that their ideas and requirements are fully understood.
2  Decide on the finished effect before starting on the perming process so that there is a very clear picture in the mind as to what is required and the best method to achieve it.
3  Before perming porous or impoverished hair always treat it with a pre-perming treatment or a restructurant to give it strength. Remember to take a test curl if in doubt.
4  Choose the correct strength of lotion for the hair type: if it is too strong the hair will frizz or break; if it is too weak the curl will not be strong enough.
5  Choose the technique and size of perm rods carefully to give the correct amount of curl where it is needed.
6  It is often better to apply the reagent after winding to prevent overprocessing and to give a more even curl.
7  Watch processing carefully. Over-processing will make the hair frizzy, under-processing will leave it 'floppy'.
8  Depending upon the desired result, it is often more successful to cut the hair after perming. This has the following advantages:

(a) If the finished curl is slightly tighter on the ends, this can be easily rectified when it is cut.
(b) If the hair is very short it prevents a frizzy effect by having to use too small a rod.
(c) If the perm is softer or curlier than required, the style can be made to suit the amount of curl present.

9  Do not brush or comb the hair while it is drying. Comb into place when wet then leave until dry or mould or scrunch dry with the fingers to give more lift. Use an Afro comb with wide teeth or use the fingers when the hair is dry.
10  Always advise the client on after-care. Explain that permed hair goes curlier when wet, therefore, if it should go flat during the week, redamp with water to reintroduce the curl. Advise that a conditioner be used regularly to counteract the drying properties of most permanent waves.

There are a number of ways of winding hair for a fashion permanent wave. It would be impossible to list and describe all of these but a brief summary of the most popular types of fashion wind are listed below. However, it must be stressed that a competent hairdresser can develop their own techniques by thinking carefully about what effect is to be achieved. New techniques are born by using the basic skills and experimenting with differing sizes of rods at various angles and positions.

## Root perming

This technique is used to give support and lift to shorter hairstyles. It is not usually suitable for longer hair as the weight of the hair will pull out any lift that has been obtained.

Lift at the root area only can be achieved by various methods, for example, winding the hair with water and coating the mid-lengths and ends of the hair with hair gel, then wrapping the hair in tin foil to prevent penetration of the perm into these areas. The hair should then be post damped with the perm lotion, thus allowing the root area only to be affected.

Manufacturers have now produced a gel perming lotion which is applied after winding is complete. Because of its viscous nature, this type of perm lotion does not penetrate through the hair mesh and is therefore active on the root area only.

However it must be remembered that the intended effect of a root perm is to give support and *not* curl to the hair. It is therefore suitable only for certain types of hairstyles and is not advisable for clients who require a substantial amount of curl or body in their hair.

## Directional winding

Directional winding is used mainly on shorter hair. The hair is wound in the direction of the style, therefore it would be impossible to give any definite method of winding as the variations are limitless. By alternating or mixing the size of the rods a mixed curl strength can also be achieved.

Figure 14.33 shows an example of directional winding. The top hair is wound sideways, curving across the top of the head with plastic pins inserted to prevent the rod rubbers from marking or digging into the hair. They also hold the rods firmly in position. The front fringe area is dragged down at the root and wound to the side to give curl on the ends of the hair only and to prevent the fringe from 'springing' up when the hair is dry.

Note how the short hair at the side of the head has been moulded into position then pincurled flat to give a slight movement with no lift (*see* Fig 14.34).

## Edge or perimeter winding

This puts curl on the ends of shorter or longer hair. This wind is usually used on hair that does not require height or lift on top. The hair is dragged at the root and wound sideways giving curl at the ends of the hair.

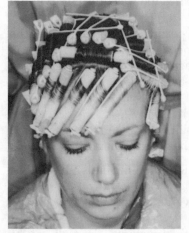

Fig 14.33

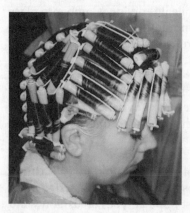

Fig 14.34

This is a useful type of wind to use in conjunction with other methods, e.g. edge wind on the fringe area to keep the fringe low on to the face while the remaining hair is wound as required.

Figure 14.35 shows the whole of the crown area edge wound which will result in no lift on top of the head but volume and curl around the edges.

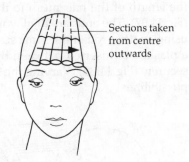
Sections taken from centre outwards

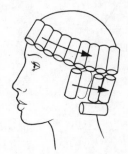

**Fig 14.35**

## Partial winding

As the name suggests, only some parts or areas of the head are permed to create volume and texture where required. This can either be to a small area of the style or to the majority of the area leaving only a small area unpermed. There are unlimited variations to this type of wind and it is a method that can be used on long or short hair.

Figure 14.36 (a) shows a partial wind at the front of the head to create volume at this area. The rods can be placed in any direction that may be required by the style.

Figure 14.36 (b) shows the top and fringe area left straight with the back and side areas permed. Again, the rods may be placed in any direction or indeed, wound by any method depending upon the required finished effect.

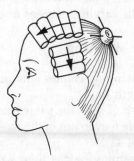

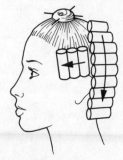

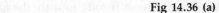

**Fig 14.36 (a)**                    **Fig 14.36 (b)**

## Piggyback winding

This is used on long hair (usually over 15–20 cm/6–8″) to give an even curl movement along the length of the hair. It also allows a more even penetration of both the reagent and the oxidiser, which is always a problem when perming very long hair.

Taking normal partings, the hair is wound from mid-way down the length of the hair mesh to the root, leaving the end unwound (Fig 14.37). The ends are then wound down to the centre of the mesh using another rod of the same size (Fig 14.38), which is secured with a plastic pin inserted between the bands of the rods to hold them securely (Fig 14.39). Varying the sizes of the rods can create endless possibilities.

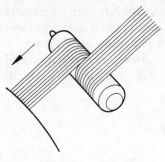

Fig 14.36

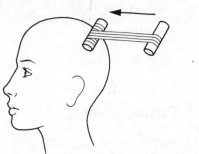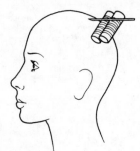

Fig 14.38                    Fig 14.39

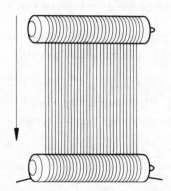

Fig 14.40

Another use of piggyback winding is to give extra volume and curl to shorter hair. In this case, a mesh of hair, the same size as the curler, is sectioned off and then divided into two lengthwise. The division can either be straight or woven. The lower half of the mesh is wound around the rod down to the root.

The remaining hair from the top half of the mesh is then wound down using another rod of the same size (*see* Fig 14.40).

This second rod is forced to lie on top of the first one as the size of the mesh will only accommodate one of the rods. By varying the sizes of the rods different effects can be achieved, e.g. a large rod at the root, small rod on top will create a looser movement at the root with varying degrees of curl throughout the ends.

## Weave winding

Weave winding creates a natural undisciplined effect on shorter or mid-length hair.

A mesh of hair, the same size as the rod is taken and fine strands of hair are woven out of the mesh and clipped out of the way (shown in Fig 14.41).

The remaining hair is then wound as normal (*see* Fig 14.42).

This technique is used on each mesh throughout the head with

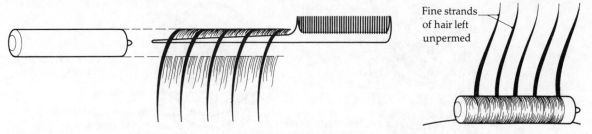

Fine strands of hair left unpermed

**Fig 14.41**                    **Fig 14.42**

the result that the bulk of the hair is permed but fine strands are left straight. Alternatively, the strands may be wound on a different sized rod; both techniques create a natural, unruly effect.

Weave winding can be done on individual areas of the head, e.g. when partial winding the top area of the head, weave winding the last few rods before the straight nape area will help to blend the permed area into the straight area without too strong a division.

Weave sectioning the hair instead of straight sectioning when using the basic perm method helps to prevent rod divisions on certain hair types although this does not necessarily mean that all hair types should be treated in this manner.

### Spiral winding

This is used on longer hair to create an even curl along its length. The hair is wound *down* the rod, usually from the roots to the points, unlike other perming techniques such as croquignole which is wound from the points to the roots.

Any short layers in the hair make it unsuitable for this type of wind as the hair must have enough length to be wound down the rod. If very long hair has been given short layers on top then it may be necessary to wind the shorter hair in a croquignole manner and only the long hair spirally.

## Sectioning the hair for spiral winding

Divide the hair off into the first major section which must be the required width usually 1.25–2.50 cm (½–1″) wide. Curve the section to run parallel with the nape hairline and pin the remaining hair firmly out of the way. (*See* Fig 14.43.)

Divide the major section into squares for the actual wind. When all the first major section has been wound, continue up the head dividing the hair into major sections before winding the square sections. (*See* Fig 14.44.)

## Winding

The winding of a spiral perm should always start on the underneath

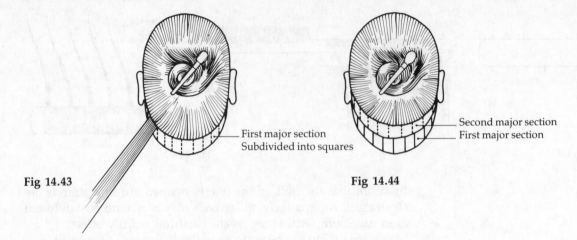

First major section
Subdivided into squares

Second major section
First major section

**Fig 14.43**

**Fig 14.44**

layers of hair, usually at the nape, as the wound rods hang down and would therefore get in the way of any unwound, underneath hair.

The sections should be square, with the size depending on the size of rod and the amount of curl required. Remember that the smaller the diameter of the rod, then the tighter the curl. Never take too large a section or the finished curl will be too loose.

## Processing and oxidising

Checking a spiral wind for development can be quite difficult as it does not always form the same type of 'S' shape as a conventional wind. Using a self-timing perm or placing a few *croquignole* wound rods, to use as test curls, in a position that is not obvious are ways that can resolve this problem.

Make sure that any heat used to cut down the development time is evenly applied, as the head when fully spirally wound is quite a size and difficult to place under a conventional dryer.

Rinsing this type of wind will usually require a longer time because of the amount of hair and number of rods. Blot the rods carefully after rinsing, it is also useful to place the client under a drier or use a hand dryer for five minutes to help remove the excess moisture before applying the oxidiser.

Again, because of the amount of hair, the application of the oxidiser must be thorough to make sure that all the hair is completely covered throughout the length of the rod.

## Rod techniques

### Rubber/foam rods

The rubber/foam rod (*see* Fig 14.45) is the most widely used rod for spiral winding and can also be used for winding conventional perms. Available in four sizes, the rod is made of either rubber or foam and usually has a wire running through its centre which allows it to bend

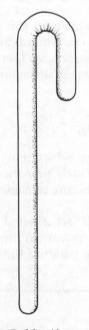

**Fig 14.45 Rubber/foam rod**

wherever needed. Twisting the hair during winding will give added volume.

Take a square section of hair. Cover hair points with an end paper then start winding down the length of the rod (*see* Fig 14.46). Secure the hair by bending the rod (*see* Fig 14.47). Adjust the amount of curl by winding close together or further apart (*see* Figs 14.48 (*a*) and (*b*)).

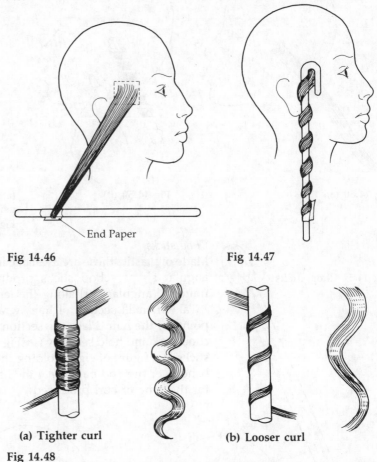

End Paper

**Fig 14.46**                                    **Fig 14.47**

(a) Tighter curl                    (b) Looser curl

**Fig 14.48**

*Spiral rods*
Spiral rods are made of plastic and are available in five sizes with left and right sloping spirals and an end securer (*see* Figs 14.49 (*a*) and (*b*)). Because of the uniform ridges along the length of the rod they produce a uniform curl down the hair shaft.

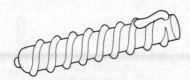

**Fig 14.49 (a) Spiral rod**                    **Fig 14.49 (b) End Securer**

Take a square section of hair approximately 1.25 cm long (½") (*see* Fig 14.50 (*a*)). Hook the section of hair on to the rod. Wind spirally down the rod then fasten with the end securer (*see* Fig 14.50 (*b*)).

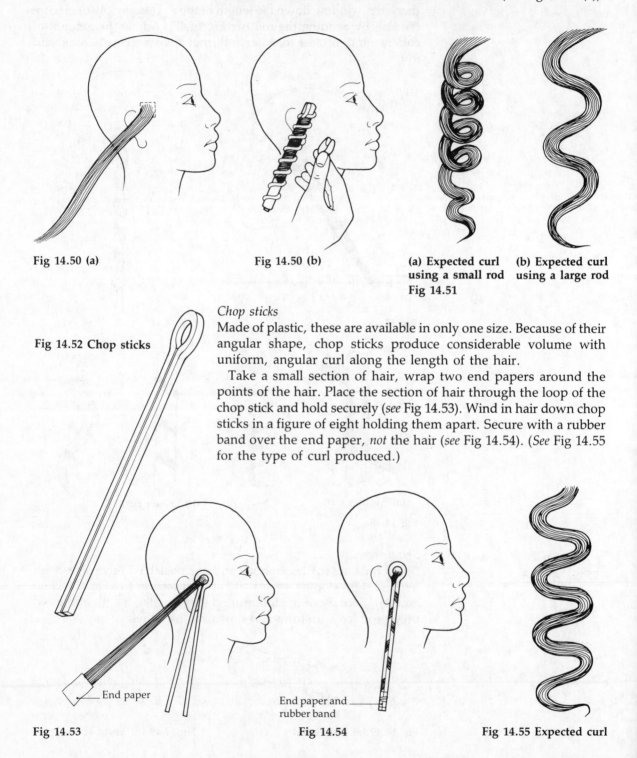

**Fig 14.50 (a)**

**Fig 14.50 (b)**

**(a) Expected curl using a small rod**
**(b) Expected curl using a large rod**
**Fig 14.51**

**Fig 14.52 Chop sticks**

*Chop sticks*
Made of plastic, these are available in only one size. Because of their angular shape, chop sticks produce considerable volume with uniform, angular curl along the length of the hair.

Take a small section of hair, wrap two end papers around the points of the hair. Place the section of hair through the loop of the chop stick and hold securely (*see* Fig 14.53). Wind in hair down chop sticks in a figure of eight holding them apart. Secure with a rubber band over the end paper, *not* the hair (*see* Fig 14.54). (*See* Fig 14.55 for the type of curl produced.)

End paper

End paper and rubber band

**Fig 14.53**

**Fig 14.54**

**Fig 14.55 Expected curl**

**Fig 14.56 U-Stick rod**

### U-stick rod

These are made of plastic and are available in three sizes. U-sticks are wound in a similar way to chop sticks but because the ends of the rods come together when wound they produce a looser curl at the roots than at the points of the hair.

Take a small section of hair and pull through the middle of the U-stick. Wind the hair in a figure of eight over A, then between the sticks, over B and repeat down the length of the stick (*see* Fig 14.57).

Place two end papers over the points of the hair and secure with a rubber band over the end papers not the hair (*see* Fig 14.58). Figure 14.59 illustrates the results of this method.

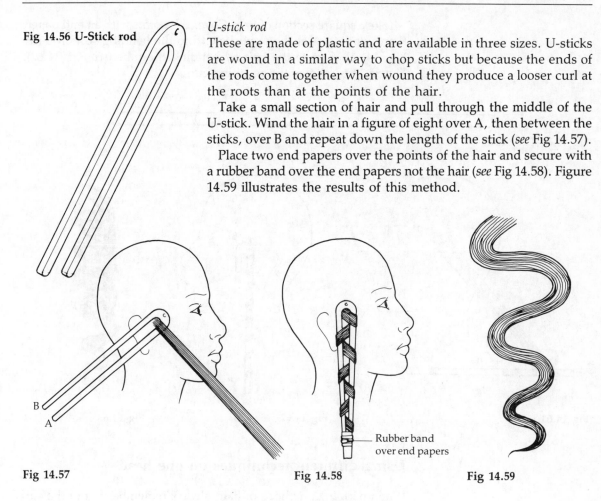

Rubber band over end papers

**Fig 14.57**

**Fig 14.58**

**Fig 14.59**

### Pen rods

Made of plastic, these are available in only one size. The degree of curl will be determined by the way the hair is wound down the rod. The closer together the hair is wound, the tighter the curl will be. The expected curl would be the same as for rubber/foam rods (*see* Fig. 14.48).

### Crystal rods

Available in two sizes, these produce an angular uniform curl because of the way in which the hair is wound behind the bars.

### Tube rods

Made of plastic and shaped like straws, tubes have a corrugated section which allows them to bend in this area (*see* Fig 14.60). Because of their small diameters they produce a tight, uniform curl throughout the length of the hair.

Take a square section of hair. Cover the points with an end paper. Start winding A at the opposite end to the bending section B (*see* Fig. 14.61). Secure the hair by bending the tube (*see* Fig. 14.62). Figure 14.63 shows the resulting curl.

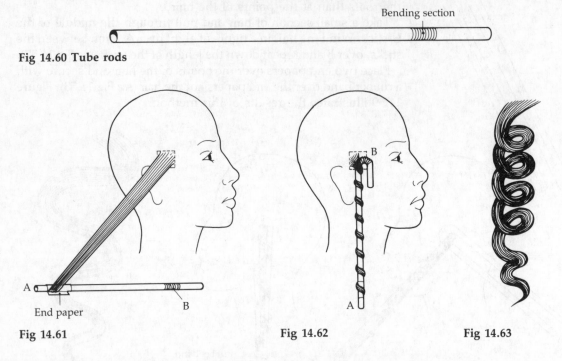

Bending section

**Fig 14.60 Tube rods**

End paper

**Fig 14.61**

**Fig 14.62**

**Fig 14.63**

## Using different techniques on one head

When perming any head of hair, always remember to put the curl or volume *where it is needed*, this may mean that a variety of techniques will have to be used on the same head to create the desired effect. Bearing this in mind, the variations and effects that can be achieved when perming the hair are limitless. By experimenting with various techniques it is possible to meet any new needs of the client as hair fashions change and also to invent new techniques by adapting the basic methods.

## Permanent waving hair previously treated with chemicals

Hair that has been previously treated with chemicals is more porous than virgin hair and will therefore absorb the perm lotion more quickly. A lotion for normal hair is too strong and can cause untold damage including breakage. It is essential to question the client carefully to find out what type of tint, bleach or other chemicals have been used on the hair, for how long they have been used and whether the hair usually feels dry or brittle.

To decide how porous the hair is follow these three steps:

**Look**  Does the hair appear dull, dry and lifeless? If so, it is probably porous.

**Feel** (tactile)  Does the hair feel rough when it is pulled between the fingers from the roots to points? This is another sign of porosity.

**Listen**  To what the client has to say. Pick up non-verbal signals as well – clients are sometimes reluctant to tell you if they have been treating their own hair.

When you have assessed the porosity of the hair, choose a suitable permanent wave lotion. All manufacturers make special lotions of various strengths and give detailed instructions on how to use them. If you are still unsure, take a small cutting of the hair, then place it in a small amount of the selected lotion. Leave for five to ten minutes then test by pulling it between the fingers. If the lotion is too strong the hair will swell, stretch like a piece of elastic and possibly break when pulled.

## Points to note

Hair that is porous may need to be wound with a pre-perm lotion or restructurant to give it protection and strengthen the cortex. It is often wiser to wind the hair without the permanent wave lotion, **post damping** it when the hair has been wound.

Do not use heat to speed up the development time as it could damage the hair and monitor the processing more frequently than for virgin hair. When the curl is fully developed, rinse the hair for a longer period than normal as the reagent is more difficult to remove from porous hair.

To show the difference between a permanent wave lotion for virgin hair and one for chemically treated hair, carry out the practical assignment at the end of this chapter.

## Perming Afro hair

1  Carry out all necessary tests to the scalp and hair. Check the client record card for any previous treatments.

2  Talk to the client to find out their requirements. With the information you have gained from the tests, record card and client consultation, select the appropriate product and read the manufacturer's instructions.

3  Assemble all equipment.

4  Protect and prepare the client and operator.

5  Gently shampoo the hair with a pre-perm shampoo.

6  Apply pre-conditioning treatment and cover with a plastic cap. Leave for ten minutes under a dryer.

7  Protect the hairline with vaseline or barrier cream.

8  Apply reagent from the nape area to the forehead, one section at a time, combing through gently, but firmly. Leave to develop for approximately 10–15 minutes.

9  When the hair is smooth, divide it into sections and begin winding it on perm rods in the direction of the style.

10  Post damp the hair with reagent making sure that the hair is thoroughly saturated. Leave to develop.

11  When it has developed fully, rinse thoroughly and oxidise in the normal way.

12  Apply pH balance conditioner and leave on the hair for five minutes.

13  Rinse thoroughly and blot dry.

14  Apply curl moisturising spray or curl activator and style hair as required.

15  Complete a client record card and advise the client on the after-care of the style.

## Straightening hair

This is the process of reducing curl or wave to make it straighter. Hair can be straightened either temporarily or permanently. Straightening the hair temporarily usually requires some form of heat if it is to be successful. The two main methods of temporarily straightening hair are:

(*a*) wet setting – such as blowdrying, roller setting, etc.

(*b*) dry setting – pulling the hair straighter using heated curling tongs, hot brushes, heated rollers or specifically designed flat irons that work on the same principle as crimping irons but trap the hair between two flat heated surfaces.

Afro-Caribbean hair can be temporarily straightened by either blowdrying using a wide toothed comb attachment which is fitted to the nozzle of the hair dryer or by using a pressing comb.

### Procedure for soft pressing Afro-Caribbean hair

Soft pressing will remove 70 per cent of the curl.

1  Protect the client with a gown and towel.

2  Check the hair and scalp for any contra-indications.

3  Shampoo the hair with a suitable shampoo then dry.

4  Divide the hair into four sections: forehead to nape and ear to ear, across the back of the head.

5  Starting at the nape, take a 1.25 cm (½″) section of hair and apply oil or conditioning cream to the mesh. Lift the hair away from the scalp at 90° (*see* Fig 14.4 p. 209) using the index finger and the thumb.

6  Check the heat of the pressing comb then insert the pressing comb teeth into the hair mesh 1.25 cm (½″) away from the scalp.

7    Slide the comb down the hair mesh, turning it so that the back of the comb is positioned on top of the hair mesh. The angle of the comb is very important as it is the back of the comb which creates the tension and actually straightens the hair.

8    Comb each mesh two or three times in this manner until the hair is straight.

9    Continue towards the front of the head taking 1.25 cm (½") sections until the whole head has been completed.

10    Apply dressing cream or oil to the hair and brush thoroughly.

11    Style the hair with curling tongs.

12    Complete a record of work and advise the client on the care of their hairstyle including any preparations that would aid the condition of the hair and add to the longevity of the hairstyle.

## Procedure for hard pressing Afro-Caribbean hair

Hard pressing will remove almost all the curl but will also weaken the hair so great caution is required when carrying out this service. Proceed as for soft pressing then either repeat the process or restraighten using Marcel waving irons.

## Precautions and considerations

1    Check that the hair is strong enough to withstand the tension and the heat needed during the process. Fine hair will require less tension and a cooler temperature than coarse hair.

2    Take special care with bleached or tinted hair. Remember that it is usually more fragile than untreated hair and will therefore require a cooler temperature and less tension to prevent breakage.

3    Always use oil, cream or conditioner on the hair before pressing. This will lubricate the hair, make it more pliable and help prevent burning and scorching.

4    Always check that the pressing comb is at the correct temperature for the type of hair. Electric pressing combs are thermostatically controlled but non-electric combs are heated by heaters and may get too hot if not properly controlled.

5    Great care *must* be taken not to touch the scalp or skin with the hot comb or burning will occur.

6    During the process, ensure that the back of the comb is pulled along the top of the hair mesh as it is this part of the comb which smooths and straightens the hair.

7    Make sure that enough tension is exerted on the hair to make it straight.

8    Advise the client that pressing is a temporary means of straightening hair and will only last between seven and ten days. Any dampness in the atmosphere will cause the hair to revert back to its curly state.

9    Do not attempt to straighten very short hair as there is a danger of burning the scalp and skin.

10   Always use a dressing cream or oil after pressing to replace some of the natural oils and give the hair shine.

## Permanently straightening the hair

Straightening the hair permanently requires the use of chemicals to alter the internal structure of the hair.

There are three main types of hair straighteners:

1   Ammonium thioglycollate – pH 9.2–9.6 (perms)
2   Ammonium sulphite – pH 7.5–8 (slower acting)
3   Sodium hydroxide (caustic soda) – pH 10–14 (Afro-Caribbean hair, fast acting)

Ammonium thioglycollate and ammonium bisulphite involve the same chemical processes as when permanently waving the hair, i.e. the cross-linkages are broken by **reduction** and reformed by **oxidation**. When sodium hydroxide is used, however, a **hydrolisis** reaction breaks the cross-linkages. These re-form after hair straightens, when an acid shampoo neutralises the alkalinity.

Some straighteners are based on a cream formula and the cream itself helps to hold the hair in the straightened position as it is being processed. The chemical process is the same as for permanent waving, the difference being that the softened hair is moulded into a straight shape rather than a curly shape.

## Application of ammonium thioglycollate (thio) straighteners

These can be applied to the whole head, combing the hair straight. Once the movement in the hair has loosened sufficiently the solution is rinsed from the head and the hair is oxidised as in permanent waving.

Alternatively, the hair can be wound on to large rollers to give a looser movement than that already in the hair. A perming cap is used for processing and when the hair is straight enough it is rinsed and oxidised.

## Ammonium sulphite straighteners

These straighteners are made to a syrupy-type or viscous liquid consistency. They have a nearly neutral pH of 7–7.5. They are slower acting but tend to be kinder to the hair. Special weaker preparations are manufactured for use on hair which has previously been chemically treated. The straightening process should never be carried out on hair immediately after it has been either tinted or lightened. The procedure of application is similar to that given for 'thio' straighteners unless straight planks are used (see Figs 14.64 and 14.65). Straight planks are used to straighten curly or wavy hair when using a chemical relaxer.

Take a section of hair 1.25 cm deep and no wider than the width of the plank (*see* Fig 14.65).

Comb hair straight along the plank and push the end of the plank against the scalp. Apply relaxer process and rinse following manufacturer's instructions.

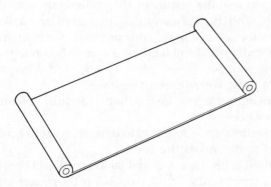

Fig 14.64

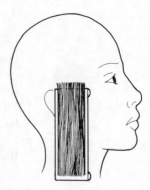

Fig 14.65

## Sodium hydroxide straighteners (relaxer cream)

These are the fastest and most effective chemical hair straightening products. They are made from caustic soda and are extremely alkaline, having a pH of 10–14. They are most suitable for use on Afro-Caribbean or very crinkly hair.

*Dangers of using sodium hydroxide*

- the hair may become brittle and break off
- if left longer than ten minutes the hair may dissolve
- can cause severe burning of the skin
- if sodium hydroxide is left on too long the hair may turn red.

A strand test should be carried out before any straightening process because of the high alkalinity of the relaxer cream.

Take a few strands of hair and apply a small amount of relaxer cream evenly along the hair lengths. Do not leave the relaxer in contact with the hair longer than recommended by the manufacturer and observe constantly. Assess the relaxation of the hair or any damage that may have been sustained. If the test shows any signs of hair breakage or excessive elasticity, postpone the treatment until the hair has been conditioned and retested at a later date. Record the results of the strand test.

*Application of sodium hydroxide straighteners*

1  Check the client's record card for any previous treatments.
2  Examine the scalp for any cuts, abrasions or inflammation – if any disorders are present postpone the treatment.

3   Examine the hair for

- tightness of curl
- elasticity and tensile strength
- texture and porosity
- any breakage.

4   Examine and assess the results of the preliminary strand test.

5   Make sure that the client is adequately protected by a gown and towel. Apply protective cream (vaseline usually) evenly in order to cover the scalp and around the hairline. Do not shampoo the hair or rub/brush the scalp.

6   The operator must wear protective gloves.

7   Read the manufacturer's instructions carefully before the treatment commences.

8   Section the hair into six – forehead to nape then ear to ear across the top and ear to ear across the back.

9   Start application at the nape area and taking small sections, apply sufficient relaxer cream to the hair. Do not allow the relaxer to touch the scalp. Work methodically in small sections towards the front.

10   With previously straightened hair, apply to the regrowth only.

11   When application is complete, use a gentle smoothing technique to straighten the hair starting where the cream was first applied. It is important that the hair should *not be pulled or stretched* during the application.

12   The approximate time for straightening hair is as follows:

(*a*) for fine hair – two to three minutes
(*b*) for medium hair – three to five minutes
(*c*) for coarse hair – five to seven minutes.

The maximum time for even the most resistant hair should not exceed eight minutes.

13   Rinse at a backwash with a strong force of warm water. Start at the hairline and hold the hose 10–12.5 cm (4–5″) from the head. Do not use hands to remove the cream from the hairline; let the force of the water remove it.

14   Use a neutralising shampoo to thoroughly shampoo the hair. On the second shampoo, gently but firmly comb the hair straight and leave for five minutes then rinse.

15   Remove excess moisture from the hair by blotting; do not rub the hair. Apply a pH moisturising conditioner as a treatment and leave for at least ten minutes before rinsing thoroughly.

16   Complete a record of work.

17   When styling the hair after straightening do not use high heated implements, e.g. hot brushes, etc.

## Contra-indications when permanently straightening hair

Do not start a straightening process in any of the following cases:

- cuts, abrasions or inflammation on the scalp
- the hair is coated with incompatible chemicals
- fragile or broken hair
- hair has been chemically damaged, in particular bleached hair
- hair or scalp with an infectious or contagious disease
- on children under ten years of age.

## Precautions and considerations when permanently straightening hair

1  Always carry out a preliminary strand test.

2  Carry out an incompatibility test if necessary.

3  Read the manufacturer's instructions very carefully and use only as directed.

4  Examine the hair and scalp carefully to determine the correct strength of relaxer. If in doubt, choose a weaker type.

5  Protect the skin and scalp with a protective cream.

6  The operator must always wear protective gloves.

7  Do not allow the relaxer cream to come into contact with the scalp or any part of the skin.

8  Do not pull or stretch the hair during the application; it could break.

9  Do not use hot brushes, heated curling tongs or any other heated implements on the hair either during or after straightening.

10  If the cream relaxer enters the eyes, rinse immediately with water and seek medical aid. Sodium hydroxide could cause blindness.

11  If the cream relaxer causes skin irritation, rinse off immediately and shampoo the hair with a non-alkaline shampoo. If irritation persists, seek medical aid.

12  Use a timer when processing to prevent the relaxer being left in contact with the hair too long.

13  Test frequently for development. Do not exceed the maximum time permitted by the manufacturer.

14  When rinsing the relaxer cream from the hair, great care must be taken to see that the chemical does not run into the eyes or ears by careless directing of the water.

15  Do not use the hands to remove the cream, use the force of the water instead.

16  Always complete a record card giving full details of the treatment carried out.

17  Advise client on after-care and the importance of conditioning treatments after straightening.

## Summary

Perming hair involves three main stages:

1  breaking some of the sulphur cross-linkage between the polypeptide chains of the hair keratin
2  moulding the hair
3  fixing the hair.

In cold permanent waving, the breaking of the sulphur linkages occurs due to a chemical process called reduction caused by the perm reagent acting as a reducing agent. In traditional alkaline perms (pH 9.5), this reagent is ammonium thioglycollate in acid perms (pH 2), the reagent is glycerol thioglycollate.

Moulding the hair is usually around rollers to produce a wave or curl (or by combing straight to straighten curly hair).

Fixing the perm is produced by an oxidation reaction using hydrogen peroxide which 'rebuilds' the broken sulphur linkages.

In heat perming, the sulphur linkages are broken by hydrolysis using heated water and no fixing agent is used.

Care must be taken during perming to avoid:

(a) reagents splashing or running onto skin or into the eyes
(b) a number of considerations which influence the final wave and hair condition.

Record cards for each client should be completed.

There are a variety of techniques available for use in perming (often called 'fashion' techniques), i.e. stack winding, directional winding, spiral winding, etc.

There are also practical techniques for straightening (relaxing) both European (Caucasian) and Afro-Caribbean hair.

## Self-assessment questions

1  Name the chemical process occurring during the first, softening stage in cold perming.
2  What is the main ingredient in acid perms?
3  What is the chemical meaning of the term 'neutralisation'?
4  What is meant by 'pre-saturation'?
5  What is a depilatory?
6  What can happen if the rod rubbers are twisted on the hair?
7  How often should perming development be checked?
8  When neutralising, why must the hair be thoroughly blotted after rinsing to remove the excess moisture?
9  What factors can cause an excessively long processing time?
10  What chemical action is used to straighten ('relax') naturally curly hair?

**Practical assignment – perming**

*You will need:*

- tuition head and clamp
- sectioning clips
- wide toothed tail comb
- rods of uniform size and end papers
- permanent waving lotion and oxidiser for normal hair with applicator bottles
- permanent waving lotion and oxidiser for treated hair with applicator bottles
- cotton wool and towel
- water spray.

## Task

(a)   Wet the tuition head thoroughly with water, remove excess moisture with the towel.

(b)   Divide the hair into three sections, forehead to crown (the width of a rod), then from ear to ear at either side. Pin the remaining hair out of the way.

(c)   Wind both the front two sections using the same size rods. When they are wound, place cotton wool around them to protect the other hair.

(d)   Apply the permanent wave lotion for normal hair to the left side section and apply the lotion for treated hair to the right side section.

(e)   Leave to develop until an 'S' shape curl is formed, giving both sides the same processing time.

(f)   Rinse thoroughly in tepid water, then blot dry and place cotton wool around the rods.

(g)   Apply the oxidiser and leave for five minutes (or according to manufacturer's instructions). Remove the rods and apply more oxidiser to the ends. Leave for a further five minutes then remove from the hair by rinsing thoroughly in tepid water.

(h)   Towel dry the hair and comb through.

*Answer the following questions*

When looking at the finished curl, which side of the tuition head is the curliest?

Which lotion was used on this side?

Which side of the tuition head developed the most quickly?

Carry out a porosity test. Which side of the tuition head *feels* the least porous?

Take a small strand from each side and test the elasticity of each by pulling gently between the fingers. Which side feels stronger?

From the practical work you have carried out and questions you have answered, make a comparison of the results.

# 15 COLOURING

## Hair colour

Tints are dyes which are used to add colour to the hair. This is the opposite of bleaching, where the aim is to remove the hair colour by decolourising it.

Two major hair pigments are:

- black/brown **melanin**
- red/yellow **pheomelanin**,

both of which are found mostly in the cortex, with a small amount in the cuticle. The hair appears to be a certain colour to the eye because the colour pigments in the hair absorb certain colours from the light falling on to it and reflect others. Only those pigments that are reflected reach the eye, so a blue object appears blue because blue light is reflected and the other colours are absorbed. Black objects absorb all the light falling on to them and white objects reflect all the light. In the shades or hues which are visible a mixing of the colours takes place. This mixing of reflected colours is complicated, but depends on the three primary colours from which other colours can be produced. This mixing effect is of great importance in tinting hair because of the way pigments are added to those already present in the hair. Colour triangles can be used to work out the combinations of pigments needed to obtain a particular shade.

When tinting hair the hairdresser must also take the light quality into account. This can be a problem in that the mix of colours in artificial light is slightly different from that in daylight.

## Hair dyes

Hair dyes work by adding coloured pigment molecules to the hair which alter the mix of colours reflected to the eye and thus the hair colour. The pigment molecules are added to the hair in two main ways:

1 the pigment coats the cuticle, that is the outside of the hair and does not penetrate into the hair cortex;

2 the pigment passes through the cuticle (often aided by making the hair swell using a steamer and/or an alkali), then into the cortex where it is deposited.

How efficiently this pigmentation happens depends on:

- the size of the pigment molecules
- the porosity of the hair – often a function of its age, the hair furthest from the scalp being the most porous – and the amount of chemical treatment the hair has received.

## Types of hair dye

There are two main methods of classifying hair dyes, which can be explained in terms of their ingredients and their permanence.

### Ingredients

The chemical nature and action of the active ingredients can be sub-divided into:

1 *Vegetable dyes* which are extracted from plants and include camomile and henna. Camomile, for example, is a golden-yellow dye obtained from the flower of the camomile plant. This dye has large molecules which will not penetrate the hair shaft and therefore coat the cuticle. It can be used to add golden tones to faded blondes.

2 *Metallic (or inorganic) dyes* which contain the metal salts of metals like lead, copper and iron.

3 *Synthetic organic dyes* which are 'man-made' substances and the most common ingredient in salon tints. A number of different chemicals come under this heading including the 'para' group.

### Permanence

The permanence or length of time the dye will last on the hair can also be sub-divided into:

1 *Non-permanent dyes* which last until the hair is next wet, e.g. at the next shampoo, and then wash out. Other types last longer (six to eight shampoos) but eventually wash out as well.

2 *Permanent dyes* which last until the tinted hair grows out.

The following section is based on the permanent classification, with details of the ingredients and their actions, where appropriate.

# Non-permanent colouring

Non-permanent colouring techniques include:

- temporary rinses
- temporary lighteners
- temporary colour sprays and paints
- semi-permanent colours.

## Temporary rinses

These consist of an acid dye which is rinsed through the hair, then dried on during setting or blowdrying. Acid dyes all share the properties of working at a pH below 7 and having some degree of negative charge on the molecule, that is, the same parts of the molecule can either pick up a negatively charged particle (an electron) or lose a positively charged particle (a proton). Therefore, they will not form a strong link to hair (as hair is negatively charged and like charges repel and will be easy to wash out.

A common acid dye used in temporary tinting is an '**azo**' dye (e.g. parahydroxy*azo*benzene). The acid used is an organic acid (citric or tartaric) and has a pH of between 2.5–4.0. Acid dyes have large, coloured molecules which do not penetrate the cortex but form a coating round the cuticle. They are soluble in water and are therefore easily removed by shampooing. A temporary rinse adds colour to the hair, but will not lighten the natural colour.

## Types of temporary rinses

Temporary rinses may be obtained in the following forms:

1 *Water rinse.* A few drops of concentrated colour are mixed with hot water.
2 *Coloured setting lotion.* Obtained ready mixed, this contains synthetic resin, polyvinylpyrrolidone (PVP) and alcohol to which a suitable acid dye, often an 'azo' dye, is added. On drying, the alcohol evaporates leaving a coloured, plastic film on the hair.
3 *Temporary toners.* Also obtained ready mixed, these are usually used on bleached hair to correct golden tones. They often contain a mild conditioning agent to which a suitable acid dye is added.
4 *Coloured mousse and gel.* Normal mousse or setting gel to which a suitable colouring pigment has been added.

## Uses of temporary rinses in the salon

1 As an introduction to colour, particularly useful for younger clients.
2 To brighten dull or faded hair. May also be used between permanent dye retouches to counteract any fading.

3  To tone bleached hair or to temporarily rectify a colour fault.
4  To enhance grey hair. It must be remembered, however, that these rinses will not completely cover the grey hairs.
5  To darken natural coloured hair.
6  To add multi or partial colouring to the hair.

## Method of application for a temporary rinse (wet method)

Temporary rinses are simple to apply. The hair is shampooed then towel dried to remove any excess moisture. If ready mixed, the rinse may be applied straight from the bottle by sprinkling on to the roots of the hair (as these are less porous), rubbing through the hair with the fingers and finally combing the hair thoroughly to ensure an even distrubution. Coloured mousses and gels are applied to the hair as normal following manufacturer's instructions but extra care must be taken to ensure that the application is even throughout the head.

Porous hair requires extra care as it will absorb the rinse very quickly, causing the resultant colour to be too dark and uneven. Applying the rinse with a tinting brush instead of straight from the bottle allows the operator greater control and enables the rinse to be applied evenly and where necessary, thus reducing the likelihood of a patchy result.

## Precautions and considerations

1  When using concentrated rinses, always mix with the recommended amount of water. Too strong a mixture acts as a semi-permanent tint, which cannot be easily removed by normal shampooing.
2  Always protect the client's clothing, particularly at the nape, by tucking a dark towel well down over any collars, etc.
3  Assess the texture and porosity of the hair before commencing the application of the temporary rinse.
4  Pre-towel dry the hair thoroughly to prevent dilution of the rinse.
5  Never choose a temporary colour a shade lighter than the natural colour of the hair – it will not have any effect.
6  Do not apply strong red shades to hair that contains a degree of white hair, particularly on the front hairline.
7  When applying temporary colours to freshly bleached hair, ensure that an antioxidant cream rinse is applied beforehand. Any hydrogen peroxide left in the hair could cause a bleach-out of the colour rinse.
8  For hair with an uneven or high degree of porosity, either apply a good hair conditioner/restructurant or leave the hair wet, by not towel drying thoroughly prior to the application of the rinse.
9  Do not use cotton wool to apply the rinse. Cotton wool can sometimes absorb certain colour granules, distorting the true colour of the rinse.

10   Use only a fine hairspray when dressing out after a temporary rinse has been used. Heavy lacquering could re-dissolve the colour and give a patchy effect.

11   Do not display temporary coloured setting lotions near sunlight or heat, as either can cause deterioration and colour distortion.

## Temporary lighteners

These are often sold to salons as if they were rinses but they are totally mis-named as they are, in reality, weak bleaches and any lightening of the hair by bleaching is permanent.

They are in fact oxidising agents, commonly hydrogen peroxide, incorporated in a setting medium which gradually and progressively lightens the hair over a period of two to three days. They must not be used too frequently otherwise they will over-lighten the hair and there will be a noticeable regrowth. When perming hair that has been lightened with a 'temporary' lightener, the hair must be treated as bleached hair. Therefore, a reagent for bleached hair should be used to prevent dryness and over-curly results.

## Temporary colour sprays and paints

There are two types of temporary colour sprays. First, a colour in a lacquer-type base (a plastic resin) used in aerosol-can form and second, the puff-on, of a powdery consistency. Both types coat the cuticle.

Hair paints can be obtained in a variety of colours – some extremely bright. The colour is brushed on to dry hair with a painting brush wherever it is required.

Both hair paints and colour sprays are ideal for special effects. They are the most temporary of the hair colourings and wear off quickly. They can be easily removed by brushing the hair thoroughly (although brightly coloured hair paints usually have to be washed out of the hair).

## Precautions

Metallic gold or silver temporary sprays or powder must be completely removed from the hair before perming, tinting or bleaching as these will react with the hydrogen peroxide used in these processes, causing rapid decomposition of the peroxide and consequently, hair damage. In other words, they are incompatible with the peroxide used in other processes.

## Semi-permanent colours

These dyes consist mainly of synthetic, organic dyes known as 'nitro' dyes, for example 2-*nitro*-1, 4-phenylenediamine, which gives a red colour. Nitro dyes are small coloured molecules which can pass through the cuticle into the cortex. Because they are small they can be gradually washed out.

Nitro dyes do not dissolve easily in water, so the benzyl alcohol is used as a solvent to allow the dye to penetrate deeper into the hair cortex. A detergent, such as sodium lauryl sulphate, is also added to the dye to produce a foam and improve the contact between the hair and the dye.

Semi-permanent dyes consist of small coloured molecules which are able to penetrate further into the hair shaft than a temporary rinse. Thus, a semi-permanent dye will usually last through approximately six to eight shampoos.

Diluted 'para'-dyes, which are oxidised to develop their colour either by the air, or more usually, by 10 vol. (3%) hydrogen peroxide are also sometimes used for semi-permanent colouration.

Semi-permanent dyes have a limited colour range and can be subject to colour build-up if used frequently. They will not actually lighten the hair and rely considerably on the base shade of the client. They produce darker tones than a temporary rinse and care should be taken when used on a client with a large percentage of white hair; an auburn colour (red), for example, is totally unsuitable for use on white or greying hair.

Individual heads vary considerably in structure, texture and porosity and these points should be taken into consideration before applying a semi-permanent dye. The larger the volume of hair, the darker and more intense the colour will appear. Porous hair will absorb the dye more readily but will also fade more quickly. If the hair is excessively porous it is often necessary to leave the hair wet, instead of towel drying, prior to the application; alternatively, apply a specially formulated pre-treatment restructurant.

## Uses of semi-permanent colours

1   To brighten dull or faded hair.
2   To tone bleached hair.
3   To enhance grey hair (but will not completely cover the white).
4   For use on clients who are allergic to 'para' dyes.
5   To rectify colour faults, e.g. a green discolouration can be rectified by red.
6   For preliminary pigmentation when returning bleached hair to its natural colour.
7   In conjunction with bleach to give subtle or striking effects to the hair (depending upon the colour of the semi-permanent used). For example, streaking or scrunch bleaching the hair, then applying a semi-permanent over the whole head will give lighter and darker tones of the semi-permanent colour.

## Method of application

Semi-permanent dyes are applied to damp hair that has been

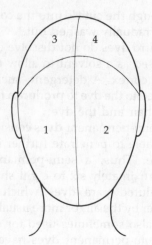

Fig 15.1 (a)

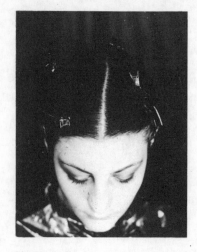

Fig 15.1 (b)

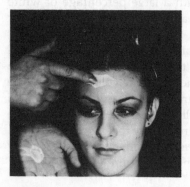

Fig 15.2

shampooed with a mild shampoo and then towel dried, unless instructed otherwise by the manufacturer.

1   Ensure that the client is adequately protected with a tinting gown, dark towel (tucked well down into the nape) and preferably a disposable plastic cape to cover the whole of the client and the chair.

2   The head is to be sectioned into four main sections (forehead to nape and ear to ear across the crown). (*See* Figs 15.1 (*a*), (*b*).)

3   Apply barrier cream around the hairline to prevent skin from staining. Care must be taken to ensure that it is applied to the skin only (*see* Fig 15.2).

4   Commence application at the nape and apply semi-permanent with a brush (or sponge or applicator bottle) to the roots and along the hair shaft (*see* Figs 15.3 (*a*), (*b*).)

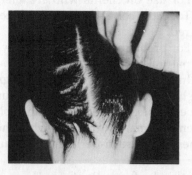

Fig 15.3 (a) Application to the roots

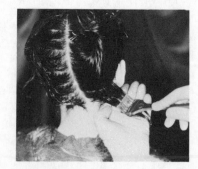

Fig 15.3 (b) Application of semi-permanent tint along the hair shaft

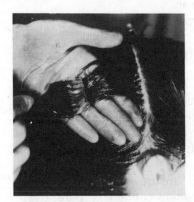

Fig 15.4

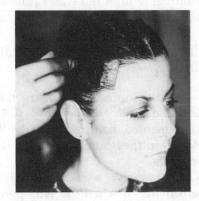

Fig 15.5

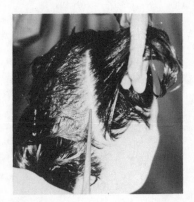

Fig 15.6

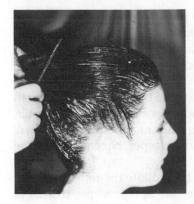

Fig 15.7 Combing hair after tint

5   Continue application towards the front hairline with the front two sections. Take the sub-sections back and away from the face to prevent the semi-permanent running on to the face (*see* Fig 15.4).

6   Apply the semi-permanent carefully to the last 1 cm (½″) of the hairline. This is best done with a brush, even when using a sponge or applicator bottle on the remainder of the hair. A brush gives more control and helps to avoid skin staining on the face and neck (*see* Fig 15.5).

7   Cross-check the application by taking sections *across* the previous sub-sections (*see* Fig 15.6). Ensure that the application is thorough and that the semi-permanent dye is evenly distributed along the hair shaft.

8   Comb the hair thoroughly up towards the crown (Fig 15.7).

9   Remove any staining to the skin with cotton wool (Fig 15.8).

10   Leave to develop for about 10–20 minutes, or according to the manufacturer's instructions (*see* Fig 15.9).

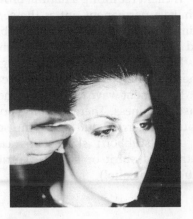

Fig 15.8

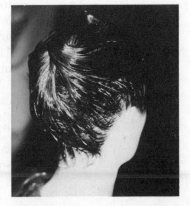

Fig 15.9 Leaving tint to process

11   When developed, add tepid water and massage the head. Rinse thoroughly until the water runs clear.

12   Complete a record of work carried out.

## Precautions and considerations for semi-permanent tinting

1   Read manufacturer's instructions carefully *before* application.

2   Some semi-permanent tints will cover up to 50 per cent of white, unpigmented hair, particularly if the pigmented hair is dark. However, they cannot cover white hair where it is concentrated in one area.

3   Always give a skin test when unsure of the client's skin sensitivity, or when the semi-permanent contains a 'para' dye.

4   Extra care should be taken when applying the liquid forms of semi-permanent tints. Although they have better penetration they are more liable to run.

5   Do not use bleach to remove an unwanted semi-permanent – it could cause complications. Instead, apply an alkaline soap shampoo (or toilet soap) which will open the cuticle scales.

Apply a second, soapless shampoo, to remove any soap scum deposit then a conditioner.

6   Poor shampooing, or lacquer left on the hair prior to application, prevents penetration of the colour and gives an unsatisfactory result.

7   Use hot water when shampooing prior to application. This will open and swell the cuticle and allow deeper penetration of the colour.

8   When dealing with extra porous hair, dilute the tint with water or reduce the development time or apply a pre-treatment restructurant.

9   If a regrowth appears on very porous hair, apply semi-permanent to the roots. Leave ten minutes, then apply to the lengths of the hair and comb through, leave for a further five to ten minutes. This will produce an even result.

10   A client requiring a natural brown shade may be better advised to have a permanent tint as the semi-permanent range of browns is limited. Also, a semi-permanent brown colour is difficult to obtain and has to be made up from a mixture of colours.

11   Do not leave the tint on for longer than the recommended time, otherwise the colour result will be too harsh and deep.

12   Permanent wave lotion will remove some of the colour and could cause patchiness. Therefore, when perming and colouring, the perm should be carried out before the semi-permanent tinting.

13   Any stubborn skin stains can be removed by industrial methylated spirit or surgical spirit (semi-permanent colours are soluble in alcohol).

# Permanent hair colouring

There are three main types of permanent dyes:

1 natural vegetable dyes
2 inorganic dyes
3 synthetic organic dyes.

## Natural vegetable dyes

Originally, all colouring materials for the hair were obtained from plants, the main one being henna.

Henna is a natural vegetable dye, also known as Lawsone. It is produced from the crushed, dried leaves of the Egyptian privet plant which grows in Iran, Egypt and along the Mediterranean coast. It is a non-toxic dye which is mixed with water and does not require a skin or patch test before application.

Pure henna imparts red pigment to the hair and the shades vary slightly according to the country of origin. The depth of red depends on the length of time that it is left in contact with the hair, i.e. the longer the development time, the more red pigment is imparted to the hair. The shade of red also depends on the base shade of the client, i.e. the lighter the base shade, the lighter the red produced.

Henna colours often have other additives to produce variations. It can now be obtained in powder form or ready mixed, but it should not be used on hair containing over ten per cent of scattered white hair, nor should it be used on highly bleached hair, as in both these cases the result would be too bright and harsh.

Henna is known as a coating dye, as it does not penetrate the natural pigment. Instead, it stains the hair shaft by adhering to the cuticle.

## Inorganic dyes

There are two main types of hair tints usually placed in this group. They are:

1 metallic dyes (including 'hair colour restorers').
2 compound henna (which is a mixture of the natural vegetable dye, henna, with a metallic dye).

## Metallic dyes

These work by depositing **metal salts** in the hair cortex and on the hair cuticle, which dulls the hair. There are three main types:

1 *Sulphide dyes* – here the hair is first coated in sodium sulphide and then with a metallic salt. A chemical reaction occurs between the two as follows:

*Sodium sulphide + Metal salt* → *Metal sulphide + Sodium salt*
*(deposited on*
*and in the hair)*

2  *Reduction dyes* – here a metal salt is converted to just the metal by a reducing agent, e.g. pyragallol. The minute particles of metal are deposited in and on the hair, thus colouring it.

3  *'Hair colour restorers'* – these are not usually used in the salon but can be bought by the public from chemists. The idea is to tint the hair in order to darken unpigmented white hair. They contain lead acetate and sodium thiosulphate which react very slowly together and darken the hair by depositing lead sulphide in the cortex and on the cuticle.

## Disadvantages of metallic dyes

- They dull the hair.
- They can colour the skin as well as the hair.
- Some metals used in metallic dyes act as a catalyst (i.e. they speed up the rate of the chemical reaction) on the breakdown of hydrogen peroxide. This effect is particularly strong if metallic dyes have been used for some time. It means that when peroxide is used during bleaching, perming or tinting, there is a risk of very rapid breakdown triggered by the metal on the hair; heat is then produced and this may damage the hair. To check whether metallic tints have been used, it is necessary to carry out an incompatibility test.

## Compound henna

This is a vegetable henna with a 'reduction' type metallic dye added. It coats the cuticle of the hair shaft only and does not penetrate into the cortex. It has a colour range of blonde to black but because of its metallic content it tends to give a dull effect.

Compound henna is not used in salons any more. Because of its metallic content it reacts with hydrogen peroxide causing rapid breakdown and heat damage to the hair, thereby limiting the other services that a salon has to offer.

It must be remembered that inorganic dyes such as metallic dyes and compound henna are not skin irritants and therefore do not require a skin test before application.

## Incompatibility test

Always test hair for the presence of any metallic salts before perming, tinting or bleaching the hair if there is any uncertainty as to what the client has had on their hair. This test is known as an incompatibility test.

*Method*

1  Take a small cutting of the hair from the crown area or the front (if the client has been tinting their own hair this will have the highest concentration of tint present).

2  Mix a simple bleach, which is a mixture of hydrogen peroxide and ammonia.

3  Immerse the cutting in the simple bleach.

4  If incompatible chemicals are present on the hair a reaction will occur.

5  Bubbles of gas (oxygen) being given off can be observed. Steam rises and heat is given off. The hair elasticity is increased and breakage occurs until the hair is completely destroyed.

## Synthetic organic dyes (oxidation dyes)

Modern permanent dyes are synthetic organic dyes consisting of solutions of *para*-phenylenediamine, or similar 'para' compounds, together with other substances, such as conditioners and antioxidants to prolong shelf-life. 'Para' compounds are a derivative of coal tar and can also be called synthetic analine dyes.

Modern 'para' dyes are used to cover white, grey or most natural hair colour and have a vast colour range. Indeed, it is possible to obtain almost any shade, from natural right through to exotic greens, reds, blues or purples.

'Para' dyes are manufactured in three forms: cream, liquid and gel. All forms must be mixed with hydrogen peroxide before application. Without the addition of hydrogen peroxide they are completely ineffective.

These dyes are water soluble and have comparatively small molecules (at this point it is often colourless) which will penetrate the cuticle and enter the cortex. When mixed with hydrogen peroxide, the oxygen released makes the small colourless molecules join together to form larger, coloured, insoluble molecules, which are then trapped in the cortex. They are too large to pass through the cuticle and therefore do not wash out easily. In this way they mimic the natural colouring pigments (*see* Fig 15.10). For an efficient tint, 20 vol. (6%) hydrogen peroxide is used, unless tints lighter than the natural shade are required, in which case, 30 vol. (9%) is used. Ammonia solution is used in 'para' dyes (as in bleaching) to speed up the breakdown of hydrogen peroxide.

Permanent oxidation dyes ('para' dyes) can be divided into two categories on the basis of how they are used. These are:

1  lightening dyes
2  covering dyes.

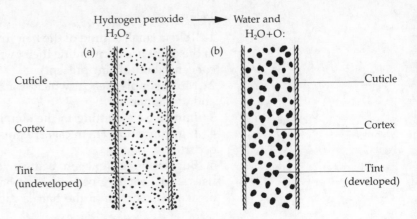

Fig 15.10 Development of the colour of an oxidation tint

## Lightening dyes

This type of dye consists of tinting the base shade of the hair lighter than the original colour.

To obtain a colour lighter than the base shade it is necessary to mix the para dye with hydrogen peroxide of a higher strength than that required to react with the para compounds. This is important because the nascent oxygen from the hydrogen peroxide combines with the para molecules to convert them to large coloured molecules; thus, any additional nascent oxygen attaches itself to the hair's natural colour pigment; making it lighter. The strength of hydrogen peroxide is usually 30 vol. (9%) unless a higher volume is recommended by the manufacturer.

It is useful to note that a higher volume strength of hydrogen peroxide sometimes throws up a golden tone. Therefore, when tinting the hair to pale ash shade (where no gold is required) some manufacturers recommend using 20 vol. (6%) hydrogen peroxide but in a greater proportion when mixing. In other words, the additional oxygen is obtained by adding more hydrogen peroxide. However, these proportions are only for certain tints and all manufacturers' instructions should be followed very carefully. Thus, correct mixing of the tint in relation to the hydrogen peroxide is extremely important to obtain the shade required.

## Covering dyes

This type of dye consists of tinting the hair darker or a similar shade to the natural base colour, or matching white hair to the natural base colour.

The para dye is mixed with 20 vol. (6%) hydrogen peroxide as this releases enough nascent oxygen to react with the para compounds without additional oxygen to bleach the natural colour pigment.

Where maximum depth of colour is required, e.g. very dark or black hair or toning after bleaching, 10 vol. (3%) hydrogen peroxide may be used.

To summarise, the base colour of the hair determines the volume strength of the hydrogen peroxide to be used. The lighter the colour required, the stronger the strength (or higher the volume) of hydrogen peroxide. The darker the colour required then the weaker the strength (or lower the volume) of hydrogen peroxide. (*See* Table 15.1 for quantities.)

**Table 15.1**

| Volume strength of hydrogen peroxide | Purpose |
| --- | --- |
| 10 vol ( 3%) | Gives maximum depth of colour. |
| 20 vol ( 6%) | For normal tinting. |
| 30 vol ( 9%) ⎤ | Lifting peroxides for lightening. |
| 40 vol (12%) ⎦ | |

Never use a higher volume of peroxide than necessary, as this causes hair damage and incorrect colour. As a general rule, 30 vol. (9%) hydrogen peroxide is the highest strength that can be safely used on the scalp and 40 vol. (12%) hydrogen peroxide is the highest strength that can be safely used on the hair. Sixty vol. (18%) hydrogen peroxide should only be used with specially designed tints and the manufacturer's instructions should be strictly followed.

## Preparation for para tinting: skin testing

Para dyes are toxic dyes in that they can produce para poisoning in some clients. This para poisoning is known as **allergic dermatitis.** The symptoms are unpleasant, with itching and a blotchy appearance on the skin of the face and neck. In severe cases, the face becomes so grotesquely swollen that the eyes cannot be opened and the mouth and lips swell to such an extent that swallowing and speaking become difficult. The skin may erupt and 'weep' over the whole of the body. These symptoms are often accompanied by a violent headache, shivering and a high temperature and it may be many months before a full recovery is made.

It is important, therefore, that the skin is tested for a reaction before each application of a para dye, as even a client who has had regular para dyes can still develop an allergic reaction (often called 'becoming sensitised'). A skin test should be carried out 24–48 hours prior to the tint application and although this may often be inconvenient, to both the client and the hairdresser, it is very much a case of 'better safe than sorry'.

## Method of applying a skin test

1 Clean a small area, either behind the ear or in the crook of the arm, with surgical spirit.
2 Mix a small amount of a dark shade of the tint to be used (the darker shades contain more para compound and are, therefore, more likely to produce a reaction) with hydrogen peroxide (as in the manufacturer's instructions).
3 Apply the tint to the clean area, about the size of a one pence piece, and leave it to dry.
4 To protect the area, cover with collodion and leave to dry.
5 Leave for 24–48 hours without disturbing.
6 If no irritation occurs, the test is negative and it is safe to proceed with the tint.
7 If irritation does occur, the test is positive and it is dangerous to proceed with the tint.

*NB* A skin test can also be called a patch test, allergy test, hypersensitivity test, predisposition test, idiosyncrasy test or Sabourand-Rousseau test.

## Strand test or test cuttings

These are taken before a full head tint, complete change of colour or whenever the hairdresser is unsure of the outcome of the tint through hair porosity, base shade, etc. It is simplest to take a small cutting of the client's hair when they book an appointment, so that the hair can be tested before the actual tint application is carried out. In the long term, a strand test can save a lot of unnecessary time and expense through choosing the wrong shade, peroxide strength, etc. It also gives the client a feeling of confidence, knowing that the hairdresser cares about them as an individual.

A strand test will ascertain the following:

- final shade of colour
- strength of hydrogen peroxide necessary
- approximate development time
- durability of the hair, i.e. breakage and tensile strength (stretching or elasticity)
- whether pre-bleaching or softening of the hair is necessary
- porosity of the hair.

*Method*

1 Take a small cutting of the hair from the front or nape area. (If the hair is white in one area in particular, take a cutting from there also.)
2 Mix a small amount of the tint and peroxide to be used in a bowl.
3 Place the cutting in the tint. To keep the cutting together, bind the ends with a small piece of sellotape.
4 Await development.

5  When the tint has developed, rinse the hair and test for durability by pulling between the fingers.

6  Dry and assess the results.

7  Record the results, together with the test cutting on the client's record card as follows:

(a) tint and shade used
(b) strength of peroxide
(c) durability of the hair
(d) development time.

*NB* The development time of the test cutting should only be used as a rough guide, as warmth or heat will make the tint act more quickly. therefore, even the temperature in the salon can have an effect on the length of the development time when actually carrying out the tint application.

8  Discuss the effect and final result with the client.

## Colour selection

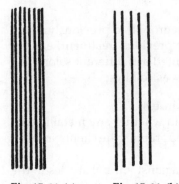

Fig 15.11 (a)    Fig 15.11 (b)

Human hair consists of two major groups of pigment which are deposited in the hair as it grows: melanin (brown or black) and pheomelanin (reddish yellow).

Each head of hair has a different distribution of these pigments and depending on the reflection of light and the density of the hair, the base shades of the hair will be different on each head. If the hair is in good condition, i.e. has a smooth cuticle, it will reflect more light and will, therefore, appear lighter. If the hair is thick and abundant, it will be more dense and the colour will appeaar darker. This phenomenon can be easily shown by the black lines in Fig. 15.11, where diagram (a) appears darker than diagram (b).

The colour of the hair also reflects on to the face of the client and this too should be taken into consideration when choosing a colour.

Colouring preparations can be divided into two groups:

1  *cold shades* – all ashen and matt shades (blues, greens, etc)
2  *warm shades* – all red or golden shades.

The cold shades will give the illusion of a darker colour, while warm shades will give the illusion of a lighter colour.

A shade chart should be used when selecting a colour. A particular shade of colour is very difficult to describe and the use of a shade chart prevents unnecessary mistakes by allowing the client to show the hairdresser exactly the shade or colour that they require.

Once the shade of colour has been chosen, the hairdresser must then take into consideration the base shade of the client as this will determine the strength of hydrogen peroxide to be used. The porosity of the hair is also an important factor. If the hair is excessively porous it is often advisable to choose a shade lighter to counteract the darkening tendency of this type of hair. The amount of white hair present on the head often creates a problem. It is sometimes necessary to use two different shades or two different peroxide strengths on one head to achieve a uniform shade, e.g. when hair is white at the front of the head and dark at the back.

In brief, the points to consider when selecting a colour are:

- client's requirements, i.e. warm or cold colour (most clients require a subtle colour change only)
- complexion, skin colouring and age of client
- lightening or covering
- base shade of the client
- texture and density of the hair
- tensile strength of the hair
- condition and porosity of the hair
- amount of white hair present.

Always remember that each client is an individual and if in any doubt, you should take a strand test.

## Matching a regrowth

It is sometimes necessary to match a regrowth to previously tinted hair without having any record of the previous treatment, e.g. for a new client who has had their hair tinted at a different salon. The procedure for matching a regrowth is as follows:

1  Ensure non-allergy to 'para' by skin test.
2  Take incompatibility test to ascertain whether any metallic salts are present on the hair (particularly important if the client has been tinting their own hair).
3  Check base shade of the regrowth against natural shades in the shade chart.
4  Check base shade of the remaining, tinted hair.
5  Check the percentage of grey.
6  Choose the shade nearest to the tinted hair, deciding if the tone is lighter, darker, warmer or cooler than the regrowth base shade.
7  Choose correct volume strength of hydrogen peroxide.
*Normal rules:*

- 30 vol strength when lifting more than two shades if there is not much grey to be covered.
- 20 vol for the average tint, i.e. the same or similar tone, slightly lighter or slightly darker, with or without grey.
- 10–15 vol for maximum coverage with no warmth or lift, e.g. black tints.

8  If undecided between two shades of colour, always choose the lighter as it is far easier to apply a darker shade afterwards than to strip out unwanted colour.
9  If in doubt as to which volume of peroxide to use, always choose 20 vol for safety.

# Permanent tinting practice

## Preparation of the operator

A tinting apron should be worn over the overall to prevent staining; an overall with long sleeves should have them turned back to prevent staining the cuffs. Rubber gloves should be worn to protect the hands, not only from unsightly stains but also to prevent dermatitis, which can be caused by constant contact with para.

## Preparation of the client

It is very important to protect the client's clothing at all times during the tinting process. Any stains to the clothing can be difficult to remove and the hairdresser may have to replace a spoilt garment which could cause embarrassment to all concerned. A tinting gown should be placed around the client to cover all their clothing and, preferably, it should be large enough to cover the chair also. This will prevent any tint from splashing on to the chair and perhaps staining another client's clothing later. Dark towels should be used, for obvious reasons, and these should be tucked down firmly at the nape to prevent them from slipping. A neck strip or strip of cotton wool placed around the nape is also a precautionary measure. Special plastic, disposable capes can also be placed at the back, over the gown and the towel to help to protect the towels and chair, etc.

To prevent staining of the skin, barrier cream should be applied around the hairline, but care must be taken not to allow the cream to coat the hair. If the tint application is carried out carefully and controlled, there should never be any risk of skin staining, but sometimes with the darker, particularly blue-black shades, it is very difficult not to stain the skin.

## Preparation of materials and equipment

All necessary equipment and materials should be assembled before commencement of the application, to prevent rushing backwards and forwards across the salon during and after the application. A competent apprentice/trainee can assemble all materials and equipment ready for the operator, thus aiding the efficiency of the salon and freeing the operator for the more skilful tasks.

The equipment should be assembled on the flat top of a trolley that can be easily wiped clean afterwards.

## Preparation of a para dye

Para dyes are usually mixed with an equal quantity of hydrogen peroxide, in the ratio 1:1. This is a simple procedure with liquid and semi-viscous forms, but with the cream form of tint, the manufacturers clearly state the amount of hydrogen peroxide to be used. There are one or two exceptions to the 1:1 ratio, but again, this is clearly stated in the manufacturer's instructions.

To mix the tint, squeeze the tube (from the bottom and roll up to prevent oxidation, by the air, of the remaining tint if only using part of the tube) or empty the contents of the bottle into a non-metallic bowl. If more than one colour is used to produce a particular shade they should be thoroughly mixed together in the bowl before adding the peroxide. Next, mix the correct amount of hydrogen peroxide with the tint, adding it very slowly to form a thick, creamy mixture. If the peroxide is added too quickly, the mixture becomes lumpy and the resultant colouration will be uneven.

## Application of a para dye regrowth

The application of para should always be done methodically, carefully and as quickly as possible. The method of applying a para dye can be varied, depending upon the porosity of the hair and the degree of white hair present. It must be remembered that the more resistant the hair, the longer it will take for the colour molecules to penetrate into the cortex; therefore, resistant areas should be treated first. Generally, the nape area is the most resistant as it does not get the same 'weathering' as the front area and is therefore not usually as porous.

## Method of application

1  Assemble equipment and materials, then check that the client's skin test is negative.
2  Protect the client's clothing with dark gown, towels, etc. Ensure that the towel is tucked firmly down into the nape (Fig 15.12).
3  Disentangle the hair and check the scalp for cuts and abrasions. If minor, protect with petroleum jelly, if major, postpone the treatment.
4  Divide the head into six major sections, forehead to nape, ear to ear across the top of the head and ear to ear across the back (Figs 15.13(a), (b)). If the hair is excessively greasy, wash with a mild, soapless shampoo, then thoroughly dry before sectioning. This is to prevent the excess sebum from forming a barrier on the hair shaft.
5  Apply barrier cream around the hairline, ensuring that it is applied to the skin only.
6  Mix the tint according to the manufacturer's instructions, then commence application at the nape, unless more resistant elsewhere. Apply the tint evenly with the tinting brush to the regrowth area around the outline of the first major nape section (see Fig. 15.14).
7  The size of the regrowth determines the size of the sub-sections: for small regrowth – small sub-section; large regrowth – large sub-section. However, sub-sections should not normally exceed 1 cm (½"). To ensure a thorough application, the tint should penetrate through to the next sub-section, but make sure you do not overlap

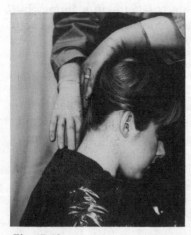

Fig 15.12

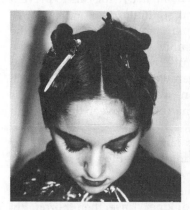

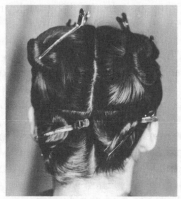

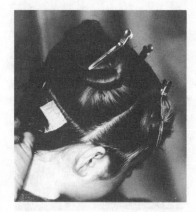

**Fig 15.13 (a) Sectioning for permanent tinting**

**Fig 15.13 (b)**

**Fig 15.14**

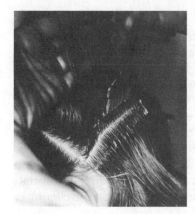

**Fig 15.15**

on to the previously tinted hair. The brush is stroked in the direction of the hair.

8   Then stroke up and across the sub-section (*see* Fig 15.15).

9   Continue to apply the tint until the front sections are reached. Tint around the outline of the front section, ensuring that all wispy hairline hairs are covered (*see* Fig 15.16). Figure 15.19 shows the final result of the tint – note the tinted wispy hairline hairs.

10   The front sub-sections may be taken towards the front hairline or down from the centre parting (*see* Fig 15.17).

11   Check the application by cross-checking across the sub-sections to ensure that the application is even and thorough (*see* Fig 15.18).

12   Remove any stains to the skin carefully with cotton wool.

13   Lift the hair away from the scalp carefully with the tail end of the tinting brush to allow the air (and oxygen in the air) to circulate freely.

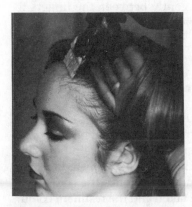

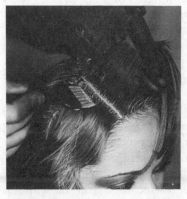

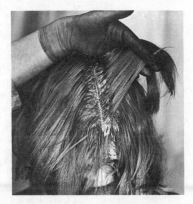

**Fig 15.16 Ensuring all hairline sections are covered**

**Fig 15.17 Applying tint to sub-sections**

**Fig 15.18 Checking the sub-sections**

14   Cotton wool may be placed behind and above the ears to prevent the tinted hair from falling back and staining them.

15   Await tint development. Heat may be applied to quicken the process either with the aid of a steamer or an accelerator.

16   Check the development frequently by removing the tint from a small mesh of hair with a piece of damp cotton wool. Dry the mesh with another, dry, piece of cotton wool. The development is complete when there is no line of demarcation between the regrowth and the previously tinted hair.

17   When developed, add a small amount of water to loosen colour and massage the head. Rinse off the tint thoroughly with tepid water until the water runs clear. Apply a cream or acid balance shampoo, massage gently, then rinse. Apply a second shampoo if necessary.

18   Apply an acid or pH balance conditioner, rinse, then thoroughly towel dry.

19   Complete a record of work carried out.

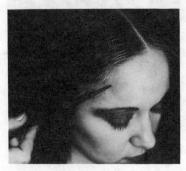

**Fig 15.19 Final result**

## Combing through

It is not necessary to comb through the lengths of the hair for every tint retouch. Tints do tend to fade and lighten slightly due to the ultraviolet rays present in the sunlight. However, if the undiluted tint is repeatedly combed through the hair it will damage the cuticle scales, making it more porous at each successive treatment. A vicious circle is produced, whereby the more porous the hair becomes, the more quickly it fades! Acid balance shampoos and conditioners help to counteract fading by tightening the cuticle layers. If fading does occur, the tint should be diluted with water or a liquid shampoo before applying to the lengths of the hair. Combing through undiluted tint is used only very occasionally or when the client has a colour change.

It is important when combing through either undiluted or diluted tint to ensure that the tint is applied to each strand of hair, otherwise the result will be very patchy. When the tint has been applied to the lengths of the hair, rub the hair gently between the fingers to distribute the tint evenly. Do not remove the tint from the roots by dragging it down the lengths of the hair to the points, this again can produce an uneven result.

## Full head application of a para compound

Clients are often reluctant to say if they have used any products on their hair, so before carrying out a full head application it is wise to take an incompatibility test to ensure that there are no metallic salts present on the hair shaft. The client should be tested for any allergy to para by giving them a skin test and once the colour has been selected, a strand test should be taken and the resultant colour of the hair cuttings shown to the client. This enables any adjustments to be made before the application. Remember that the test cuttings will appear slightly lighter than the finished colour because of the density of the hair on the head. When all the tests are found to be satisfactory it is safe to proceed with the application.

The first-time application of a covering, darkening dye is quite straightforward. Section the head as for a retouch and commence application at the most resistant area. Apply the tint carefully to the roots and lengths of the hair shaft. The application must be thorough to ensure that every hair is evenly coated throughout its entire length. If the points of the hair are very porous, apply the tint to the roots and mid-lengths first and the points of the hair last.

The full head application of strong reds, purples, light reds and lightening dyes must take into account the effect of body heat. The roots of the hair are closest to the scalp and the heat from the scalp activates the tint more quickly in this area; therefore, the application to the mesh begins approximately 10 mm (½″) from the scalp. When application to all mid-lengths and points of the hair has been completed, the tint is left to develop approximately to the half-way stage or over. In the case of high lift tinting it is sometimes beneficial to protect the root area with strips of cotton wool placed along the sub-sections; this prevents the tinted hair from accidentally touching the roots. Fresh tint is then mixed and applied to the root area and left to develop until the colour is even from root to point.

When tinting long hair, allowance must be made for not only the effect of body heat, but also for the varying degree of porosity throughout the hair length. The hair points are the most porous due to wear and weather, while the mid-lengths are usually the most resistant and will absorb the tint more slowly. Application should, therefore, be made first to the mid-lengths, then the points and finally to the roots.

## Record cards

It is essential to complete a record of work done for each client after every application of tint. The professional hair colourist may find it necessary to mix any number of colours to produce a certain shade of colour and it is very difficult, if not impossible, to remember exactly what has been used on every head. A record card should record the colour/s used and in what quantity, the strength of hydrogen peroxide, the date of each skin test and the result, the development time and any remarks concerning the finished colour result. Any faults should also be recorded for further reference (*see* Fig. 15.20 for an example of a typical record card).

## Contra-indications for permanent para tinting

Do not proceed with the tinting when:
1 The client suffers from a contagious disease of the hair and/or scalp, e.g. ringworm.

| Name: ............................ | Base shade: ........................ |
| Address: ............................ | % white: ........................ |
| ............................ | Hair texture: ........................ |
| Tel No: ............................ | Hair condition: ........................ |

| Date | Skin test | Tint | Strength peroxide | Development time | Remarks |
|------|-----------|------|-------------------|------------------|---------|
|      |           |      |                   |                  |         |

Fig 15.20 Sample record card

2  Incompatible chemicals are present on the hair shaft as shown by an incompatibility test.
3  You get a positive reaction to a skin test.
4  A lighter shade of tint is to be applied over a dark dye. The previous dye should first be removed or lightened, otherwise the new lighter shade will not show.
5  Hair is very weak and fragile. This type of hair should always be tested for tensile strength (*see* Strand test, p. 255) particularly if a full head tint lightener is required. Only if these tests prove satisfactory should the tint lightener be attempted.

## Precautions and considerations for para tinting

1  Take a skin test before each para application.
2  If in doubt, always take tests of the hair to ensure that it can be tinted satisfactorily.
3  Regrowth should not be allowed to exceed 10 mm (½").
4  Grease or heavy lacquer on the hair can form a barrier and prevent satisfactory penetration of the tint. If this is the case, shampoo the hair with a mild, soapless shampoo, then dry under a warm drier before commencing the application.
5  Ensure adequate protection of the client and the operator.
6  Always check the scalp for cuts and abrasions. If minor, protect with petroleum jelly. If major, postpone treatment.
7  Check carefully that the correct shade of tint is mixed with the correct volume strength of hydrogen peroxide. In a busy salon it is an easy mistake to put a tube or bottle of tint back in the wrong box, with disastrous results.

8  Mix the correct amount of hydrogen peroxide with the tint, usually a 1:1 ratio.

9  Never use a higher strength of hydrogen peroxide than necessary.

10  Only mix the tint when ready to apply, otherwise the colour molecules will become too large to enter the cortex and result in poor coverage.

11  Commence application at the most resistant area.

12  Always work as quickly as possible. Remember that the colour molecules are being oxidised as soon as the tint is mixed.

13  When a regrowth is too wide, in excess of 10 mm (½"), and the hair is being lightened, it may be necessary to pre-soften the middle band of untreated hair with 20 or 30 volume hydrogen peroxide, then dry under a warm hairdryer. Proceed with the root application as normal, overlapping the middle band. This will counteract the effect of body heat on the 10 mm (½") nearest to the scalp. Be careful: this is a difficult procedure and should only be attempted by experienced operators.

14  Always check the application by cross-checking, to ensure that no area is inadvertently missed and that the application is even throughout the whole of the head.

15  Remove any stains to the skin after the application and before development. They are much easier to remove at this stage.

16  Lift the hair away from the scalp when the application is complete. This allows the air to circulate more freely.

17  Do not remove the tint before it is fully developed. All the colour molecules should be completely oxidised to give a satisfactory result.

18  Never repeatedly comb through undiluted tint, it can make the ends of the hair very porous and cause colour fade.

19  When perming tinted hair, remember that it is more porous than untreated hair and will, therefore, require a special, weaker perming solution.

20  Always advise the client on the after-care of tinted hair. Explain the importance of regular retouching of the regrowth and the use of conditioning treatments.

# Hair discolouration and unwanted colour tones

An unwanted discolouration of the hair can often be masked by the addition of another colour. This is because brown hair colour is made up of three primary colours (blue, yellow and red).

By mixing the primary colours it is possible to produce the secondary colours.

These three secondary colours are produced as follows:

| Primary | | Secondary |
|---------|---|-----------|
| Blue + Yellow | = | Green |
| Yellow + Red | = | Orange |
| Red + Blue | = | Purple |

If all the three primary colours are mixed together, they produce brown, which is a neutral or *tertiary* colour.

**Blue + Yellow + Red = Brown**

Using this fact, any peculiar discolouration of the hair can be masked and brought to a neutral brown colour by the addition of the missing colour. For example, a green discolouration can be brought to brown by the addition of red. This is shown as follows:

**Green = Yellow + Blue**
**but Yellow + Blue + Red = Brown**

By drawing two triangles, one with the primary colours and the other with the secondary colours, then superimposing the two triangles to form a star, it is possible to see quite easily which colour can be masked by the addition of another colour (*see* Fig 15.21).

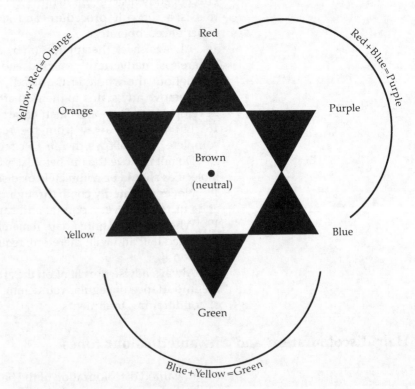

**Fig 15.21 Colour mixing triangles**

Manufacturers take the characters from around the colour star and add them to various depths to create a range of shades.

From Fig 15.22, it is possible to see that any discolouration can be masked by the opposite contrasting colour. Thus:

- *Orange* discolouration is masked by *blue*
- *Yellow* discolouration is masked by *purple* (mauve)

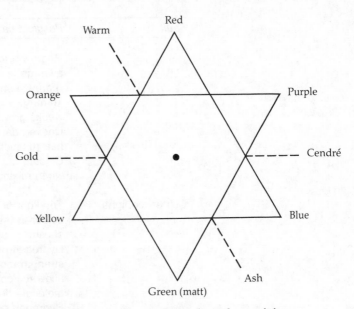

**Fig 15.22 Producing a range of shades by colour mixing**

- *Red* discolouration is masked by *green* (matt)
- *Gold* discolouration is masked by *cendré*
- *Warm tones* are masked by *ash*.

*NB* When masking unwanted colour tones by adding a contrasting colour, remember that the depth of both colours must be the same, e.g. pale yellow can be masked by pale purple (mauve) to produce pale brown (beige).

## Rectifying colour faults

Several unsatisfactory outcomes can result from hair colouring. The following is a summary of the main ones with their causes and remedies.

**Table 15.2**

| Fault | Possible cause | Action required |
|---|---|---|
| Patchy and uneven colour after tint application | Insufficient application or covering of tint Overlapping, causing colour build-up in parts Underprocessing, i.e. not allowing full colour to develop Use of spirit setting lotions which may remove colour | Correct by spot tinting, applied to light areas |

| Fault | Possible cause | Action required |
|---|---|---|
| | Regrowth too wide – average length of regrowth should be 10 mm (½″) or 4–6 weeks growth<br>Uneven damage to the hair (uneven porosity)<br>Colours not blended when mixing | |
| Colour too light | Too light or insufficient colour in the shade chosen<br>Hydrogen peroxide strength too low to allow full colour molecule development<br>Hydrogen peroxide strength too high for degree of lift required<br>Underprocessing or hair too porous to hold the colour | Retint, using the correct shade of colour with the correct volume strength of hydrogen peroxide for the correct length of time |
| Colour fade after two or three shampoos | Underprocessing, i.e. colour molecules not fully developed<br>Poor condition, hair too porous<br>Unnecessary combing through of undiluted tint<br>Wrong shampoo used after application | Retint, mixing the tint as a semi-permanent colour bath to add colour only. Watch development carefully. If the hair is highly porous use a special restructurant before tinting. |
| Colour too dark after application | Colour choice too dark<br>Poor condition – porous hair will sometimes take up too much colour<br>Possibly incompatible chemicals present, e.g. metallic dyes | Test the hair for incompatible chemicals. If test is positive do not treat hair with other chemicals. If negative condition, then correct by using a colour reducer, following the manufacturer's instructions, or use a mild bleach to lighten the colour. Always test tinted hair before using either a reducer or bleach. |

| Fault | Possible cause | Action required |
|-------|----------------|-----------------|
| Hair too red or brassy | Peroxide strength too high<br>Insufficient development, not all colour molecules have developed<br>Natural colour base too warm for chosen colour<br>If pre-bleached, wrong choice of neutralising colour or not bleached light enough | Apply a matt or green colour to mask the unwanted red or a purple/mauve to mask the yellow, brassy tones |
| Unexpected discolouration of the hair | Poor condition, too porous to hold the colour<br>Repeated combing of undiluted tint through the hair<br>Possible reaction to incompatible chemicals | Test the hair for incompatible chemicals. Recondition and restructure porous hair if test is negative. Counteract any unwanted discolouration with a contrasting colour or remove colour with colour reducers or a mild bleach. |
| Colour build-up | Overlapping during application<br>Combing undiluted tint through the hair unnecessarily | Apply a simple bleach or colour reducer, then condition the hair thoroughly |
| Roots too light | Failure to allow for body heat when lightening<br>Strength of hydrogen peroxide too high<br>Wrong colour choice when matching a regrowth | Retint the roots using a mixture of tint and 10 vol (3%) strength of hydrogen peroxide or one shade darker tint. Check carefully for development |
| Hair resistant to tint or poor coverage | Closely packed cuticle scales – often strong white hairs are resistant to tint<br>Tint and hydrogen peroxide mixed too soon before application, thus colour molecules have become too large to | Retint, using correct shade of tint with 20 vol (6%) hydrogen peroxide for coverage. If the hair is resistant, because of first cause given on left, then correct by pre-bleaching to open the cuticle scales, |

| Fault | Possible cause | Action required |
|---|---|---|
| | enter the cortex <br> Wrong product or colour shade used <br> Incorrect application <br> Not enough product used <br> Insufficient development <br> Too weak peroxide strength to oxidise fully the colour molecules | lengthen the development time and use a darker shade of tint. Moist heat will also help to swell the cuticle scales. |
| Insufficient lift | Wrong strength of hydrogen peroxide used <br> Wrong quantities of tint and hydrogen peroxide mixed <br> Insufficient product used <br> Insufficient development <br> Natural base shade too dark for chosen colour | Retint with correct colour and volume strength of hydrogen peroxide. Allow sufficient development. Pre-bleaching may be required if the natural base shade is too dark. |

# Colour removal (decolouring)

Women often like to change their hair colour, even if it is already tinted, but sometimes the tinting results are not successful. Some of the worst cases of unwanted colour tones are caused by home hairdressing and, in such cases, partial or complete removal of the original tint followed by recolouring may be necessary. Sometimes, the colour can be improved with only a slight correction (see Table 15.2), but when more drastic treatment is needed it can be a long, slow, painstaking process that may also cause considerable hair damage.

Colour removal should always be carried out methodically and with extreme care. Every head is particular to each individual and so creates different problems; therefore, strand tests must be taken to ensure that the colour can be successfully removed. The results of the tests should be shown to the client so that they will know in advance what to expect.

Thorough consultation with the client is very important in order to find out what products have been previously used on the hair. If the client has practised 'home tinting', an incompatibility test is necessary to ensure that the product they have used does not contain any metallic salts. If the client has had it tinted by another hairdresser, try to ascertain the manufacturer of the previous tint as most colouring manufacturers have an advisory service and can give valuable assistance to the hairdresser.

Do not take details of a previous treatment at face value. Clients are often reluctant to admit what they have actually used on their hair, particularly when the results have been unsatisfactory. They also do not realise that a permanent product applied to the hair several months previously could still be present on the ends of the hair; therefore, it is extremely important to check all the facts thoroughly before deciding upon the best method of colour correction to use.

Before commencing any form of colour removal the following information must be assimilated and assessed.

- condition of the hair and the scalp
- porosity of the hair
- history of any skin troubles
- make and type of the previous treatment(s)
- shade of the previous tint(s)
- general colour state – patchy, dull, multicoloured, etc.
- final colour shade required.

If the condition of the hair and skin is satisfactory, a skin test, incompatibility test and strand test should be taken. When all these tests have been completed and it is shown that the hair colour can be removed satisfactorily, with no adverse effects to the hair or the client, it is safe to proceed with the colour removal.

There are two basic methods of colour removal:

1 reduction (colour reducers)
2 oxidation (bleaching).

## Reduction

This is an acid removal which involves the chemical process known as 'reduction'. The oxygen is removed from the converted colour molecules which are then converted into colourless **leuco-compounds**. This means that only the artificial colour pigment is removed and that the natural colour pigment is left unlightened, it also means that the lightening power of the reducers is limited.

Colour reducers, or reducers as they are sometimes known, are usually in liquid or powder form and may be mixed with either water or peroxide. They must be used in strict accordance with the manufacturer's instructions. For simple cases the reducer is mixed with water and this will take the hair colour down by approximately one shade. If the hair is dark through colour build-up and requires more lightening, the reducer is mixed with 10 or 20 vol (3 or 6 per cent) hydrogen peroxide. Occasionally, for very dark shades and dramatic removal, 30 vol (9 per cent) hydrogen peroxide may be used, but never stronger than this.

It is not possible to obtain cold or flat shades when reducing as some of the red pigment will stay in the hair. A toning shade of matt will therefore be necessary to mask any unwanted warm shades.

Colour reducers make the hair more porous; therefore, a tint applied after reducing is likely to process more quickly or produce a deeper shade than required. To counteract this it is advisable to use a tint a shade lighter than the one required to achieve the best results.

The condition of the hair is also affected by colour reducers. Thus, it is important to condition the hair thoroughly after the treatment and extra care should be taken when perming decoloured hair.

## Method of removal by reduction

1  Check all tests to ensure that they are satisfactory.

2  Protect the client's clothing with dark gown, towels, etc.

3  Check the scalp for cuts and abrasions.

4  Divide the hair into four major sections (forehead to nape and ear to ear across the top of the head).

5  Mix the reducer in a non-metallic bowl (do not allow the mixture to come into contact with metal comb or clips).

6  Commence application with a sponge or tinting brush, taking intersecting partings across the crown.

7  Application must be done speedily and thoroughly. Apply the mixture to the tinted hair only, and avoid the root section if there is a natural colour regrowth. The natural regrowth can be blocked out with cotton wool strips if necessary.

8  When the application is complete, comb through thoroughly to ensure complete penetration of the meshes, but do not allow the reducer to come into contact with the root area. Pay particular attention to the front hairline and the ends of the hair as this usually has the highest concentration of tint.

9  Leave to develop, usually up to 50 minutes, but check with the manufacturer's instructions.

10  When development time is complete, check that the hair has sufficiently lightened, then rinse thoroughly and shampoo.

11  Rinse hair with a stabilising solution of 10 vol (3 per cent) hydrogen peroxide and comb through gently. This will show whether all the colour pigment has been removed from the hair.

12  If the hair redarkens after combing through, it means that the pigment has not been successfully removed and it will be necessary to repeat the application.

13  Dry the hair to check the colour. If patchy, re-apply the reducer to the patches. If the colour is even but the shade is too orange, red or brassy, tone out with a semi-permanent or permanent tint in the usual manner.

14 Condition the hair well.
15 Complete a record of work carried out.
16 Advise on after-care conditioning treatments.

## Oxidation

This is an alkaline method of removal done with bleaching preparations. It will lighten both the artificial and natural colour pigments. The bleach mixture is applied to the tinted area of the hair only, in the same manner as a reducer. It may, however, be necessary to bleach the hair a shade or two lighter than the required colour to allow for corrective tinting afterwards. When an even, bleached base has been achieved a permanent tint can then be applied to obtain the colour that is required.

It is very important when carrying out colour removal to test the hair for breakage and tensile strength during the processing (this is done by pulling the hair between the fingers). Remember that the hair is probably in a very porous state before colour removal and the addition of still more chemicals to the hair can be very damaging. The importance of strand tests prior to the application cannot be stressed too strongly nor too often. The client will also require advice on after-care conditioning treatments to counteract the damaging effect of the chemicals.

## Contra-indications for colour removal

Do not proceed with colour removal in any of the following cases:

- contagious/infectious disease of the hair and/or scalp
- excessively weak and porous hair
- incompatible chemicals present on the hair shaft
- adverse reaction to the strand test
- adverse reaction to the skin test (if using para after the decolouring) in which case it may be necessary to mask any unwanted colour tones with a semi-permanent colour that does not contain para
- highly sensitive scalp
- build-up of very dark products that are impossible to remove.

## Precautions and considerations for colour removal

1 Always check the client's final requirements thoroughly. It may not be possible to achieve the exact desired colour due to the previous treatments, and the client should be made aware of this fact.
2 Always test the hair before commencing a decolouring process.
3 Ensure that the hair is in reasonable condition before strong colour stripping.

4  Do not allow anything metallic to touch either the reducer or the bleach mixture.

5  Do check the hair thoroughly for uneven porosity and tensile strength before beginning the application.

6  Always work methodically and quickly.

7  Never allow the reducer or the bleach to run on to the natural regrowth as this can often prove harder to correct than the actual colour correction!

8  Check the application thoroughly. Ensure that the reducer is applied to all the tinted hair. Rubbing the meshes gently between the fingers helps to ensure even penetration through the meshes.

9  Avoid using the steamer for processing. The reducer or bleach may run down the hair shaft and on to the natural colour regrowth.

10  If some areas begin to develop too rapidly, it may be necessary to remove the product from these areas with wet cotton wool to prevent them from becoming too light.

11  When decolouring just patches of tinted hair, block out all the other areas with strips of cotton wool or oil.

12  Always watch the development carefully and check the hair frequently, not only for development, but also for breakage.

13  When rinsing the hair, remember that it will now be in a much weaker state and that the scalp may also be more sensitive. Therefore, treat both the hair and the scalp gently at this stage.

14  Conditioning is very important after decolouring. The client should be given advice on after-care conditioning treatments that may be carried out either in the salon or at home.

15  When decolouring, the hair often goes through traumatic colour changes (bright reds and oranges, etc.) that can be distressing for the client if they are not forewarned. If possible, seat the client away from a mirror while the decolouring process is being carried out.

16  Finally, remember that the client has spent many months or maybe years obtaining their present colour. It takes time and very careful pre-planning to remove it in one day.

## Fashion colouring techniques

Fashion colouring techniques are usually used to improve the look of a hairstyle or haircut. Colour can emphasise a shape, give the illusion of increasing weight or of lightening heaviness, depending upon how and where it is applied. Most important of all, fashion colouring techniques can be fun. The more outrageous or different the equipment and methods used, the more interest is stimulated. Clients are often unaware of the many effects that can be achieved using colour, so it is the responsibility of the hairdresser to suggest various techniques that can be used to improve the hairstyle of the client. Most clients want to improve their image and once made aware of the subtle effects that can be achieved on their hair are prompted to do something positive.

Fashion colouring techniques are a natural progression from the basic colouring techniques. Once the hairdresser has become skilled in the art of hair colouring, with a little imagination and the confidence to try out new ideas, the opportunities and variations of colour are endless.

Recent trends in hair colouring are to use more than one colour or partial colouring in one form or another, on one head. Most colour shades are intermixable and when used in conjunction with bleach or lightening agents allow complete freedom to achieve anything from the subtlest form of colouration to the most outrageous. With confidence and experience it is possible for the hairdresser to create personal techniques to achieve the effect desired.

A few of the popular techniques are indicated below.

## Block colouring

This is a good technique to emphasise short hairstyles. Two, three or even four colours can be used to emphasise the hairstyle, but there should be at least two shades difference between the colours. The darkest shade is usually used at the nape, graduating to the lighter shade at the front. Zig-zag the partings or divisions to prevent a hard line between the shades. Cotton wool/foil strips can be used to block out each section as it is completed to prevent the colours from touching each other, although a more subtle effect is created if the tint is carefully combed together up from the nape to the crown when application is complete.

Subtle effects are created by using similar colour tones to the client's own hair. Dramatic effects can be created by using contrasting colours, e.g. dark brown at the nape graduating to bright red-orange at the front.

## Points to remember

1  When tinting lighter, allow for the effect of body heat at the scalp; the mid-lengths and ends must be tinted before the roots. When tinting darker, the tint can be applied from the roots through to the ends. It may, therefore, be necessary to use both techniques on one head when block tinting.
2  The hair is naturally lighter at the front and crown area because of the effect of sunlight etc.; by using lighter shades in these areas a more natural effect is achieved. To give a very dramatic effect, reverse the colours, i.e. darker shades at the front and lighter shades at the nape.
3  Darker shades make the hair appear more dense and, therefore, heavier. Lighter shades give the illusion of less weight. This is a useful fact to bear in mind when emphasising a hairstyle with colour.

## Painted lights (flying colours)

This technique adds colour and depth to a particular hairstyle. The hair is combed into shape and a decision is made as to where the style needs accentuating. This may be at the nape, sides or crown. A semi-permanent colour or permanent tint is then painted on to the hair using a vent brush, a wide toothed comb or a fine artist's paint brush. Apply the tint in the direction of the style but try not to work in straight lines as this can give a heavy effect.

## Points to remember

1   A number of shades can be used throughout the head. Lighter shades at the front and darker shades at the sides and nape will give a shimmering effect.
2   This is a good method to add interest to dark hair. Paint the hair with strong red or burgundy shades of tint.
3   A tinting gun can be used instead of a vent brush etc.; this creates interest in the salon but it requires plenty of practice so handle it with caution.
4   Painted lights are a very quick method of adding colour and are an invaluable way of using up odd quarter tubes of tint etc., but remember not to get too enthusiastic. Applying too much tint (particularly tint lightener) in too great an area can defeat the object of the method and give a patchy result.

## Shimmer lights

This has the same effect as painted lights. Shampoo and towel dry the hair thoroughly then comb into the desired style with gel, using a wide toothed comb. This will create 'tram-lines' in the direction of the hairstyle. Using a tint at least two shades lighter and of a brighter tone than the natural colour, apply carefully along the raised lines with a fine artist's brush or a tinting gun.

   This method can be used all over the head or just on certain areas, depending upon the effect desired.

## Colour flashes

This technique can be used on its own or in conjunction with other techniques. it is equally effective on long, short, curly or straight hair.

   A fine or thick band around the front hairline is lightened with a tint lightener. If a bright colour is required the band is pre-bleached to the degree of lightness required and then a permanent tint is applied to this area. Similarly, after banding, a semi-permanent colour can be applied all over the whole head to brighten all of the hair and create a lighter tone of the same colour at the front.

## Points to remember

1  Use zig-zag partings to soften the demarcation line.
2  Colour flashes can be used in conjunction with fine highlights of the same colour through the back of the head to give added interest or to emphasise and soften the front hairline.
3  Another use of colour flashing is to lighten the weight of a heavy forward fringe. Take out a section at the front hairline of the fringe (zig-zag parting) about 10–20 mm (⅜–¾") wide, and use a tint lightener in this area. When all of the fringe is combed forward, the darker back section of the fringe will blend with the front section, creating a wispier, lighter effect.

## Scrunching

This gives a good effect on either long or short curly hairstyles but is not suitable for long straight styles. This quick and easy technique adds colour and depth to the ends of the hair, thus emphasising the outline of the hairstyle.

   The hair is shampooed then rough-dried into shape. Mix the desired shade of tint (usually tint lightener). The operator must wear rubber gloves. The tint is then spread evenly onto the palms of the rubber gloves and the ends of the hair are squeezed or 'scrunched' between the fingers; this deposits the tint on the ends of the hair only. Apply throughout the head, or wherever required.

## Points to remember

1  If the hair is longer and tends to flop, backcomb the hair thoroughly at the root in the areas that require scrunching, then carefully lacquer the roots with a fine hairspray. This will prevent the tint from running or flopping on to the root area.
2  More than one shade of tint can be used, depending upon the result required.
3  Bleach may also be used in preference to tint, but care must be taken only to lighten a few shades. When bleach is developed and removed, a semi-permanent tint can be applied over the whole head to give light and darker tones of the same colour (*see* p 304).
4  This method is excellent for the client who enjoys changing their hair colour frequently or for brightening dull hair during the winter months. Because only the ends of the hair are tinted or bleached lighter, they are soon removed by cutting.

## Highlighting

Highlighting gives a very natural effect, particularly on lighter hair. Fine streaks are pulled through a streaking cap and bleach is applied. When the hair has been lifted sufficiently, the bleach is removed and a full head permanent or semi-permanent tint is applied. An alternative method after removing the bleach is to weave out more fine strands of hair over both the previously bleached and the natural, virgin hair. A tint lightener is applied to these strands which are then wrapped in tin foil or plastic. This method produces a much lighter overall result.

## Lowlights

In this case, a number of lighter and/or darker colours than the natural base shade are used on fine streaks of hair to produce a natural colour movement. It is particularly useful on grey hair as an alternative to a full head permanent tint. Lowlights blend the white hairs with the natural coloured hair and eliminate the need to retouch the roots every four weeks as with permanent tints, it is also much easier to return the client to their natural colour if they so wish.

Lowlighting can also produce good results on bleached or very light hair using toning colours to put darker toning lights in the hair.

One to three colours can be used and they are applied either using a streaking cap or tin foil in the same manner as for highlighting.

## Points to remember

*When highlighting/lowlighting with tin foil*
1 The tint should be at least two shades lighter than the natural base shade when a lighter result is required.
2 Two shades of tint may be used instead of one, in which case the colours are alternated up the sections.
3 For subtle effects, the colours should tone and complement each other.
4 Faded red hair is given new vibrancy if gold and bright red shades (mixed as tint lighteners) are used to lowlight the hair. The colours may appear extremely bright on the shade chart, but as they are only applied to fine strands of hair they blend with the natural hair colour to give a brighter but subtle effect.
5 The tin foil/plastic method of highlighting/lowlighting is more time-consuming but it gives a far superior result on long hair.

*When highlighting/lowlighting with the cap*
1 Remember to comb the hair in the direction of the finished hairstyle before placing the cap on the head.
2 Take only fine strands of hair, otherwise the final result could be striped.
3 Check that there is no seepage of bleach (or tint) through the holes of the cap onto the scalp, otherwise the result will be patchy.

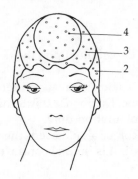

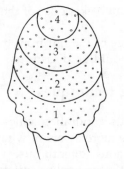

**Fig 15.23**

# Tortoiseshell lowlights

This technique gives a richer effect than the usual lowlights and is suitable for any length of hair.

Three to four different colours are used, ranging from one shade darker to two to three shades lighter than the natural base shade. The different colours are applied separately and alternately to fine woven streaks of hair that have either been pulled through a streaking cap or woven with foil. A variation on this method, although it does not give the same effect, is to use the shades in bands of colour from the nape up towards the front (*see* Fig 15.23). The lightest shade is usually used on the front and the darkest shade at the nape.

# Glimmering (polishing)

This is a very quick technique for any length of hair, but particularly good on very short nape hair where it is difficult to use other techniques.

Comb the hair into style. Take a piece of tin foil or cellophane and paint the surface with the chosen shade of tint. Hold the tin foil or cellophane in both hands and allow it to touch the ends of the hair, then gently stroke backwards and forwards in a polishing motion in the direction of the style. Pull away and repeat over the whole head or just the areas that will emphasise the style.

## Points to remember

1  Do not be afraid to use bold colours as this technique gives a subtle effect.
2  Do not become too enthusiastic and cover all of the hair – it is usually just the ends of the hair that are tinted.
3  Polish the hair gently otherwise the tint may be inadvertently placed where it is not required.

## Slicing or tramming

A very dramatic effect can be produced with this technique and it is a very bold method of colouration.

Comb the hair into style and decide which area of the head requires emphasising (slicing usually looks more effective on the front section of the head). Section the remaining hair away from this area. Take a mesh of hair about the size of a perm rod from the area to be coloured and apply the tint to the mesh. Wrap in tin foil or cling film then leave out a fine 5 mm (¼") section and take the next section in the same manner as before. Continue across the area to be covered, tinting a section and leaving a section until completed. Leave to develop.

## Points to remember

1 More than one colour may be used depending upon the desired result.

2 Because the hair is not woven the colour is far more dense in certain areas and therefore more dramatic. Do not use this technique on clients who wish to have subtle colouration only.

3 The brighter and more vibrant the colour shade used, the more dramatic the effect will be, particularly if it is in total contrast with the client's own hair.

4 Work methodically from one side of the area to the other. The fine sections that do not require tinting can be kept out of the way by winding on a perm rod.

5 Always ensure that there is no seepage of the tint from the tin foil or cling film, otherwise the results could be disastrous.

## Precautions for fashion colouring techniques

1 Introduce the client to colour with subtle colouration. Once they have gained confidence they will become more aware of what the salon has to offer and be willing to be more adventurous.

2 Use colour as an extension of the client's personality, but do not use too bright or very dark colours on older clients, it can be ageing.

3 When a subtle effect is required always look at the natural base shade carefully, there are usually golden or reddish glints to be seen that can be emphasised and highlighted. When using two or more colours on the hair try to keep within the same colour tones and use different depths of these tones, e.g. red tones, gold tones, beige tones etc. This will produce a more natural effect.

4 Do not be afraid to experiment with more than one technique on one head. With confidence, the operator will develop his/her own personal techniques.

5 When using tin foil to add lights to the hair, ensure that there is no seepage at the roots by wrapping a doubled strip of tin foil round the packet at the root.

6 Always discard rubber streaking caps when holes become too large. The bleach or tint can seep through these holes onto the scalp and hair with disastrous results.

7 Some of the fashion tinting techniques are so quick that it is a great temptation to tint more of the hair than necessary. Remember that it is better to apply to too few areas than too many. More highlights, slices, etc., can be added but they could prove time-consuming to remove.

8 The main mistake when highlighting hair is to weave or pull the meshes of hair too thickly. This can give an unsightly striped effect and make the hair so light overall that a regrowth can soon be seen.

9 Always advise the client on the after-care of their colouration. The condition of the hair is of prime importance, as tinted hair only looks good when it is healthy. The client will also need advice on

the upkeep of their colour and on how often salon visits will be necessary.

## Summary

The natural colour of hair is determined by the colour mixture of the light it reflects. Tinting hair involves using the colouring pigments in hair dyes to alter the hair colour. The pigment molecules coat the hair shaft and are relatively easy to wash away. They can penetrate the hair cortex and produce a permanent (or semi-permanent) tint. There are a variety of different hair dyes which can be grouped into non-permanent and permanent dyes.

*Non-permanent types include:*

Temporary rinses, which only coat the cuticle, commonly contain an 'azo' dye, e.g. parahydroxyazobenzene, and are produced as a concentrated liquid, coloured setting lotions, gels and mousses and temporary toners. They are all easy to apply but extra care is required with porous hair, and it is important that the client's clothing be protected.

Temporary lighteners are often classed as dyes, but in reality these are weak bleaches which gradually lighten the hair. Temporary rinses may be applied by aerosol (and these often contain minute metal particles). Care must be taken, as these metals may be incompatible with hydrogen peroxide.

Semi-permanent dyes last about six to eight shampoos and contain 'nitro' compounds, e.g. 2-nitro 1,4-phenylenediamine. Semi-permanent dyes have a limited colour range but have a variety of uses in the salon and are widely used. The client should be protected by a tinting gown and dark towel, and by the use of barrier cream around the hairline. If a 'para' compound is being applied then a skin test should be carried out.

Permanent dyes include the vegetable, inorganic and the synthetic organic types of dye. The inorganic, metallic dyes coat the hair with a metal deposit. A major problem is that some of the metals act as a catalyst on hydrogen peroxide when this is used in another hairdressing operation. The very rapid decomposition of the peroxide produces heat and can seriously damage the hair. It is important, therefore, to carry out an incompatibility test on a small sample of the client's hair before carrying out any operation which involves hydrogen peroxide.

The synthetic organic group include the 'para' dyes, e.g. paraphenylenediamine, and these work by small, colourless dye molecules passing through the hair cuticle into the cortex. These are then 'developed' into larger, coloured molecules by oxidation with hydrogen peroxide. These large molecules are trapped in the hair shaft and produce a permanent colour change. These dyes are used both in tint lightener and covering techniques. Due to the possibility of sensitisation to the 'para' compounds producing contact dermatitis, it is important that the client has a skin test 24–48 hours before the dye is used and that the hairdresser wears protective rubber gloves. A strand test (or test cutting) can be used to assess hair condition and the action of the dye on a sample of hair.

Colour selection should be carried out using a shade chart and a number of factors, e.g. porosity and quantity of white hair present need to be considered. This is important in matching a regrowth on previously tinted hair, and in a full-head application. When unwanted colour tones are produced, a knowledge of adding other colours to mask this discolouration is important. Colour triangles can be used to select suitable colours. There are a number of faults that can occur in tinting and a series of practical steps that can be taken to remedy these.

With colour removal, reduction or oxidation methods may be used. It is important to carry out a strand test before commencing this operation.

Fashion colouring techniques are a progression from the basic techniques and include:

- block colouring
- painted lights (flying colours)
- shimmer lights
- colour flashes
- scrunching
- highlighting (with foil or cap)
- tortoiseshell highlights
- lowlights
- glimmering
- slicing (tramming).

## Self-assessment questions

1  Name two natural vegetable dyes. What advantages do these dyes have over other types of hair dye?
2  List two methods used to allow dyes to penetrate more rapidly into the hair cortex.
3  Why is the hair porosity an important factor when using a colour rinse?
4  What is meant by a dye being 'incompatible' with hydrogen peroxide?
5  Why is it inadvisable to use either a semi-permanent or temporary rinse that is lighter in colour than the client's natural base shade?
6  If a client requires both a perm and a semi-permanent tint why is it necessary to perm the hair before carrying out the tint?
7  What is 'compound' henna?

8 Outline the theory of the action of oxidation dyes.
9 List the factors important in making a colour selection.
10 Name two methods used in colour removal (decolouring).

## Practical assignment – Tinting

Calculating the percentage of white in the client's hair is quite difficult and requires practice. To help you to understand what each percentage looks like you are going to make a **percentage of white** chart.
   You will need:

- white wool and brown wool of any thickness
- large piece of card
- sellotape, pens and scissors.

(a) At the top of the card rule off a section for the heading then rule the remainder into 11 equal spaces. Label each space from 0% through to 100% as shown.

Percentage of white chart

| 0% | 10% | 20% | 30% | 40% | 50% | 60% | 70% | 80% | 90% | 100% |
|----|-----|-----|-----|-----|-----|-----|-----|-----|-----|------|
|    |     |     |     |     |     |     |     |     |     |      |

(b) Cut the wool into 5 cm (2") lengths. You will need 10 pieces of wool for each space and the pieces will be mixed to indicate the percentages of white.
(c) In the 0% column tape 10 pieces of brown wool. In 10% column tape 9 pieces of brown wool and 1 white, increasing the amount of white in each column to show the percentage e.g. 70% will be 7 pieces of white wool and 3 pieces of brown etc. Therefore in the 100% column you will have 10 pieces of white wool.
(d) Make sure that you mix the white and brown wools together before taping them flat into place so that you can easily see and count the percentages.

# 16 BLEACHING

Bleaching is a process which lightens the shade of the hair by lightening or decolourising the colouring pigments in the hair shaft. The two main pigments are melanin and pheomelanin, which are found as tiny granules, mostly in the hair cortex, but some are in the outer hair cuticle. The bleaching process is a permanent lightening of these natural pigments and cannot be removed by shampooing.

## Basic chemistry of bleaching

### Decolourising the hair pigments

The two major pigments are melanin (which is a dark brown to black colour) and pheomelanin (which is a yellow to red colour). Melanin in particular (pheomelanin is more resistant) can be lightened in shade by the action of atoms of oxygen. Oxygen gas in the air consists of molecules of oxygen (symbol: $O_2$). Each of these molecules is made up of two atoms of oxygen joined together by chemical bonds. The type of oxygen which produces bleaching consists of single atoms of oxygen, not the molecules of oxygen gas. These single atoms are very reactive, and oxygen in this form is called nascent oxygen (symbol: O:). Nascent oxygen will link to any substance capable of accepting it and this adding of oxygen to a substance is called oxidation. The substance providing the nascent oxygen is known as the oxidising agent and whatever accepts this oxygen is described as having been oxidised. In bleaches of all types the oxidising agent is the active ingredient in the bleach and it is the hair pigments which are oxidised.

The bleaching process in chemical terms is shown in Fig 16.1 and can be summarised as:

1 the oxidising agent(s) in the bleach break down, releasing nascent oxygen (*see* Fig 16.1 (*a*))

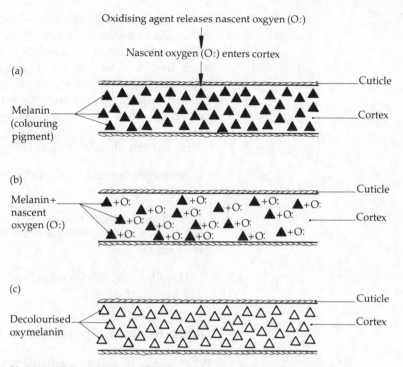

Fig 16.1 The sequence of events in chemical bleaching of the hair

2  this nascent oxygen penetrates the hair shaft and decolourises the pigments as follows (*see* Fig 16.1 (*b*), (*c*))

*Melanin*     +  *Nascent oxygen*  →  *Oxidised melanin*
*(natural*         *(from oxidising*      *(which, if*
*hair*             *agents in*            *sufficiently oxidised,*
*pigment)*         *bleach)*              *becomes colourless)*

This decolourisation can be seen when bleaching black hair, as a series of colour changes as the pigment is increasingly oxidised. These are:

*Black → Brown → Red → Orange → Yellow → Pale yellow → White*

The main oxidising agent used in bleaches is hydrogen peroxide (formula: $H_2O_2$), which can break down (or decompose) to release nascent oxygen.

## Hydrogen peroxide ($H_2O_2$)

This is an effective bleaching agent which releases nascent oxygen which can then bind to the hair pigments and lighten their colour. This ability to act as an oxidising agent is also used in:

1  'neutralising' or 'normalising' perms, where the nascent oxygen rebuilds the disulphide linkages in the hair, thus 'fixing' the perm;

2 developing oxidation tints, where the nascent oxygen converts the small, colourless tint molecules into larger, coloured ones.

Hydrogen peroxide is colourless and odourless and looks very much like its close relative, water ($H_2O$). The difference is that hydrogen peroxide has an 'extra' atom of oxygen in its molecule making it $H_2O_2$, compared with water which is $H_2O$. Because of this 'extra' atom of oxygen, the hydrogen peroxide molecule is unstable and will easily break down or decompose and release the 'extra' oxygen atom as nascent oxygen, this is written out as:

$$Hydrogen\ peroxide \rightarrow Water + Nascent\ oxygen$$
$$H_2O_2 \rightarrow H_2O + O:$$

The nascent oxygen released will either link on to a substance and oxidise it, or will link with another atom of oxygen to form oxygen gas. That is:

$$O: + O: \rightarrow O_2\ (Oxygen\ gas)$$
$$2\ atoms\ of\ oxygen$$

## Using hydrogen peroxide in the salon

When using hydrogen peroxide it is important to know:

(*a*) the routine precautions
(*b*) how to dilute hydrogen peroxide to the strength needed in a particular operation.

## Routine precautions

Because of its chemical structure, hydrogen peroxide is an unstable chemical which will spontaneously (i.e. 'on its own') break down into water and oxygen gas. Manufactured hydrogen peroxide is made more stable by adding some acid to the reagent (salicylic or phosphoric acid) to give a final pH of about 5. Despite this, hydrogen peroxide is still unstable and will break down or decompose. This process happens rapidly in the presence of:

1 *Dust* – the tiny particles of dust in the air can cause rapid breakdown of hydrogen peroxide. To prevent this, the top of the container should be replaced immediately after use.
2 *Ultraviolet light and heat* – these accelerate the breakdown and, as both are present in sunlight, hydrogen peroxide should never be stored in a place liable to direct sunlight. A dark, cool place is recommended.
3 *Alkalis* – that is, soluble substances which produce a solution with a pH above 7. Alkalis are deliberately used to speed up the release of oxygen by hydrogen peroxide (ammonium hydroxide is often used). But if a strong alkali is mixed with strong hydrogen peroxide there is an explosively fast release of oxygen.

Other important precautions are:

4  Take care to keep the reagent off the skin, clothing and eyes. If it is splashed on to the skin or clothes, wash off immediately with lots of water. Similarly, if hydrogen peroxide gets into the eyes, wash out with lots of water and get medical help as soon as possible. Always wear rubber gloves when using hydrogen peroxide or preparations containing it. Take all precautions to protect the client.

5  Hydrogen peroxide reacts with metals and chemicals containing metallic salts, e.g. some hair dyes. Because of this, hydrogen peroxide should never be used on hair tinted with a metal-containing dye, and it is important to check a client's hair for this with an incompatibility test (*see* p 252). What happens is that the metal acts as a **catalyst** and causes a very rapid breakdown of hydrogen peroxide. The rapid oxidising action and the heat produced by this chemical reaction can seriously damage the hair.

6  When diluting hydrogen peroxide use **distilled** or **deionised** water (i.e. water with the chemicals normally found in ordinary tap water removed). These chemicals may cause the peroxide to break down rapidly and thus release its oxygen too quickly.

## Diluting hydrogen peroxide

Dilute means to 'water down', that is, to reduce the **strength** or **concentration** of a solution.

A solution is a substance (or substances) dissolved in a liquid. The substance which dissolves is called the **solute** and the liquid in which it dissolves is called the **solvent.** In most solutions used in hairdressing the solvent is water. The strength or concentration of a solution depends on how much solute is dissolved in a certain amount (or more properly a certain volume) of the solvent. A common method of expressing the concentration is a percentage (%), that is, the number of parts of solute (measured as a weight or volume) in 100 parts of solvent.

## Strength or concentration of hydrogen peroxide

There are two alternative methods of expressing the strength, or more properly, the concentration of hydrogen peroxide solutions. These are:

- volume strength (or vol. strength); the units are vols
- percentage strength expressed as a '% solution'.

### Volume strength

This refers to the amount or volume of oxygen gas which will be released if a particular amount of hydrogen peroxide is completely broken down to oxygen and water. The stronger the solution the more oxygen it can release, so the higher the vol. strength. This method of expressing the concentration is closely linked to the use of hydrogen peroxide as an oxidising agent because the higher the vol. strength the more nascent oxygen it can release, so the faster and more complete the oxidation.

To calculate the amount of oxygen that could be released, the amount of hydrogen peroxide involved is multiplied by its volume strength. For example:

(*a*) How much oxygen will be released by the complete breakdown of 5 ml of 20 vol. hydrogen peroxide?

$$\textit{Amount of oxygen (ml)} = \textit{Amount of peroxide} \times \textit{Vol. strength}$$
$$= 5 \times 20$$
$$= 100 \textit{ ml of oxygen}$$

(*b*) What volume of oxygen will be released by the complete decomposition of 10 ml of 60 vol. hydrogen peroxide?

$$\textit{Volume of oxygen (ml)} = \textit{Volume of peroxide} \times \textit{Vol. strength}$$
$$= 10 \times 60$$
$$= 600 \textit{ ml of oxygen}$$

Try to solve the following (answers on p. 289):
What volume of oxygen will be released by the complete decomposition of:

1   6 ml of 10 vol. peroxide?
2   15 ml of 40 vol. peroxide?

## Percentage strength

This refers to the quantity of hydrogen peroxide as a percentage (%) of the total volume of the solution, the rest being water. There is a relationship between 'volume' and percentage strength as laid out in Table 16.1 below.

**Table 16.1**

| Volume strength (vol.) | Percentage strength (%) |
| --- | --- |
| 100 | 30 |
| 60 | 18 |
| 40 | 12 |
| 20 | 6 |
| 10 | 3 |

If one of these can be remembered, perhaps that 10 vol. = 3%, then the others can be calculated from this reference. For example, 60 vol. is six times stronger than 10. 10 vol. = 3%, therefore 60 vol. = 6 × 3 = 18%.

## Peroxometer

This is used to measure directly the strength of a peroxide solution (but cannot be used for cream peroxide) if there are doubts as to its actual strength, e.g. after a long period of storage. The peroxometer consists of a weighted float with the strength of peroxide marked on it as a scale. The stronger the peroxide the higher the float rises, because the density of the liquid is higher.

# How to dilute hydrogen peroxide

Hydrogen peroxide is often supplied to salons in strengths far greater than that required for hairdressing operations. It can often be 60 vol. (18%); this is far too strong to use on hair and will cause burns on the skin. Therefore, hydrogen peroxide must be diluted before use and it is important that the dilution is carried out accurately in order to finish with the correct strength and volume needed.

The strength of the solution to be diluted is known; so what needs to be worked out is how much (or what volume) of this original solution needs to be mixed with how much (or what volume) of water to finish with the strength and amount of peroxide required.

The method for doing this is broken down into steps using the following example: a hairdresser wishes to make 120 ml of 20 vol. (6%) hydrogen peroxide from a 60 vol. (18%) solution. How much 60 vol. (18%) peroxide and how much water must be mixed?

*Step 1*

$$\text{\textit{Fraction of final solution which will be original solution}} = \frac{\text{\textit{Strength of final solution}}}{\text{\textit{Strength of original solution}}}$$

$$\textit{Fraction} = \frac{20}{60} \left(\text{\textit{or}} \ \frac{6}{18} \ \textit{if \% used}\right) = \frac{1}{3}$$

Therefore, one-third (or one part in three) of the final solution will be the original, 60 vol. (18%) solution.

*Step 2*

*Volume of original = Fraction from Step 1 × Final volume required solution to use*

$$\textit{Volume} = \frac{1}{3} \times 120 = \frac{120}{3} = 40 \ ml$$

So, 40 ml of 60 vol. (18%) peroxide is needed.

*Step 3*

$$\text{\textit{Volume of water needed for dilution (ml)}} = \text{\textit{Final volume of solution (ml)}} - \text{\textit{Volume of original solution to use (ml)}}$$

$$\text{\textit{Volume of water (ml)}} = 120 - 40 = 80 \ ml$$

So, to make 120 ml of 20 vol. (6%) solution from a 60 vol. (18%)

solution, the hairdresser must mix 80 ml of water with 40 ml of 60 vol. (18%) peroxide solution.

Try this method to calculate the following (answers below).

(a) A hairdresser has 60 vol. (18%) hydrogen peroxide as a stock solution and wishes to make 100 ml of 15 vol. (4½%) solution. What volume of the stock solution and what volume of water should they use?

(b) What volume of 60 vol. (18%) hydrogen peroxide solution is needed to make up 240 ml of a 10 vol. (3%) solution?

*Answers*
p. 287

1  $6 \times 10 = 60$ ml oxygen gas
2  $15 \times 40 = 600$ ml oxygen gas

(a)  $\dfrac{6 \times \overset{1}{\cancel{100}}}{\underset{1}{\cancel{100}}} = 6$ ml hydrogen peroxide

(b)  $\dfrac{9 \times \overset{3}{\cancel{150}}}{\underset{2}{\cancel{100}}} = \dfrac{27}{2} = 13½$ ml hydrogen peroxide

(c)  $\dfrac{3 \times \overset{3}{\cancel{300}}}{\underset{1}{\cancel{100}}} = 9$ ml hydrogen peroxide

(a) Step 1: $\dfrac{15}{60}$ (or if % used $\dfrac{4½}{18}$) $= \dfrac{1}{4}$

Step 2: $\dfrac{1}{4} \times 100 = 25$ ml

Step 3: $100 - 25 = 75$ ml
Therefore use 25 ml original solution and 75 ml water.

(b) Step 1: $\dfrac{10}{60}$ (or if % used $\dfrac{3}{18}$) $= \dfrac{1}{6}$

Step 2: $\dfrac{1}{6} \times 240 = 20$ ml

There is no need for step 3 as the problem only asks for the volume of peroxide to be used. The answer is 20 ml of original solution.

# Types of bleach

Bleaches can be divided into two categories:

1  brighteners or brightening shampoos
2  alkaline bleaches, which include:

(*a*)  simple bleach
(*b*)  oil bleach
(*c*)  powder bleach
(*d*)  emulsion or gel bleach.

All types contain an oxidising agent or agents, mainly hydrogen peroxide, and work by the oxidising agent releasing nascent oxygen which then binds to the melanin pigment in the hair and lightens (or 'lifts' or decolourises) the pigment. 'Boosters' or 'activators' as they are sometimes called can be used to supply additional nascent oxygen and this speeds up and makes more complete the bleaching action.

## Boosters or activators

These can be used with emulsion bleaches. They increase the speed of the bleaching as they are oxidising agents which can release extra nascent oxygen which adds to that being produced by the hydrogen peroxide. Chemically, the active ingredients are usually a mixture of ammonium and potassium persulphate. Ammonium persulphate breaks down rapidly releasing its nascent oxygen and is therefore fast acting. Potassium persulphate breaks down more slowly and therefore acts more slowly.

Boosters or activators can only be used with hydrogen peroxide because they cannot physically break up the pigment granules in the hair. Hydrogen peroxide can do this and the boosters then speed the **decolourisation** of the pigment once the granules break up.

## Brighteners or brightening shampoos

These will lighten the hair a few shades only and are used to:

- lighten blond hair that has grown darker with age
- brighten 'mousy' hair
- make resistant hair more likely to tint.

It is applied over the whole head and the rate of lightening is sensitive to body heat, that is, the nearer the scalp, the warmer the conditions, so the faster the bleaching action. Consequently, it must be removed before any appreciable lift of colour is obtained, otherwise the hair nearest the scalp will be lighter than that further away. The bleaching action takes place mostly in the cuticle, where there are relatively few pigment granules (most being in the cortex), so the amount of lightening is relatively small. Approximately 10 vol. (3%) hydrogen peroxide is used and a typical list of ingredients is:

- 20 ml of 20 vol. (6%) hydrogen peroxide
- 20 ml of hot or warm water
- 10 ml of shampoo.

The shampoo is added to improve the contact by breaking the surface tension between the solution and the hair and to condition the hair.

Commercially produced lighteners contain an organic acid (e.g. tartaric acid) which stabilises the preparation and gives a pH of 4.0 to 4.5.

## Method of application

1 Shampoo the hair as normal.
2 Apply the solution in a second shampoo. Lather up and leave for approximately ten minutes.
3 Rinse thoroughly.

## Alkaline bleaches

These are usually made up immediately before use, the alkali used being **ammonium hydroxide** (often called **ammonia solution**) in most types of alkaline bleaches.

## Ammonium hydroxide (ammonia solution)

This is supplied to salons in a concentration (or strength) of 35% (that is 35 parts of ammonia in 100 parts of the solution). This is often expressed as the density of the liquid and this solution has a density value of 0.880 – this is described as 'eight-eighty ammonia.'

*Precautions*
(*a*) Ammonia solution, especially when heated, will give off large amounts of choking ammonia fumes.
(*b*) If 0.880 ammonia solution is mixed with 100 vol. (30%) hydrogen peroxide, oxygen is given off explosively quickly.

*Disadvantages*
(*a*) Excess ammonia creates too much swelling of the hair shaft leaving it in a porous, weakened state.
(*b*) Traces of the alkali left in the hair cortex may result in a continued bleaching action which lasts for 3–4 months, with a continual deterioration in the hair strength and condition. This process, called **creeping oxidation** can eventually result in a large amount of hair breakage. It can be rectified by applying mild acid cream conditioning rinse, where the acid penetrates into the cortex and neutralises the remaining alkali.

## Action of the alkalis used in bleaching

The alkaline pH produced by mixing the alkali with the oxidising agent has two main effects:

1 It causes the hair to swell which helps the nascent oxygen released by the oxidising agent to penetrate the cortex and decolourise the melanin granules.

2 It neutralises the acids added to hydrogen peroxide which makes this chemical break down rapidly, releasing nascent oxygen. In addition, ammonium hydroxide acts as a catalyst and therefore accelerates further the breakdown of hydrogen peroxide.

## Types of alkaline bleaches

1 *Simple bleach* – will lighten the hair a few shades but tends to leave the hair appearing 'brassy', the final colour being dependent on the amount of the red/yellow natural pigment, pheomelanin, in the hair. Care must be taken when mixing because, if mixed incorrectly, the high pH value can cause hair breakage and burns. This type of bleach was originally used for pre-bleaching prior to tinting as it does not leave a chemical deposit on the hair, so the tint could be applied without first removing the bleach.

Modern tint lighteners have almost eliminated the need for pre-bleaching, except in the case of very resistant hair.

A simple bleach consists of 20 vol. (6%) hydrogen peroxide mixed with a few drops of 0.880 ammonia solution.

2 *Oil bleach* – is produced as a liquid, and really the name is inaccurate because modern 'oil' bleaches contain no oil or bleach. Originally, an oil called 'Turkey red oil' was used, but this has been replaced by a **thickener** which has the ability to form a viscous gel when mixed with hydrogen peroxide (which actually does the bleaching). This can then change into a mobile liquid during brushing on to the hair and then change back into the viscous gel to prevent dripping once applied to the hair (this is the same principle as used in 'non-drip' paints). Despite these changes, these bleaches may run down the hair shaft during the application and make overlapping when carrying out a retouch almost inevitable. In addition to the thickener, an ammonia solution is present in an oil bleach and has functions as described on p. 291.

Oil bleaches lift the hair colour by relatively few shades and tend to produce 'golden' tones in the hair.

3 *Powder bleach* – consists of two powders, one being **magnesium carbonate**, which forms the paste but does not take part in the bleaching process; the other being **ammonium carbonate** or **sodium acetate** which makes the pH slightly alkaline at a value of 8.5. The powder is mixed with hydrogen peroxide to form a creamy 'paste-like' mixture. If the mixture is too thick, however, it will not coat the hair evenly and will not penetrate the hair meshes. While the mixture is developing, a crust is formed on the bleach which slows down evaporation and allows more action of natural heat from the scalp.

Modern powder bleaches are now mainly used for bleached

streaks and highlights as they have a high degree of lift and will usually lighten dark hair to blond.

4 *Emulsion bleach* – is used in conjunction with boosters/activators and also has a high degree of 'lift'. When mixed, the emulsion bleach has a gel-like consistency which makes it easier to apply for a full-head bleach. The emulsion itself contains an alkali, a thickening agent, conditioners and modifiers.

Table 16.2 gives a summary of the different types of bleach.

**Table 16.2**

| Bleach type | Ingredients | Degree of lift |
|---|---|---|
| Simple bleach | Hydrogen peroxide + ammonia 0.880 | 1–3 shades |
| Brightener shampoo | 20 vol. (6%) hydrogen peroxide + water + liquid shampoo | 1–2 shades |
| Oil bleach | Ammonium hydroxide + thickener (mixed with hydrogen peroxide) | 2–4 shades |
| Powder bleach | Magnesium carbonate + ammonium carbonate (or sodium acetate) mixed with hydrogen peroxide | Will usually lighten from dark to blond |
| Emulsion/gel bleach | Alkali + thickeners + conditioners + modifiers, used in conjunction with activators (mixed with hydrogen peroxide) | Will usually lighten from dark to blond |

## Uses of bleaching

1  to lighten previously unbleached hair;
2  to pre-lighten prior to tinting;
3  to lighten or remove tint from hair;
4  to lift the cuticle scales slightly and make the hair more porous – therefore, resistant hair becomes more susceptible to tinting as it can penetrate into the cortex more easily;
5  to break down any resistant patches before a tint is applied;
6  to give highlights and streaks to the hair;
7  in conjunction with tint to produce extra hair colouring techniques.

# Preparation for bleaching

Before commencing a full-head bleach it is often wiser and safer to take a strand test of the hair when the client books the appointment, particularly if it is a new client whose hair is unfamiliar to the operator. A strand test taken and completed before the commencement of the bleach application can divert many disasters and also gives the client confidence in the operator's professionalism.

The strand test is taken from the front, crown and nape areas, as these areas can vary in porosity. If the client has been treating their own hair with chemicals, these may not have been evenly applied to the hair or may be incompatible with the bleaching agent to be used.

## Strand test method for bleach

A small amount of the chosen type of bleach is mixed with the required strength of hydrogen peroxide and is then applied to the hair cuttings. Always choose the mildest bleach and the lowest strength of peroxide possible to achieve the degree of lift required, as the final condition of the hair must be of paramount importance to the operator. The cuttings are then left to develop until the desired amount of lift has been achieved. Carefully rinse the cuttings then dry them and assess the results.

Record the results on a record card to ascertain:

1  the development time
2  the final elasticity and tensile strength of the treated hair
3  that the correct type of bleach has been used for the required amount of lift
4  that the correct volume strength of hydrogen peroxide has been used for the required amount to lift
5  that there are no incompatible chemicals present on the hair shaft
6  that the required amount of lift has and may be achieved.

A skin test is not required before bleaching unless the client has an extremely sensitive skin (strong bleach mixtures can burn sensitive skin), or in rare cases, the client may have an allergy to ammonia. If in any doubt, apply a skin test as for tinting, but using bleach instead of tint.

## Preparation of operator and client

Bleaching agents will remove colour from clothing; therefore, adequate measures must be taken to protect both the operator and the client.

The operator should wear rubber gloves to protect the hands and a tinting apron to protect the salon dress or overall.

The client's clothing should be protected in the same manner as for tinting, with a tinting gown to cover the clothing and preferably the chair also. The towel should be tucked firmly into the nape to protect collars etc., and also to prevent the towel from slipping during the bleaching process. A cotton wool strip or neck strip placed at the nape is an added protection. A disposable plastic cape to cover the gown, towel and back of the chair prevents any bleach splashing on to these areas and removing the colour.

## Preparation of materials and equipment

All materials and equipment should be assembled, prior to the bleaching application, on the flat top of a trolley that can easily be wiped clean afterwards.

## Preparation of the bleach

Bleach is usually mixed with hydrogen peroxide in a 2:1 ratio, i.e. 2 parts hydrogen peroxide to 1 part bleach, unless otherwise stated by the manufacturer. Measure out the required amount of bleach into a non-metallic bowl then add the hydrogen peroxide slowly while mixing. Always follow the manufacturer's instructions.

## Application of a full-head bleach

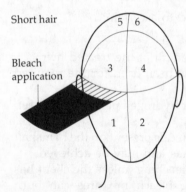

Short hair

Bleach application

Long hair

Bleach application

Fig 16.2

1  Assemble equipment and materials.
2  Protect the client's clothing with tinting gown, towels, etc. Ensure that the towel is tucked firmly into the nape.
3  Disentangle the hair and check scalp for cuts and abrasions.
4  Ensure that the client's hair is free from grease or heavy lacquer. If this is so, shampoo gently with a mild soapless (or lacquer removing) shampoo, then dry.
5  Divide the head into six major sections (forehead to nape, ear to ear across the top and ear to ear across the back).
6  Apply barrier cream around the hairline, ensuring that it is applied to the skin only.
7  Mix the bleach with the hydrogen peroxide, according to the manufacturer's instructions.
8  Commence application at the nape (unless more resistant elsewhere) and apply the bleach mixture evenly to the mid-lengths and points, if the hair is short, mid-lengths only if the hair is long (see Fig 16.2). Allow approximately 10 mm (½") untreated hair at the roots to counteract the body heat which will develop the bleach more quickly. In the case of long hair, the points are usually more porous and will therefore develop more quickly.
9  Continue applying the bleach in this manner through from sections 1 to 6, in the correct order. Care must be taken to prevent the bleached areas touching the roots, otherwise the result will be patchy. To avoid this, strips of cotton wool may be placed between the sub-sections.

10   When the application is complete, gently work the bleach into the hair with the fingers to ensure that the bleach has penetrated each mesh. Extreme care must be taken at this stage to prevent the bleach touching the root area. In the case of long hair the bleach is now applied to the points of the hair in the same order as before, i.e. commencing at the nape through to the front area, unless the hair is more resistant elsewhere.

11   Check through the application to ensure that all meshes are evenly and thoroughly covered.

12   Await bleach development, checking frequently by removing the bleach from a small strand of hair with a piece of damp cotton wool. If the hair is not the correct shade, re-apply bleach to the strand of hair that has been checked. When the desired shade has almost been reached, mix up a fresh bleach and apply to the root areas as quickly as possible (work in the same order as previously).

13   Check that all the hair has been completely and evenly covered by cross-checking across the sections. Gently lift the hair out from the head to allow the air to circulate.

14   Await development, checking frequently using the same method as before.

15   When the hair is an even shade throughout the entire length of the hair shaft, remove the bleach by rinsing thoroughly in tepid water. It is very important that all the bleach is completely removed from the hair.

16   Apply a mild acid balance or cream shampoo and massage the head gently. Rinse the hair thoroughly and repeat. Remember that the scalp may be very tender at this stage and excessive massage will cause discomfort to the client.

17   Apply a mild acid balance conditioner to counteract the alkalinity of the bleach and prevent the creeping oxidation described on p. 291. Rinse the hair thoroughly using warm water.

18   Towel dry the hair and disentangle. Treat the hair carefully at this stage because of its increased porosity and elasticity.

19   Apply a temporary rinse or toner to neutralise any unwanted golden or brassy tones. If a toner containing a 'para' compound is used the client must have had a skin test 24–48 hours previously to ensure that there is no allergy to this type of tint.

20   Complete a record of work carried out and advise the client on after-care.

## Bleaching a regrowth

The bleaching of a regrowth requires far more skill and attention than the colouring of a regrowth because of the excessive damage that can be caused to the hair by bleaching agents incorrectly applied.

When carrying out a bleach retouch, the operator must take extra care not to overlap the bleach onto the previously treated hair as this could, at best, give a striped effect, and at worst could cause breakage of the hair.

The bleach must be applied quickly and evenly if an even result is to be achieved and must be forced well down to the scalp to prevent the appearance of tiny black pin-pricks at the roots. Each hair must be thoroughly covered with the bleach as any areas that are missed or overlooked will be clearly visible on the finished result.

Body heat has the effect of increasing the chemical activity close to the scalp; therefore the regrowth should not be allowed to exceed 10 mm (½"). This means that the client will require a retouch every three to four weeks, depending on the rate of hair growth. If the regrowth is greater than 10 mm (½") it is very difficult to achieve an even shade throughout the length of the hair shaft and it often results in a striped effect which is difficult to rectify.

## Method of application for a bleach retouch

Proceed as for a full-head bleach application, but apply the bleach to the regrowth area only. Do not overlap onto the previously bleached hair. When application is complete, check carefully across the sections to ensure an even coverage. Await development (this is complete when there is no demarcation line between the regrowth and the remaining hair). When the hair is the same shade throughout the length of the hair shaft, remove the bleach by rinsing thoroughly in warm water and applying a mild acid balance shampoo then a mild acid balance conditioner. Complete a record of the work carried out.

Special attention must be paid at all times to the sensitivity of the scalp, the porosity and elasticity of the hair both during and after bleaching. The application of heat to shorten the development time should be approached with caution as it could cause extra damage to the hair and scalp by opening the skin pores and swelling the hair too much.

## Contra-indications when bleaching

Do not proceed with the bleaching process in the following cases:

1 when the hair has been coated with a metallic substance, e.g. compound henna, hair colour restorers

2 if hair is overprocessed or excessively damaged, e.g. after over-perming

3 if the hair is extremely fine or fragile – use a very mild bleach only and test hair carefully beforehand

4 when any contagious or infectious diseases are present on the hair or scalp

5 when there are any severe cuts or abrasions on the scalp.

## Precautions and considerations when bleaching

1 Always take into consideration the porosity and tensile strength

of the hair before bleaching. Bleaching agents are strong chemicals that can damage the hair if used incorrectly, and the hair must be strong enough to withstand the treatment. If in doubt do a strand test.

2   Never use too high a volume strength of hydrogen peroxide on the hair, it can cause unnecessary damage.

3   Do not allow the regrowth to exceed 10 mm (½″), otherwise the result could be 'stripy', because of the effect of body heat at the scalp.

4   Use barrier cream around the hairline if the skin appears sensitive.

5   Remember to allow for the effect of body heat at the roots when commencing a full-head bleach application.

6   Work quickly and methodically when bleaching the hair – the quicker the application the more even the result (providing that the application is thorough and even).

7   Always check the application thoroughly by cross-checking the hair.

8   The application of heat, particularly a steamer, during processing should be approached with caution as it can make the bleach 'runny' and it could run down the hair shaft on to previously bleached hair.

9   Remove all the bleach when fully developed. Any traces of the bleach (an alkali) left on the hair could cause creeping oxidation.

10   Bleached hair is less elastic and more porous than untreated hair; therefore, it will require far more attention when conditioning, perming or tinting.

# Bleach toners

These are used to neutralise any unwanted golden tones produced by the bleaching process.

It is important to remember that even careful bleaching will damage the cuticle scales and in some cases creates a highly porous state. The biggest problem is that after bleaching the hair may have an *uneven* porosity, either along the hair, or throughout the entire head. Toners must therefore be applied with extra care, following the manufacturer's instructions, to avoid a patchy and uneven result.

## Types of toners

There are three main types:

- temporary
- semi-permanent
- permanent.

## Temporary toners

These are rinses that are applied to the hair after shampooing (*see* p 244). They usually last from one shampoo to the next. However, because of the highly porous nature of bleached hair there is often a colour build-up if these rinses are used continuously over a period of time. To correct this fault, apply the rinse to the root area only until the colour fades from the ends of the hair. it is preferable to apply the rinse with a tinting brush to ensure an even coverage.

## Semi-permanent toners

These toners last from one bleach retouch to the next, although when applied to bleached hair they can fade more quickly than when applied to untreated hair. Application should be made with a brush to the roots of the hair first as they are not as porous as the points of the hair. The manufacturer's instructions should be carefully followed (some manufacturers produce semi-permanent tints specifically designed for bleached hair).

Check the development of the application carefully. Because of the damage to the cuticle scales by the bleach, the toner is absorbed quickly but is also easily removed; therefore development may appear complete, but on rinsing the colour may be almost removed! Alternatively, the development may be rapid and if the toner is left in contact with the hair too long the finished result will be too dark.

A semi-permanent toner used regularly after each bleach retouch may create a colour build-up on the ends of the hair after a period of time. To rectify this, apply the toner to the root area only, then comb through to the ends of the hair, if and when necessary.

## Permanent toners

No toner used on bleached hair can be truly permanent. The degree of porosity of bleached hair causes any toner to fade quite quickly.

A permanent toner is usually a 'para' dye, which is mixed with 10 volume (3%) hydrogen peroxide. If this type of toner is used, a skin test is necessary because of the possibility of a reaction to the 'para' compound. Care must be taken not to damage the hair still further by the use of too high a volume strength of hydrogen peroxide with the tint.

# Highlighting

This gives a very natural effect and is far kinder to the hair than bleaching the full head. Retouching should only be required after three months and then only at the crown, front hairline and any parting. After a further three months, highlighting should be repeated on the roots of the entire head. Avoid the ends of the hair if it is already highlighted, otherwise the effect will be an overall bleached look.

There are many ways of highlighting the hair, depending on the base shade, length of hair and the hairstyle. Bleach can be streaked or painted onto the hair wherever a lighter effect is required. However, the two main methods for achieving an allover highlighted effect are the traditional cap method and weaving the hair with aluminium (tin) foil.

### Traditional cap method

Although this method does not have the accuracy of the weaving method, it has the advantage of being less time-consuming and is therefore a popular method with busy salons.

### Method of application

1  Assemble equipment and materials.
2  Comb hair into the position it is normally worn (if the hair is excessively greasy or heavily lacquered, shampoo it then dry thoroughly).
3  Fix the highlighting cap firmly over the head by pulling it over the head from the front.
4  Pull fine strands of hair through the holes in the cap with the crochet hook, starting at the front hairline and working through to the nape (*see* Fig 16.3).
5  When enough strands of hair have been pulled through, comb the strands gently with a wide toothed comb to ensure that no strand of hair is tangled or overlaps another.
6  Mix the bleach with the hydrogen peroxide to form a stiff paste to prevent the bleach from running down through the holes and causing 'spotting' at the roots.
7  Apply generously and evenly to the hair, but do not press the bleach onto the cap – it could be forced through the holes (*see* Fig 16.4).
8  Cover with a plastic, disposable cap to retain the body heat and await development. Apply heat if necessary to decrease the development time.
9  When the desired degree of lift is obtained, rinse thoroughly. Apply a small amount of conditioner to the highlights as this will allow the highlighting cap to be removed more easily.
10  Remove the highlighting cap. Shampoo the hair, rinse thoroughly and apply a mild acid balance conditioner.
11  Complete a record of the work carried out.

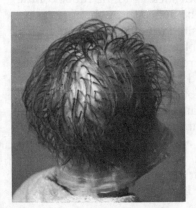

**Fig 16.3**

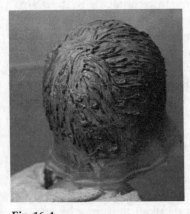

**Fig 16.4**

### Toning the hair after highlighting

When toning the hair after highlighting with a toner that is mixed with hydrogen peroxide, remember that the hydrogen peroxide could alter the natural base shade of the client. To prevent this, apply the toner to the highlights before the highlighting cap is removed, thus colouring only the highlights.

If using a semi-permanent toner without hydrogen peroxide, apply in same manner as above or remove the highlighting cap and apply the toner to the whole head.

## Precautions when highlighting with a cap

1  It is usual to pull only fine strands of hair through the cap. If the strands are too thick, it can give a striped effect, or alternatively the finished result can be too light, causing a definite regrowth to be seen within a few weeks.

2  Sprinkle talcum powder inside the cap before placing it over the client's head. It prevents the hair from sticking to the rubber of the cap and allows the strands of hair to be pulled through more easily.

3  Think carefully about the final desired result before commencing the application. It is possible to use bleach in conjunction with tint lighteners, e.g. the strands may be treated with bleach at the front of the head and a tint lightener used on the strands of hair at the back of the head to give a more subtle, shaded effect.

4  Do not highlight or streak the hair along any definite partings in the hairstyle. If the client does wear their hair with a parting, take a fine mesh of hair along this parting and section this area off before placing the cap over the head.

5  After pulling the strands of hair through the cap, comb the strands carefully to ensure that the hair is not tangled or bent at the roots.

6  A stronger solution of hydrogen proxide can be used for highlighting as the bleach does not come into contact with the scalp. The highest volume that can be safely used on the hair is 40 volume (12%), unless otherwise stated by the manufacturer.

7  Do not use a 'runny' bleach for highlighting as it can seep through the holes in the cap and cause 'spotting' at the roots.

8  Stroke the bleach on to the strands of hair, do not dab or force the bleach down on to the cap – the bleach could be forced through the holes.

9  Always discard any highlighting cap that has become perished, or when the holes become too large, otherwise the bleach will seep through the holes.

10  Always ensure that all the bleach is removed from the hair to prevent creeping oxidation. An acid balance conditioner used after rinsing helps to neutralise any traces of alkali that may be left on the hair.

11  Advise the client on the after-care of the highlights. The bleached strands of hair will be drier and more porous than the untreated hair; this must be allowed for if the client requires other chemical processes on the hair, e.g. perming.

## Weaving with aluminium (tin) foil

This method requires more time and effort, but the finished result is far more subtle than the cap method. The whole head can be woven with foil, or just certain areas (partial weaving) can be woven to accentuate and lighten specific parts of the head, e.g. crown or front areas.

The work should be completed as quickly as possible to prevent the first sections woven from becoming lighter than the other sections. If this should happen, remove the foil from the sections that are developed sufficiently and remove the bleach with water. The use of tint lighteners in place of bleach often gives a more subtle result − they do not lighten as quickly, nor do they take the hair as light as bleach.

## Sectioning the hair

Sectioning the hair prior to the application is very important as it allows the operator to work quickly and methodically through the head in the correct order. The hair is usually divided into fourteen sections but this depends on individual preference.

## Method of application for full-head highlights

1  Assess hair and scalp. Protect client's clothing and assemble equipment and materials.
2  Section the hair, making sure the partings are clean and accurate (*see* Fig 16.5 (*a*), (*b*)).
3  Mix the hydrogen peroxide with the bleach to form a stiff paste.
4  Starting at the nape, weave in and out of a fine mesh of hair with the tail end of the tail comb or pin-tail comb (*see* Fig 16.6).

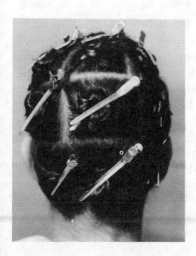

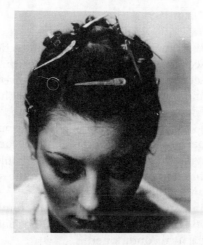

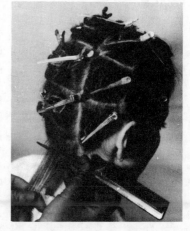

Fig 16.5 (a)          Fig 16.5 (b)          Fig 16.6

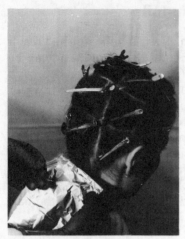

**Fig 16.7**

5   Place a strip of aluminium foil, non-shiny side next to and beneath the woven hair (*see* Fig 16.7).

6   Brush the bleach evenly on to the woven hair, making sure that all the strands are completely covered (*see* Fig 16.8).

7   Using the tail end of the tail comb, crease the foil then fold it over towards the root hair (*see* Fig 16.9).

8   Fold both sides of the foil in towards the centre, creasing the foil with the tail comb first, making a parcel (*see* Fig 16.10).

9   If necessary, fold another piece of foil into a long strip and wrap around the base of the parcel to prevent it slipping.

10   Continue weaving and wrapping up from the nape to the front of the hair frequently checking the first wrapped parcel for development.

11   The number of parcels depends on the thickness of the hair and the effect required. For the best results, the woven strands of hair should be very fine; if they are too thick it will give a striped effect.

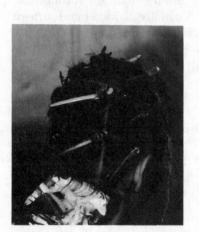

**Fig 16.8**

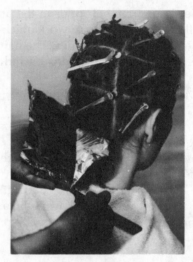

**Fig 16.9**

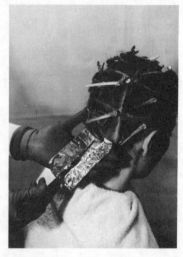

**Fig 16.10**

12   When weaving the front sections (*see* Fig 16.11) take a fine section of hair at the hairline, then weave the hair behind this section. If the actual hairline is woven the effect could be striped and there will be an obvious growth to be seen almost immediately. Figure 16.12 shows the completed application.

13   When the weaving and wrapping are complete, check the first parcel wrapped, and depending upon the length of time taken to wrap the rest of the head, this should now be lightened sufficiently.

14   Remove the foil parcels in the same order as they were placed on the head.

15   Rinse the hair thoroughly, removing every trace of the bleach.

16   Shampoo with a mild acid balance shampoo and apply mild acid balance conditioner.

17   Complete a record of work carried out.

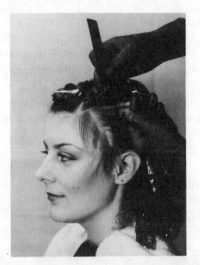

Fig 16.11

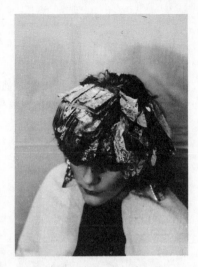

Fig 16.12

# Scrunch bleaching

This is a very quick and commercial method of adding lighter glints to the hair and is suitable for thicker hair, usually with some movement to the style.

Scrunch bleaching does not give the same effect as highlighting, since the hair is only lightened at the points and not throughout the length, but it can look very effective on darker as well as lighter hair, especially if used in conjunction with semi-permanent colours. No retouching is necessary – the bleached area has usually been cut from the hair after a couple of months when retouching would normally become necessary.

## Method of application

There are two main methods of application, one using two tinting brushes, the other using the hands only.

### Method 1 (two tinting brushes)

1  Assemble materials and equipment.
2  Comb the hair into style. On short hair it is usually the crown and front areas that require scrunching. On longer hair the entire head is usually scrunched, although this depends on the client's personal preference.
3  Backcomb thoroughly the areas to be scrunched (*see* Fig 16.13), pushing the hair well down to the roots to prevent the hair falling back on itself when the bleach is applied. Backcombing the hair also makes the final result less dense as some of the hair points will be omitted from the bleach.

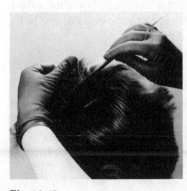

Fig 16.13

Figure 16.14 shows the completed area backcombed.

4 Using a fine hairspray, lacquer the roots of the backcombed hair.

5 Mix the hydrogen peroxide with the bleach to form a stiff paste.

6 Using two tinting brushes, apply the bleach to the points of the hair, making sure that both sides of the meshes are completely covered (*see* Fig 16.15).

Figure 16.16 shows the points of the hair coated with the bleach.

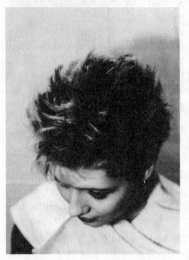

Fig 16.14

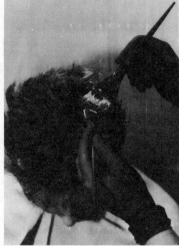
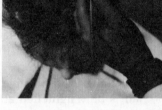
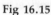

Fig 16.15

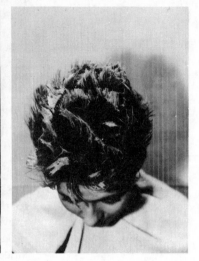

Fig 16.16

7 Allow the bleach to develop naturally, without heat. Do not allow the bleach to go too light, otherwise the contrast between the darker and the bleached hair will be too great.

8 When the hair has lightened sufficiently, gently comb out the backcombing and rinse the hair thoroughly. Apply an acid balance shampoo, rinse and condition with a mild acid balance conditioner.

9 If a semi-permanent colour is required, this should now be applied to the whole head in the normal manner. The final effect of this gives lighter tones of the same colour to the ends of the hair.

10 Complete a record of the work carried out.

## Method 2 (without brushes)

Proceed as for Method 1 but instead of applying the bleach with two tinting brushes, evenly spread the bleach onto the palms of the operator's gloves. Then scrunch the points of the hair where required with the fingers, imparting the bleach from the gloves onto the points of the hair. It is important to ensure that the points of the hair are kept lifted out from the scalp away from the root area.

Await bleach development and then proceed as for Method 1.

# Returning bleached hair to a natural colour (prepigmentation)

This is not as simple nor as straightforward as returning tinted hair to its natural colour.

During the bleaching process, the chemical action of the nascent oxygen liberated from the hydrogen peroxide causes the hair to progress through several colour changes, from the base shade of the hair to pale yellow or white. However, the red shade of pigment (produced by pheomelanin) is the most difficult colour to convert and there is usually a lot of this colour pigment present in the hair shaft. If brown pigment, which is a mixture of red + blue + yellow is added to the bleached hair, the hair absorbs the red from the brown pigment, leaving a green (blue + yellow) discolouration of the hair.

To avoid this discolouration, **prepigmentation** of the hair is necessary, using red colour particles.

## Method of prepigmentation

1  Take a strand test of the hair.
2  Ensure that the client has had a skin test if using a 'para' dye.
3  Assemble materials and equipment. Protect client's and operator's clothing.
4  Disentangle the hair and check for cuts and abrasions on the scalp.
5  Section hair into six major sections as for permanent tinting.
6  Apply a red semi-permanent tint using a brush, for greater precision, to the bleached areas only. It is preferable to use a semi-permanent that does not require the addition of hydrogen peroxide so that the hair is damaged as little as possible.
7  When the application is complete, check that the semi-permanent is evenly and thoroughly applied to all the bleached areas.
8  Leave to develop according to the manufacturer's instructions but check the development frequently with a swab of damp cotton wool.
9  When the development is complete, rinse the semi-permanent from the hair with warm water until the water runs clear.
10  Dry the hair and re-section into six as before.
11  Proceed then as for a normal full-head tint, using the shade of tint required but applying to the pre-pigmented areas only.
12  Complete a record of work carried out.
13  Advise the client on the after-care of the hair. Although the hair may appear to be the client's natural colour it must be emphasised that the hair will now probably be in a highly porous state due to all the chemicals that it has been subjected to. It will be necessary to treat the hair with conditioning and/or restructurant preparations until the treated hair has been removed by cutting. This could take 6–12 months depending on how short the client wears their hair. If the client requires other chemical processes on the hair, e.g.

perming, the porosity of the hair must be given due consideration when selecting the strength of reagent to use; always test the hair before embarking on perming this type of hair.

The porosity of the hair may also cause fading of the new colour after a few weeks. In this case, the tint should be re-applied but without prepigmentation.

## Bleaching faults and corrections

Even if you follow all the precautions before and during bleaching, there are still some faults that could occur, such as:

**Table 16.3**

| Fault | Causes | Remedies |
|---|---|---|
| Hair breakage | Use of too strong a bleach mixture Overlapping when retouching the roots Incompatible chemicals present on the hair prior to bleaching, e.g. metallic dyes Bleaching of hair that is already in a porous and weakened state Overprocessing Use of other strong chemicals over the bleached hair, e.g. permanent wave reagent Unnecessary application of heat during processing | Condition the hair and apply restructurant |
| Scalp irritation or inflammation | Sensitive skin Use of too strong a bleach mixture Cuts and abrasions present on the scalp prior to bleaching | Seek medical aid |
| Hair feels slimy and slippery when wet and takes a long time to dry | Hair in a highly porous state Use of too strong a bleach mixture Overprocessing Use of other strong chemicals over the bleached hair | Condition the hair and use restructurant |

| Fault | Causes | Remedies |
| --- | --- | --- |
| Tiny dark pin-pricks at the root of the hair | Bleach not pressed into the root area firmly enough | Leave, but the client will require a retouch application sooner than normal |
| Uneven colour along the length of the hair shaft | Underprocessed retouch<br>Overprocessed retouch<br>No allowance made for the effect of body heat on a full-head application<br>Uneven application<br>Overlapping<br>Regrowth allowed to exceed 1.25 cm (½″) | Spot bleach darker areas. Rebleach if underprocessed. Tone lighter areas if overprocessed |
| Uneven colour throughout the whole head | Commencing application at the most porous area instead of the most resistant – this causes hair to be lighter in some areas than others<br>Uneven application<br>Application too slow<br>Sections too large | Spot bleach or rebleach darker areas |
| Finished result has an orangy-red cast | Base colour too dark for strength of bleach mixture used<br>Excessive amount of red pigment present in the hair shaft<br>Use of too weak a bleach mixture<br>Too much ammonia present in the bleach mixture | Test hair for strength and porosity. If satisfactory, rebleach, if unsatisfactory, apply a green or matt toner |
| Hair too yellow or brassy | Underprocessed;<br>Incorrect choice of bleach for the base shade<br>Incorrect choice of volume strength of hydrogen peroxide | Apply a violet/mauve corrective toner |

## Summary

Bleaching hair involves the decolourisation of the natural hair pigment granules in the hair shaft. This produces the lightening of the hair and is carried out by using an oxidising agent, mainly hydrogen peroxide ($H_2O_2$), although in emulsion bleaches other oxodising agents are also used; they are called 'boosters'.

Hydrogen peroxide is an unstable compound which breaks down (decomposes) easily to release nascent oxygen. The nascent oxygen then oxidises the pigments in the hair. The breakdown of hydrogen peroxide occurs rapidly in the presence of heat, ultraviolet light, dust, and catalysts (alkalis, e.g. ammonium hydroxide and certain metals, some of which are used in hair dyes). The strength of hydrogen peroxide is expressed as a 'volume strength' or as a percentage. Using hydrogen peroxide often involves dilution with water and the amount of the original solution and the volume of water mixed with it can be worked out depending on the type of hair and the colour required. Because hydrogen peroxide is a strong oxidising agent and is chemically unstable, care needs to be taken during its use and storage.

There are two main categories of bleach commonly used in salons:

1 brighteners (brightening shampoos), which are applied as a second shampoo and lift the colour by a few tones only;
2 alkaline bleaches, which mostly use ammonium hydroxide (0.880 ammonia solution) as a catalyst. This category includes:

(a) simple bleach (hydrogen peroxide and a few drops of ammonia solution);
(b) oil bleach (which in modern preparations do not contain oil);
(c) powder bleach (which produces a high degree of lift);
(d) emulsion bleach (produces high lift, but with less drying to the hair than powder bleaches).

Before bleaching, a strand test should be carried out to check:

(a) the physical state of the client's hair;
(b) the presence of incompatible chemicals (metallic dyes) on the hair.

The hairdresser should be protected by rubber gloves and the client by a gown and cotton wool at the nape.

## Self-assessment questions

1 What do manufacturers add to hydrogen peroxide to slow down the decomposition, thereby giving a longer shelf-life?

2  Why must hydrogen peroxide be diluted with distilled water in preference to tap water?

3  At what strength is ammonium hydroxide used in the salon?

4  When mixing bleach, what is the usual ratio of bleach to hydrogen peroxide?

5  When bleaching a full head of natural hair, why is it necessary to apply the bleach mixture to the root area last?

6  What is the desired maximum length of a regrowth for bleaching?

7  What volume strength hydrogen peroxide is generally used with a permanent toner?

8  Which toners require a skin test?

9  What is the correct term for the process of bleaching?

10  How can 'creeping oxidation' be prevented?

## Practical assignment – Bleaching

There are a variety of bleaching agents available for use on the hair and knowing which product to select for the effect you need can be difficult at first. The following task sheet has been designed to help you to understand the degree of lift and the characteristics of the main types of bleach in current use.

You will need:

- three types of bleach; gel, powder and oil.
- hydrogen peroxide in strengths; 6%, 9% and 12%.
- cling film or easi-meche packets.
- tuition head and clamp.
- comb, tinting brushes, small mixing bowls.
- pen and paper.
- a cutting of hair.

## Task

(a) Set up the tuition head and assemble the equipment.

(b) In separate bowls, mix a *small* amount of each type of bleach with each peroxide strength.

(c) Apply the mixtures to fine meshes of hair on the tuition head using easi-meche or cling film to keep them away from the other hair. Leave to develop.

(d) When developed, rinse off the bleach, dry the hair and record the degree of lift obtained when using:

    oil bleach
    gel (emulsion) bleach
    powder bleach

(e) Take the cutting of hair then select and write down the amount of 'lift' required. Choose what you consider to be the appropriate bleach and volume strength of hydrogen peroxide to achieve this degree of lift. Mix a small amount of your chosen bleach then apply it to the cutting. Record your findings. Was your choice correct? If not, try again on another cutting.

## Practical assignment – Bleaching and tinting

The aim of this assignment is to help you to understand how bleaching and/or tinting the hair can improve the client's hairstyle by accentuating the shapes and lines within the style. It may help you to remember that where you lighten the hair it will appear finer and less dense while where you darken the hair it will appear thicker and more solid.

## Tasks

1 Analyse the following hairstyles (*see* Figs 16.17–16.19) then decide how you would accentuate the shape of each style using bleach or a combination of bleach and colour (tint).

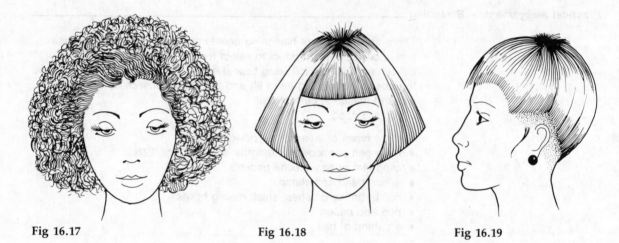

Fig 16.17          Fig 16.18          Fig 16.19

2 Using whatever medium you consider suitable, e.g. crayon, paint pastel etc., colour the hairstyles to show the finished effect that you wish to create.

3 Take cuttings of hair for each style (these can be obtained from either your workplace or tuition head) and use these cuttings to illustrate:

(a) The base shade of the hair (give the number and letter, which you can find by matching it to the hair swatches in the tint shade chart).

(b) The type of bleach and/or tint you would use.

(c) The strength of hydrogen peroxide required for each.

(d) The approximate development time.

(e) The elasticity and porosity of the hair both before and after the process.

(f) The finished effect.

4 Write out a detailed report for **each** style. Include the following information in your report:

(a) The effect you hope to achieve.

(b) Reasons for your choice of tint, bleach and hydrogen peroxide strength.

(c) A comparison of the elasticity and porosity of the hair before and after the chemical processes.

(d) Approximate development times.

5 Design a folio of fashion bleaching and colouring techniques using the above information. Include any other interesting techniques that you may find in trade journals etc.

# SECTION 4
# MORE ADVANCED WORK

# 17

# LONG HAIR

Shiny, healthy, long hair can be extremely glamorous and, in the hands of an imaginative stylist, can be far more versatile than short hair. It can be worn curly, wavy, smooth, tumbling down over the shoulders, plaited or coiled up on the head. Many stylists are inhibited by long hair and indeed, the styling of this length hair does usually take more time than the styling of short hair. However, long hair offers the stylist a whole new world of creativity and as with any other skill, the more that it is practised then the more proficient and creative the stylist will become.

Long haired blocks are ideal for practising long hair styling as they can be used whenever there is a free or quiet moment in the salon or they can be taken home to try out any new ideas.

To look its best, long hair must be shiny with no breakage or split ends therefore, the **condition** of the hair must *always* be of the utmost importance whatever service is being carried out.

There are significant differences between dealing with short and long hair and the following checklist (which is by no means complete) outlines the main areas to consider.

## Considerations when cutting long hair

1 The longer the hair, the heavier it becomes. Therefore, if the client requires height on the top it will be necessary to cut this area shorter to prevent it from flopping.

2 Hair does not grow evenly, thus, long hair will require cutting every 8–10 weeks. However, it is important not to remove too much of the length as hair only grows at approximately 1.25 cm (½") per month, therefore if the stylist removes more than 2.5 cm (1") each time the hair is cut then it will never appear to grow any longer!

3 Before layering long hair which is all the same length (e.g. bobbed) make sure that the client has been adequately informed of the likely effect and implications as it can take several years to grow

out layers if the hair is very long and the client is unhappy with the style.

4   Increased layering can often make the hair *appear* longer because it takes away the width at the sides and gives more height on top.

5   Any split ends (fragilitis crinium) should be removed by cutting them off. If they are left they will become worse and make the hair appear dull and lifeless.

6   If the hair is very long, then the client may have to stand while it is being cut. If this is the case then always make sure that the client's head is held at the correct angle while cutting the hair.

7   To ensure that the guideline at the nape/back is absolutely level and precise it may be necessary to remove or alter the position of the gown and towel around the client. However, it is still important to keep the client's clothing protected.

## Considerations when setting and drying long hair

1   A better result can be obtained by setting the hair when it is damp as the finished result tends to be over curly if it is set from wet. Use a good, suitable setting agent such as mousse to give the hair body and protection.

2   Choose the rod size carefully. Unless a lot of curl is required, it is usual to use a large rod to achieve most effects.

3   Because of its length, long hair takes a long time to dry. Therefore, before styling, near-dry the hair first to remove the excess moisture.

4   When drying the hair it is often more efficient to use the fingers instead of a brush. Aim the air-stream down the hair shaft alternating between hot and cold air to smooth the hair.

5   Do not over-dry the hair. Leave it slightly damp before using heated rollers, tongs or hot sticks. The heat from these appliances will finish the drying process.

6   Use a diffuser attachment on the blowdryer when drying long, curly hair which requires curl in the finished style. It helps to prevent frizzing.

7   Do not set the heat of a dryer too high as it can damage the hair and dry out its moisture content.

## Considerations when dressing long hair

1   Always use a dressing cream or oil, particularly on the ends of the hair to replace the natural oil and give the hair shine.

2   If the dressing requires backcombing, try to keep it to the root area only (unless the style dictates otherwise) to minimise the risk of breakage or damage to the hair.

3   Make sure that smooth styles are thoroughly brushed before dressing. However, styles which are very curly are usually dressed using only the fingers or an Afro-type comb as brushing this type

of style would create frizzing of the hair.

4  To prevent damage to the hair, use bands which are covered and grips which have covered ends, if they are needed, to put the hair up.

5  Trying to cope with a large amount of hair can be overwhelming for some stylists so decide on the overall effect to be achieved before starting then break down the task into small stages.

6  Work methodically through the dressing. Don't panic!

7  Make sure that the head is kept in the correct position while dressing. For example, if it is held to one side at an angle when putting the hair up it will alter the balance of the style.

8  Because of its weight, very long hair e.g. waist length, is often difficult to secure with hair grips and covered elastic bands. When creating chignons on this hair length it is usually easier, quicker and firmer to tie the hair *itself* into an ordinary knot then secure in position with hair grips. By sectioning the hair and knotting it in different places many different and unusual effects can be achieved.

9  When the dressing is finished, check its **shape** from all angles, particularly if the hair has been put up or drawn away from the face.

## Considerations when chemically processing long hair

1  Always remember that the ends of the hair have been there for a long time and have been subjected to much physical (e.g. brushing, heated appliances etc.) and atmospheric (e.g. sun, wind, rain etc.) influences. Therefore the ends of the hair will be far more porous than the remaining hair and will process more quickly when perming, tinting and bleaching.

2  Long hair should be regularly conditioned as the hair's natural oil of sebum does not always manage to coat the whole of the hair shaft, particularly with the trend towards frequent shampooing.

3  The client must be made fully aware of the long term implications of using potentially damaging chemicals such as perm reagent, tint and bleach on the hair. If these chemicals should damage the hair then it is extremely difficult to rectify and often the only real remedy is to remove the damaged hair by cutting. It is extremely upsetting for a client who has grown their hair over a number of years to have to have it cut off because a chemical process has damaged it.

4  Always protect the hair with restructurants, pre-chemical or post-chemical treatments.

5  Use only good quality products which will do the least damage to the hair. Do not use excessively high hydrogen peroxide strengths or harsh reagents.

6  Do *not* over-process the hair. However, when perming long hair also make sure that it is not under-processed as it is not usually advisable to reperm on this length of hair.

7  Always advise the client on how to look after their hair by protecting it from the sun, regular conditioning, using a suitable

shampoo, using oils and waxes and on the effects of over-using heated appliances such as curling tongs, hot brushes, heated rollers etc.

## Dressing long hair

### Dressing long hair into a pleat

1   Backcomb or backbrush the hair if necessary to give volume and hold the hair together (*see* Fig 17.1). The backcombing/backbrushing is usually done underneath the hair mesh at the roots and possibly mid-lengths. If the whole hair length is done then it can be very difficult to smooth over.

2   Leave out the top sections and take one side of the back section just past the centre back (*see* Fig 17.2). Secure firmly with hair grips positioned alternately up and down next to one another to prevent any hair from slipping through.

3   Brush the hair from the other side of the back section and brush towards the centre. Fold this hair under and secure firmly with hair grips making sure that they are positioned not to show (*see* Fig 17.3).

4   Smooth the top hair and blend it in with the pleated back hair either by twisting it round into a curl, as shown in Fig 17.4 or under like an envelope. Secure firmly with hair grips.

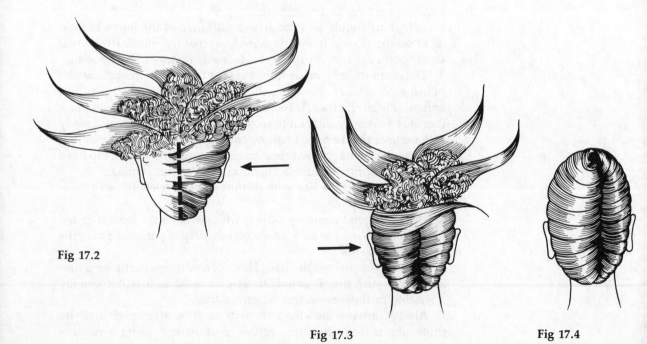

Fig 17.1

Fig 17.2

Fig 17.3

Fig 17.4

## Dressing long hair into a knot on the crown

1   Position the client's head at the appropriate angle. Brush the hair thoroughly away from the hairline and up towards the crown (*see* Fig 17.5).

2   Twist the hair in an anti-clockwise direction and secure with hair grips. (*See* Fig 17.6). Tuck the ends of the hair underneath the previously wound hair and make firm with hair grips.

Variations can be made to this method of dressing hair to produce a knot at the nape or an asymmetrical hair knot.

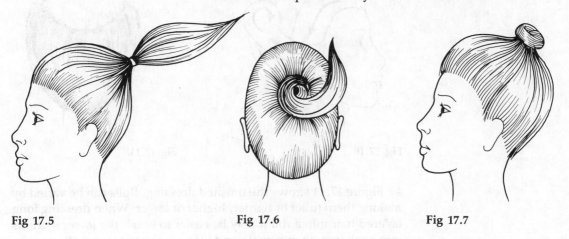

**Fig 17.5**          **Fig 17.6**          **Fig 17.7**

## Dressing long hair into a horizontal roll

1   Backcomb or backbrush the hair, if necessary, to give volume and hold the hair together (*see* Fig 17.8). Initially, the backbrushing should be placed underneath the direction in which the hair is to be dressed.

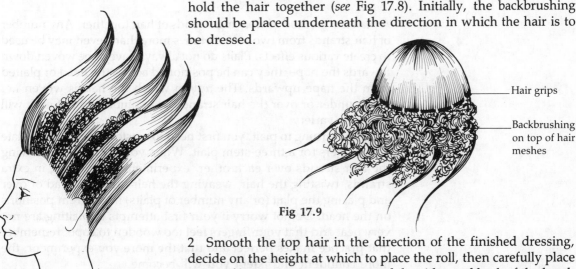

Hair grips

Backbrushing on top of hair meshes

**Fig 17.8**          **Fig 17.9**

2   Smooth the top hair in the direction of the finished dressing, decide on the height at which to place the roll, then carefully place a row of hair grips in an arc around the sides and back of the head. The hairgrips are usually placed approximately 2.5 cm (1″) below the height of the finished roll to allow for the actual rolling of the hair. *See* Fig 17.9.

3 Starting at one side of the head, the underneath hair is folded over into a roll in the direction indicated by the arrows in Fig 17.10. Work in sections round the head, securing each rolled section with a hair grip when it is thoroughly smoothed and in the correct position. Care should be taken to avoid showing any hair grips in the final dressing.

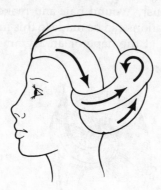 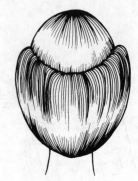

**Fig 17.10**               **Fig 17.11**

4 Figure 17.11 shows the finished dressing. Rolls can be varied by making them fuller or tighter, higher or lower. When dressing long layered hair into a roll it may be easier to brush the lower sections into a roll first, then smooth and blend in the top layers afterwards.

## Plaiting the hair

A plait is a method of weaving strands of hair together. Any number of hair strands from two to sometimes more than seven may be used to create various effects. Plaits do not always have to be woven down towards the nape, they can be positioned across the head or plaited from the nape upwards. The *way* in which the hair is woven i.e. either under or over the hair strands or a combination of each will also give variety.

When learning to plait, you first need to master how to manipulate your fingers for a three-stem plait. When you are used to weaving the hair strands over each other, experiment by bringing in extra strands, twisting the hair, weaving the hair under instead of over and placing the plait (or any number of plaits) in different positions on the head. Do not worry if your first attempts at plaiting are not very neat and that your fingers feel too wooden to cope; remember that practice makes perfect and that the more you experiment, the more confident and adept you will become.

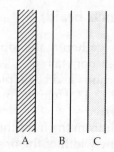

**Fig 17.12**

# Method of plaiting a three-stem plait (English plait)

1  Divide the hair into three equal strands (*see* Fig 17.12).
2  Take strand A to the right and wrap over strand B. Pull strand B in the opposite direction (left) to aid the wrapping (*see* Fig 17.13).
3  Strand C is then taken to the left and wrapped over strand A (*see* Fig 17.14).
4  Strand B is taken to the right over strand C in the same direction as strand A (*see* Fig 17.15).

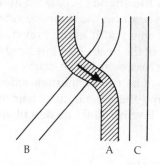

**Fig 17.13**

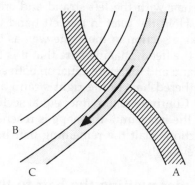

**Fig 17.14**

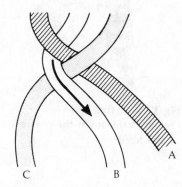

**Fig 17.15**

5  Strand A is now taken back in the opposite direction and over the centre strand B (*see* Fig 17.16).
6  Continue wrapping the strands over each other, always taking the outside strands in towards the centre, in the manner described above until all the hair has been plaited (*see* Fig 17.17). Secure the ends of the hair with a covered band or alternatively, wrap a piece of the hair tightly round then tuck in the ends securely.

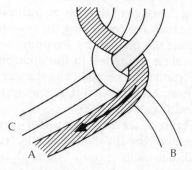

**Fig 17.16**

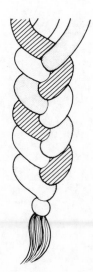

**Fig 17.17**

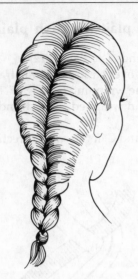

Fig 17.18 A finished
French Braid down the centre
of the head

## Plaiting the hair to the scalp (French braid)

1  To plait the hair to the scalp, begin by gathering the top hair, from the temples to the crown, into a thin ponytail.
2  Divide this hair into the three equal sections and begin plaiting in the manner described in Figs 17.12 and 17.13. Hold the braid in the right hand keeping the strands separated.
3  With the left hand, take a strand of hair from the front through to the back which is approximately half the width of the originals and draw it back towards the ponytail. Combine this new strand of hair with the left strand and cross over the centre.
4  Hold the plait in the left hand with the strands separated and take a section in the same way as before but on the opposite side of the head, making sure that it is the same width as the previous strand and therefore equal on both sides of the head. Add this newly gathered hair to the right strand and cross over to the centre.
5  Continue taking fine, equal sections of hair from alternate sides of the head until the nape is reached and there is no more hair to section. Plait the remaining hair in an English braid as described previously.

## Under-plaiting the hair to the scalp

This is carried out in almost the same way as a French braid. The hair is gathered into a fine ponytail from the temples through to the crown and is divided into the three equal sections. Commence plaiting as described previously, however, instead of wrapping the hair **over** it is taken **under**.

Fine strands of hair are then taken alternately from each side of the head and combined with the original strand of hair from that side remembering to cross each strand under the centre instead of over. The finished result is a plait which rests on top of the hair instead of being incorporated into it. Under plaiting can also be done along the edge of the hair by including sections from only one side of the hair and combining them with the plait strands on that side.

1  Start the plaiting by wrapping strand A *under* strand B. Strand B is taken to the left in the opposite direction (*see* Fig 17.19).
2  Strand C is then taken to the left under strand A (*see* Fig 17.20).
3  Strand B is taken left, in the opposite direction and then under strand C (*see* Fig 17.21).
4  Figure 17.22 shows an under-plait down the centre of the head. Note how the finished plait sits on top of the hair.
5  Under-plaiting can be done along the edge of the hair on both sides of the head. The two plaits are held together with a covered band and the ends are then turned under and secured at the nape with hairgrips (*see* Fig 17.23).

Usually referred to as **corn rowing**, this type of plaiting shown in Fig 17.24 is extremely popular for Afro-Caribbean styling. Many small plaits are used throughout the head and the ends can be

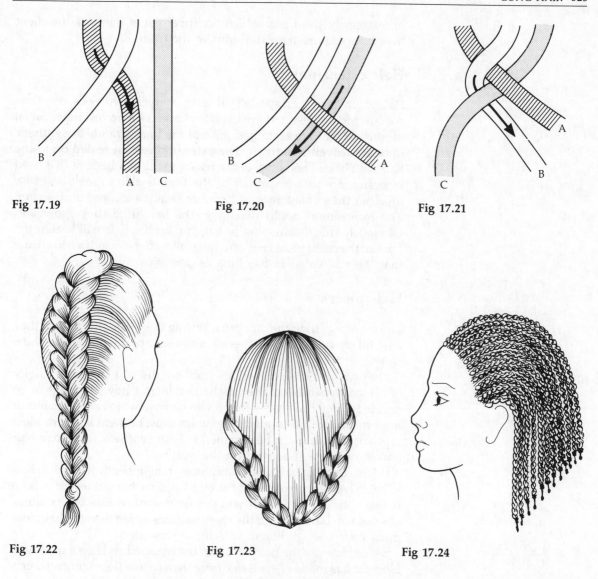

Fig 17.19

Fig 17.20

Fig 17.21

Fig 17.22

Fig 17.23

Fig 17.24

secured with cotton thread, or beads to give more decoration. The direction of the plaits create the style and the variations are almost limitless to the experienced plaiter.

## Added hair and hair pieces

Using additional hair and hair pieces can make natural hair appear longer, thicker, or almost instantly different depending on how, why and when they are used.

A popular type of added hair is **hair extensions**. These are made from synthetic fibre which is woven on to the client's natural hair either throughout the head or just where required. For example, on extremely short hair which is clipper cut at the back the client may only require the extensions at the front.

## Hair extensions

Hair extensions are a specialised service which involves a very time consuming process and are usually charged for accordingly. Small meshes of hair are sectioned off and the long strands of synthetic fibre are woven into them. The extension is then sealed on to the hair with heat. This is one of the reasons why synthetic fibre is used in preference to human hair as the fibre is able to melt and fuse together thus enabling it to be more firmly anchored and secure. The extensions should remain in the hair until they grow out. Obviously, harsh brushing or tugging on the hair will loosen the fibre so the client must be given the correct after-care advice to ensure that the extensions last as long as possible.

## Hair pieces

These were at their most popular during the 1960s and 70s but they are still useful today for special occasions, photographic or show work.

They are available in various hair lengths and sizes, the choice of which depends on the finished style and how they are to be dressed. They can have either a woven base which can be hand or machine made or a knotted base which must be hand knotted. Most types of hairpiece can be obtained in both synthetic or human hair and the price will depend on the quality.

When dressing hair using hairpieces, remember to select the most suitable type of hairpiece for the effect you wish to achieve. Postiche is like natural hair in that you can only work within the confines of what you have. Thus if the client requires a plait then the hairpiece must have enough length to achieve this effect.

Set or blowdry the hairpiece into the required style on a malleable block. If it is made of synthetic fibre then follow the manufacturer's instructions as the fibres will usually melt if any kind of heat is used. The dressing can be carried out either on the block or on the client's head.

### Attaching a hairpiece

To attach the hairpiece to the head, first brush or comb the hair in the direction of the style, decide on the position of the hairpiece on the head then section off a square mesh of hair in the centre of this position, curl it round in a pincurl and secure with two crossed hairgrips. If the base of the hairpiece has a comb this can then be pushed under the grips to hold it firm. Use hairgrips to attach the hairpiece to the scalp taking care not to harm the base. If the grips are placed correctly there should be no need to use an excessive amount, it is also useful to try to place the grips in approximately the same places each time you attach a hairpiece so that when it has to be removed you do not have to struggle to find the grips!

Backcomb/backbrush the natural hair if required (this is often done before attaching the hairpiece) then blend the hair with the hairpiece making sure that its base is camouflaged and that all hard lines and edges are also blended.

Advise the client on the care of the hairpiece and demonstrate how it is attached and removed. If the hairpiece is treated correctly it will last for many years with the minimum of upkeep.

## Using ornamentation in the hair

A client with very long hair is not usually able to achieve a change of style by having a new shape cut into the hair. Any new style must therefore be achieved by setting/blowdrying or dressing the hair in different ways. Ornamentation such as ribbons, ornamental grips, decorative combs, beads and embroidery thread, when used imaginatively can alter the effect of a hairstyle and give the client more variety.

Ornamentation has been used on the hair for centuries and is often used for special occasions, the most usual of which is a wedding. Because this is regarded as such an important day in a person's life it is essential that the ornamentation forms part of a total 'look' together with the hairstyle and the dress. This applies to all the members of the wedding party but in particular the bride and the bridesmaids. It is also important to plan carefully beforehand to ensure that the ornamentation is suitable and to the client's liking.

When creating a hairstyle for a bride it is useful to find out as much as possible about all the other accessories that she will be wearing, whether she will be wearing flowers, a bow or a headdress in her hair; for example, if a headdress is to be worn whether it will have a veil or not; the length and thickness of the veil which will be relevant to the choice of style. Finally, find out what type of person the client is. Is she introverted or extroverted? If she is the latter then go for an over-the-top style but if she is the former then her wedding is not the time for drastic changes in style!

The bride must portray a complete image from head to toe, therefore the hairstyle must also be in keeping with the wedding dress. Find out if it is to be classical, Victorian, modern etc. Obviously the texture and length of the hair will influence the final choice of hairstyle but as a general rule, high necklines such as Edwardian look better with the hair off the face and neck in a roll or knot whilst a low neckline can take a style that is loose and flowing. Tailored suits look good with a sleek style such as a bob whilst a tumble of curls can look stunning with a Pre-Raphaelite style dress.

If possible encourage the client to attend the salon prior to the wedding to condition the hair so that it will look its best on the big day. Organise any cutting and perming so that it is carried out about a month beforehand with any highlighting two weeks before to allow the hair to settle and the client to get used to managing the style. A full-head tint should be carried out approximately three days before so that there will be no regrowth but still allowing the hair time to settle.

Have a 'practice run' before the day to make sure that the client is happy with the style and that it is suitable. Make sure that the bride and any bridesmaids come to the salon as early as possible on the day to help them to relax and to make sure that you have enough time to spend on the hair. If you are going to the bride's home make sure that you allow plenty of time as the bride's house on her wedding day is usually chaotic!

## Summary

**Long hair should be shiny and healthy, whether the effect is to be curly, wavy or straight. The condition of long hair is of paramount importance so extra care must be taken when cutting, setting, drying, dressing and chemically processing the hair to ensure that it is kept in optimum condition. Make sure that the client is given adequate and suitable advice on how to look after the hair between salon visits, particularly on the damaging effects resulting from over use of electrical appliances such as curling tongs, heated rollers etc.**

**Long hair can be worn loose, plaited or twisted up on to the head in pleats or knots. Added hair such as hair extensions or other forms of postiche can make natural hair appear longer, thicker or almost instantly different. Ornamentation can also be used to alter and give different effects to a hairstyle and is often used for special occasions.**

## Self-assessment questions

1  Why is it better to set long hair from damp instead of wet?
2  Why is a diffuser used when drying long, curly hair?
3  When drying long hair, why should the dryer not be used on too high a heat?
4  Why is dressing cream or oil used when dressing the hair?
5  Why should long hair be regularly conditioned?
6  Why is it necessary to make sure that the hair is sufficiently processed when perming?
7  How would you advise the client to look after long hair?
8  When dressing the hair into a pleat, why may it be necessary to use some backcombing/brushing?
9  What is a plait?
10  What is the difference between a French braid and under-plaiting?

**Practical assignment – Long hair**

Long hair work requires flexible fingers. This assignment has therefore been devised to help you to handle strands of hair more easily and with greater confidence.

You will need:

- A4 size piece of card.
- large safety pin, scissors and stapler.
- 19 strands of very thick wool about 25 cm (10″) long.
- old cushion.

## Task

1   Take three strands of the wool, knot the ends together and attach the safety pin 2.5 cm (1″) from the ends of the wool.
2   Attach the safety pin and wool to the cushion and plait the wool into a three-stemmed plait as described on page 323. Secure the ends by twisting one strand of the wool around the others and knot. Remove the safety pin and place the plait to one side.
3   Repeat the procedure using four strands of wool, then five then seven until you have four completed plaits of differing sizes.
4   Draw or collect an illustration of a hair style for each type of plait.
5   Attach the plaits to the card with the stapler (or adhesive tape) displaying them to their best advantage together with the relevant illustration. Ornaments or dried flowers etc. may be used to emphasise the plaiting. Label each plait clearly using block letters.
6   Write a short report on how you carried out the task and any difficulties you encountered.

# 18

# MEN'S HAIRDRESSING

This section covers the key skills needed for men's hairdressing. These are:

- Razors – types and sharpening (honing) them
- Shaving
- Men's face massage
- Trimming beards and moustaches.

The use of razors in the salon carries a high risk of cutting the client (or hairdresser). It is therefore important to bear in mind the Health and Safety points given in Chapter 5.

## Razors

There are various types of razors that can be used to shave the beard and these can be categorised as either safety or open.

Traditionally open razors have been used by barbers to shave beards. However, for safety and hygienic reasons safety razors with disposable blades are now becoming much more popular as each client can have their own new, sterile blade for each shave. The most recently developed safety razor has special blades which can be inserted and removed without the operator having to handle any part of the blade at all.

For those salons that prefer to use open razors, extreme care must be taken to ensure that the razors are kept clean, sharp and sterile and that all possible precautions are taken to prevent cuts to the skin and cross infection.

### Open razors

Open razors are made of steel with a bone, vulcanite or celluloid handle. They can be either **solid** or **hollow-ground**. Hollow-ground razors are finer, more pliable and quicker to set than solid razors which are rigid and kinder to sensitive skin. Solid razors also have the advantage of being suitable for haircutting, thus making them more versatile for salon use. However, all razors vary according to steel quality, hardness, grinding and tempering.

The main categories of open razor are: **hollow-ground English, hollow-ground German** and **French** which is smaller in blade length, depth and thickness than the other two types and is known as a solid razor. The most popular open razor for salon use is the 16 mm medium full hollow-ground.

Different razors have different uses and the following table lists the advantages and disadvantages of each.

**Table 18.1**

| Type | Advantages | Disadvantages |
|------|-----------|---------------|
| English/German hollow-ground | Durable, pliable, quicker to set and lighter to handle. | Too hard for sensitive skin types. Will damage cuticle of the hair if used for hair cutting. |
| French solid | Smooth and soft to the skin therefore good for thin, fine skin. Suitable for haircutting. | Has to be ground and stropped more frequently than hollow-ground as the metal is softer. |

## Honing and stropping

When magnified, the edge of a razor is like the teeth of a carpenter's saw which becomes worn down as it is used. **Honing** restores the worn edge by creating a new row of teeth while **stropping** is used between honing to help preserve the edge for as long as possible.

The honing process is often called *setting* and is done on a stone known as a **hone**. If it is carried out correctly it will give a perfect cutting edge to the razor's blade. There are various types of hone, each of which has a specific use. Table 18.2 overleaf gives a brief summary of the various types.

## Honing (or setting) a hollow-ground razor

1  Place the hone on a tissue. Wipe the surface of the hone to ensure that it is clean and free from hair.
2  Sprinkle the selected lubricant over the surface of the hone and spread evenly with the back of the razor.
3  Stroke the razor blade diagonally across the hone, leading with the cutting edge of the razor. Start with the heel and finish with the toe. The blade should be kept flat on the surface and equal pressure exerted on the razor at all times.
4  Turn the razor on its *back* to commence the second stroke. Using

**Table 18.2**

| Type | Made from | Use | Lubricator |
|---|---|---|---|
| Californian | Fine-grained, natural stone from California set into a slate base. | General purpose. | Usually oil but lather or shampoo may also be used. |
| Water (slatestone) | Fine quality slate. | Hollow-ground razors. | A sandstone strip dipped in water then rubbed over the hone surface. |
| Carborundum | Carbon and silicon obtained in various forms. | Very coarse, used to remove any gaps or notches on the blade prior to finer honing. | Usually oil but lather or shampoo may be used. |
| Pike's | Various compositions. | Hollow-ground and French solid. | Oil lubrication. |

the fingers to roll the razor over and *not* the wrist. As the razor turns over slide it from the bottom to the top of the hone so that the heel is again on the hone.

5  Next draw the razor diagonally across the hone with the cutting edge leading.

6  Repeat this figure of eight movement until the razor is what is known as 'set' i.e. the cutting edge has been restored. The lubricant will darken during the honing process as the steel is removed from the blade.

7  After setting, wipe the blade on a tissue (along the back to avoid cutting the fingers). Clean the hone and store away carefully with the surface protected so that it does not become chipped.

## Honing a French solid razor

The steel of a French solid razor is softer than the hollow-ground and must therefore always be set on a fine grain hone with thin oil or lather as a lubricant.

The strokes should be shorter and crisper than those used for the hollow-ground with only the razor edge resting, almost flat on the hone. The strokes resemble a 'v' with the razor turned on its back at the end of each stroke. As the strokes progress they become steeper and steeper until they are almost perpendicular. (*See* Fig 18.1)
NB When honing any type of razor the edge can be blunted and damaged if the razor is turned on its edge instead of its back.

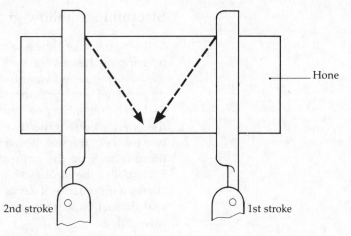

2nd stroke          1st stroke

**Fig 18.1 Honing a French solid razor**

## Testing the razor

This is done by pulling the razor across a moistened thumb nail. The different degrees of sharpness will give a different tactile sensation.

- A perfect or **keen** edge will dig into the nail with a smooth, steady grip.
- A blunt or **dull** edge will pull smoothly across the nail without dragging or cutting.
- A coarse edge will feel jerky and dig into the nail.
- An over-honed edge will stick to the nail with a harsh, grating sound.
- A nick in the razor will feel uneven as it is drawn across the nail.

## Stropping

As you have already learned, stropping is done to preserve the cutting edge of the razor between setting. It cleans debris such as soap, skin and hair from the razor's edge and also re-aligns the teeth.

Stropping is carried out on a leather strop which can be of either the hanging or solid (hand) variety. The hanging strop is flexible with leather on one side and canvas on the other, it is used for hollow-ground razors. The solid or hand strop is rigid and is used for solid French razors.

Before being used for the first time, a new strop must be treated by smearing it with plenty of oil and leaving it to soak overnight. The canvas side of a hanging strop should also be treated by rubbing soap into the canvas. After treating, both surfaces are then rubbed with a round, glass bottle until a glazed surface is obtained.

Always store strops away from dust, damp and hair cuttings as any damage to the surface of the strop will ultimately spoil the cutting edge of the razor.

## Stropping a hollow-ground razor

1   Hang the strop on a hook then hold firmly in a horizontal position by gripping the free end with the hand. Hold the razor shaft between the first finger and thumb of the other hand to allow the razor to be revolved easily during stropping.
2   Lie the razor flat and stroke it, with the back leading, away from the operator down the strop. When it has travelled approximately two thirds of the way down the strop, turn the raxor on its *back* and bring it back up the strop in the opposite direction.
3   Initially, the strokes should be slow and careful as speed only comes with practice. Twelve strokes is usually sufficient (six forward and six back). Over stropping should be avoided as it will spoil the razor edge.

## Stropping a solid razor

A solid razor is rigid and therefore does not 'give' when being stropped.

Place the solid strop in a horizontal position. Hold the razor between the thumb and the first finger, but with the back of the razor slightly off the strop with the edge resting flat and even on the strop. Use six strokes backwards and forwards as before but as the steel of the solid razor is softer than the hollow-ground the stropping will have more effect.

## Stropping a French solid razor

These razors are also very rigid and the method of stropping is therefore very similar to that of stropping solid razors. French strop paste is mildly abrasive making each stropping of the French razor a mild form of honing. The condition of the edge will determine the number of strokes required. The duller the blade then the more strokes are needed. Six strokes each way is usual for normal stropping rising to 12 strokes each way if the razor has a dull (blunt) edge.

It is important to remember that if the razor is turned on its *edge* during any type of stropping, the strop may be cut and split making it useless for further use. Making a mistake of this kind will also damage the razor's edge.

### Shaving

A good shave should not be felt by the client and should result in a smooth face. Shaving has three separate phases:

- preparation of the client
- lathering
- shaving.

## Preparation of the client

For hygienic reasons, ensure that your own hands and nails are clean and that the client's beard is clean and free from grease before commencing the shave. Any grease remaining on the beard will prevent the lather from foaming correctly.

Discuss with the client his requirements then seat him in a reclining chair with a clean paper towel placed over the headrest. Protect the client with a gown then place a towel across his chest and tuck it in firmly at the neck. Position the client's head well back so that the chin and lower face area are easily accessible, then place a paper towel, tissue or shaving square near to the neck.

Examine the face for any abnormalities, broken skin, strong or unusual beard growth patterns and length of sideboards. If everything is satisfactory then the client is now ready for the next stage.

## Lathering

This process is carried out to soften the beard and help prevent the shave from being painful. The lather is produced by soap and water. Shaving soap can be obtained in foam, powder, cream or liquid form. Block or tablet soap is not recommended because it would be unhygienic to use the same block for a large number of clients.

*Procedure*

1  Steam a sterile towel in a steamer. Place the towel over the beard area. Avoid covering the nose to allow the client to breathe. If an open razor is to be used, this is usually stropped while the face is steaming.

2  Replace the cooled towel with a second steamed towel. Fill a shaving mug or bowl with hot water.

3  Remove the towel and mix the lather by first dipping the brush into the mug of hot water then placing a small amount of the soap to be used into the centre of the brush bristles. Rotate the brush vigorously (almost like whisking an egg) in the bowl of the shaving mug or a second bowl until a lather is produced.

4  Begin lathering the face by placing the brush under the tip of the chin and rotating it over the chin, cheeks and neck until all the beard is well covered. To lather the upper lip the brush is spread by placing the finger in the centre of the bristles, this prevents the lather from going up the nose or on the lips. Use a thin, watery application at first increasing the lather later.

5  Keep the brush warm by dipping it into the hot water and remember that the better the lather the easier the beard will be to shave.

## Shaving

Any shaving will remove a fine layer of epidermal skin so it is essential that the angle of the razor and the direction of the razor strokes are correct. **Always** stretch the skin taut when stroking with the razor as this will hold the hair up to the razor and allow it to be cut more closely and will also help to prevent cuts to the skin.

When shaving, the blade of the razor must be wiped clean of hair and lather between each razor stroke. It is *very important* to wipe the razor on its back, avoiding the edge otherwise the operator may cut their fingers quite badly and blunt the razor edge.

The temperature of the water should be kept warm. Cold water will cause the razor to drag while hot water swells the face and prevents a close shave. A right-handed operator should stand and start on the right hand side while a left-handed one should stand and start on the left.

## First time over shave

The first time over shave is always done in the same direction as the hair growth i.e. *with* the grain of the hair. When stretching the skin for this shave, the finger is placed *behind* the razor instead of in front, as it is very difficult to get a firm grip on the skin when the face is slippery with the lather.

*Procedure*
1 Hold the razor loosely with the thumb on the blade. The actual position will vary with the different strokes, and dip the razor into the hot water.
2 Begin the shave on the side nearest to the operator. Always start by holding the dry, unlathered skin at the sideboard area (to prevent the fingers slipping) pulling it taut to commence the shave. It is important to start any razor stroke *before* a bony prominence to prevent cutting the client.
3 Move the razor in a slicing, scythe-like motion following the movements shown in Fig 18.2.
4 Each side of the face should be completely shaved before starting the other with the centre chin section left until last. Try to incorporate each side of the upper lip area when shaving that side of the face, thus leaving just the centre section which is then shaved upwards while pressing the tip of the nose upwards to tighten the skin. Avoid holding the nose as this can be painful to the client and could cause sneezing.
5 When one side of the face has been completed, the client's head is turned towards the operator to make it easier to shave the other side.
6 To shave the point of the chin, pull the skin tight between the finger and thumb then use the middle of the razor blade to shave *across* the chin.
7 Finish by shaving the neck area downwards.

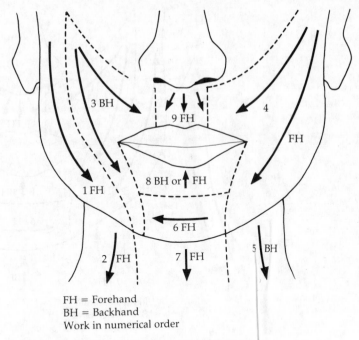

FH = Forehand
BH = Backhand
Work in numerical order

**Fig 18.2 Shaving procedure – first time ove**

## Second over shave

This shave is necessary to ensure that th hair is cut as closely as possible giving a clean finished result. T hair is cut against the growth in an upward movement.

This is usually the final shave unless th lient is very dark haired with a strong beard growth. In this case, ihay have to be followed by a sponge shave. This entails soaking a nall sponge in hot water then dragging it across the face with the azor following closely.

*Procedure*
1  Re-lather the face in the manner desoed previously.
2  Begin the shave at the collar area with e fingers again holding the dry, unlathered skin. Move upwar in backhand strokes, completing one side of the face before sting the other as for the first time over shave. *See* Fig 18.3 for the der and manner of the strokes.
*NB* Juvenile beards are quite soft and m not therefore require shaving against the growth with upwar trokes.
3  Any cuts or punctures to the skin shouhave a powder or liquid styptic applied to stop the flow of blood. Fvever, for hygienic and health reasons extreme care must be takei avoid contact with the blood, particularly if the operator has anyts or punctures to their own skin.
4  Clean the face with a damp, warm tov or sponge then gently

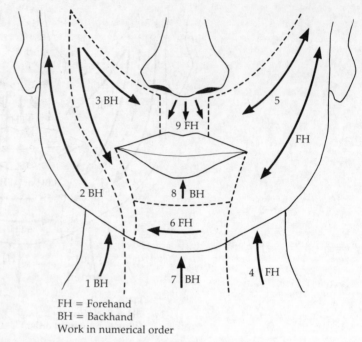

FH = Forehand
BH = Backhand
Work in numerical order

**Fig 18.3 Shaving procedure – second time over**

pat dry with another clean towel. Apply a small amount of talcum powder to ensure that the skin is thoroughly dry and to prevent chapping of the skin after the shave.
5   Finish with an after-shave lotion, which is an astringent, and will therefore close the pores and leave the skin feeling fresh and clean.

## Mens' face massaing

The massage is usually carried out after shaving to aid skin elasticity, tone the facial muscles and encourage natural excretion of waste products. However, the main benefit of a face massage is to relax the client and this point should be remembered by the operator while the massage is being carried out.

Before commencing the massage, make sure that the client's clothing and hair are well protected from the massage cream. Check that hands and nails are clean and assemble equipment.

*Procedure*
1   Steam the face with two hot towels.
2   Stand behind the client and commence the massage by placing the flat surface of the closed fingers on the forehead at the eyebrows. Stroke the fingers back towards the front hairline then across the forehead in gentle, stroking, effleurage movements until the client is relaxed.
3   Move to the corner of the eyes and rotate the skin in a petrissage

movement then continue with the same movements above the nose. Gentle tapotement (tapping movements) can be used under the eyes so that the skin is not pulled.

4  Next, stroking effleurage movements are used from the temple down and round the cheekbone to the side of the nostril base. The hands are then turned so that the backs are together with the palms facing outwards. Carry this movement on up the sides of the nose ending between the eyebrows.

5  Placing the third finger of each hand on the side of the nostrils, use small, circular movements up the sides of the nose to help to unblock the pores.

6  With the tips of the fingers held together, gently stroke from the upper lip sliding the fingers sideways and diagonally upwards towards the outer corner of the eye finishing with a circular effleurage movement around the bony part of the eye socket.

7  The lower part of the face is massaged using the flat of the hands in a circular movement from the mouth out towards the ear then from below the mouth to under the ears.

8  The top of the chin and jawline can be massaged by rotatory petrissage movements but tapotement or vibratory movements are more suitable for fleshy or double chins.

9  Finish the massage by rolling the skin upwards between the thumb and the forefinger from the chin to the forehead.

10  Complete the treatment with another hot towel followed by a cool towel and/or an astringent to close the pores and tighten the skin. Finally, a light dusting of powder, cream or lotion may be applied depending on the personal preference of the client.

## Using vibro massage

This is a mechanical massage with very strong tapotement movements. It can be used in place of a manual hand massage (*see* p. 126) but it is only suitable for the fleshy areas. Great care must be taken when using the vibro on bony areas such as the jawline and forehead as it can be very uncomfortable for the client and it must *never* be used on the nose and around the eyes.

If the vibro is used to replace some of the hand massage movements, it should be used in the same order and direction as the massage movements that it is replacing. Always be aware of the comfort of the client and use the vibro carefully and gently. If it feels too strong for the client then use the attachments over the hand.

# Trimming beards and moustaches

A beard should suit the client's face shape and balance the hairstyle giving a 'total' look. Client consultation is very important before commencing the beard trim to determine the client's requirements and overall final length of the beard.

Clippers and attachments are often used for very close beards, for example, 'designer stubble' or when a very short uniform look is required.

*Procedure*

1  Place the client in a reclined position.
2  Make sure that the client's clothing and eyes are adequately protected. This is done by placing a gown over the client's clothing and covering the eyes with a small cloth. Small, bristly beard cuttings are sharp, dangerous and can cause infection therefore it is extremely important to protect the client as much as possible.
3  Begin the trim by disentangling the beard, combing the hair in a downward direction.
4  Cut the beard using the scissor over comb method combing the beard upwards. Take small sections and keep the comb moving as you cut. Remember that the further away from the face that the comb is held then the longer it will leave the hair.
5  Take extra care when trimming under the chin and around the lips as it is easy to tickle the client and could result in cutting the skin.
6  Outline any moustache by supporting the scissors with the first finger to prevent cutting the lips.
7  When enough hair has been removed from the beard, outline the final shape using a razor/shaper or clippers.
8  Remove the beard clippings from the client with a brush and show the client the result in the mirror.

## Summary

The razors used in men's hairdressing may be of the 'safety' type with disposable blades (preferred for hygiene reasons) or the traditional open type (of various kinds) which need to be kept clean, sharp and sterile. The open razors are kept sharp by honing (or setting) which is done on a stone (the hone). There are different types of hone and varying techniques for different open razors. Stropping is carried out to preserve the sharp edge produced by honing and to clean debris from the blade. Stropping uses a length of leather (the strop) smeared with oil and there are different techniques for the various types of razor.

Shaving involves a number of practical steps and hygiene precautions. The practical steps include the use of towels, lathering the face and the use of the razor during 'first time' and 'second time' over shaving. The hygiene precautions involve ensuring that the razor is sterile and that cuts or punctures are avoided. If the face does bleed, stop the bleeding with styptic and take great care to avoid contact with the client's blood.

Men's face massage is usually carried out after shaving and the main purpose is to relax the client. There are practised techniques for this type of massage which may involve the use of a vibro massage machine.

The trimming of beards and moustaches involves careful client consultation and consideration of the balance of the 'total look'. There are practical methods for carrying out these trims.

## Self-assessment questions

1 Give the advantages and disadvantages of hollow-ground and solid open razors.
2 What does honing do to the edge of the razor?
3 List four types of hone and give their uses.
4 What will happen if the razor is turned on its edge instead of its back during honing?
5 How is the razor edge tested for sharpness?
6 What is the purpose of stropping?
7 What are the three phases of shaving?
8 What should you look for when examining the face prior to shaving?
9 Why is the face lathered before shaving?
10 Why is the skin stretched taut when stroking with the razor?
11 How often is the razor wiped clean when shaving?
12 How is the razor wiped and what could happen if it was wiped along its edge?
13 What is the main benefit of a face massage?
14 Which type of massage movement is used first to relax the client?
15 What type of movements are more suitable for fleshy or double chins?
16 What is the purpose of an astringent?
17 What is the vibro massager suitable for?
18 Where must the vibro massager never be used?
19 What can be done to aid client comfort if the vibro feels too strong for the client?
20 Why is client consultation necessary before commencing the beard trim?
21 What is often used to produce a beard with a very short uniform look?
22 How should the client be positioned for a beard trim?
23 What happens to the length of the hair when the comb is moved further away from the face?
24 What technique is used to prevent cutting the lips when outlining the moustache?
25 What is used to outline the final shape of the beard?

## Practical assignment – Men's hairdressing

Some salons use the traditional 'open' razors which need to be kept both sterile and sharp. The problem with this type of razor is that there is a chance of cross-infection between clients if not properly sterilised and considerable skill is needed to sharpen them (honing and stropping). The best kind to use are 'safety' razors where the blade is changed for a new sterile one between clients, without being touched by the hairdresser. This assignment therefore concentrates on the uses of the 'safety' type of razor.

Shaving the face is a skilled operation which improves with practice. It is, however, the hairdressing operation most likely to cause bleeding and it is important to know what to do if this occurs. This assignment is designed to help you to develop your practical skills and hygiene operations.

## Tasks

1  Using an inflated balloon of about head size, lather, and shave as you would a face. You know instantly if you have cut into it! You can use a peach instead of a balloon but this lacks the realistic size.
2  If you cut a client while shaving (or at any other time):

(a) use styptic to stop the bleeding. Put the styptic on to a tissue, give this to the client for them to hold on the cut.
(b) if any blood has fallen on to surfaces, wipe with neat bleach and wash off with plenty of water and detergent.

Explain each of the steps (a) and (b).

# 19      POSTICHE SERVICES

Wigs and hairpieces are collectively known as **postiche** and may be worn for a variety of reasons including fashion, convenience, theatrical, or to replace thinning hair and hair loss.

A client may ask you to clean or dress postiche in the salon for any of the above reasons, therefore some knowledge of the different types of hair and the construction of the various wigs and hair pieces is essential.

The following table summarises the types of hair that are used in postiche services.

**Table 19.1**

| Type of hair | Obtained from | Characteristics |
|---|---|---|
| European | Spain | Best quality dark hair |
| | Northern Italy | Best quality dark and white |
| | France | Best quality brown and auburn |
| | Germany | Best quality blond |
| Asian | China | Coarse textured dark hair |
| | Japan | Coarse textured dark hair |
| Nylon (synthetic) | | Any colour but difficult to restyle. Non-absorbent so can be hot and uncomfortable. |
| Mohair | Angora goat | Fine, white, long hair too soft for normal use but often used in competition work. |
| Yak | Ox in Tibet | Long, thick and silky |
| Virgin | | Any hair that has not been treated with chemicals |

# Wigs

Postiche can be made from human hair, animal hair or synthetic fibres which are woven or knotted into the desired shape and size either by hand or by machine. There are three main types of wig:

- machine made
- semi-machine made
- hand knotted

## Machine made

These wigs can be made from either human hair, animal hair or synthetic fibre. The hair is sewn on to long wefts which are then cycle sewn by machine on to a cotton or elasticated base. This type of wig is durable, strong but heavier to wear than the hand knotted types and because they can be mass-produced, they are usually inexpensive to buy. Most fashion wigs are machine made with synthetic fibre.

## Semi-machine made

These wigs have the crown hair sewn by machine, but the hair around the hairline is hand knotted which makes it easier to style and gives a more natural appearance. The base of the wig is often a combination of silk and cotton, making it lighter and more comfortable to wear. However, this type of wig is more expensive than a fully machine made wig.

## Hand knotted

These are the most expensive types of wigs and are usually made from the finest quality hair. Each hair is individually knotted into a silk mesh by hand. These are much easier to style, cooler and lighter to wear than the machine made variety. However, because of the individual knotting they must be carefully handled to prevent damage and they should be professionally cleaned and maintained by the salon. At one time hand knotted wigs were provided by the National Health Service to clients who required wigs because of some type of baldness. However, the recent trend is towards synthetic, machine made wigs which are less expensive and require very little upkeep.

## Measuring for a wig

If the client requires a personalised hand made wig then it must be made to measure. Because of the expense of hand made wigs, the operator must take precise, accurate measurements of the client's head to ensure a correct fit. Any mistakes at this stage can be

**Table 19.2**

| Types of postiche | Use/benefit |
|---|---|
| Switch (one-, two- or three-stem) | For coils or plaits |
| Pin curls | Small curls which can be placed anywhere |
| Diamond mesh | Various sized bases which can be bent to the head. Creates different effects depending on length |
| Crêpe pad | To give lift or bulk to the style |
| Wigs (hand knotted or machine) | Covers whole head to disguise baldness or for fashion/theatrical effects |
| Toupee | Disguises male pattern baldness |
| Hair extensions | Make the hair appear longer (see p 325) |

extremely costly and will create an unprofessional impression of the salon.

Client consultation is important to find out the exact requirements of the client before ordering to prevent any misunderstanding or future disappointment. Spend time talking to the client to find out the following information about the finished wig:

- hair colour – take hair cuttings if necessary
- hair quality
- length and style required
- amount of curl required
- any partings – note the length and position in relation to the centre of the front hairline

Measurements of the head should only be taken after carrying out a thorough consultation with the client to ensure that their needs are fully understood.

## Taking measurements for a wig

1  Assemble all relevant tools and equipment.
2  Prepare the client with a protective gown and ensure that they are comfortably seated.
3  Take and record the following measurements (*see* Fig. 19.1)
   (a) The circumference of the head
   (b) Centre front hairline to nape of neck
   (c) Ear peak to ear peak across the front of the head
   (d) Ear to ear across the top of the head
   (e) Temple peak to temple peak round the back of the head
   (f) Temple peak to temple peak across the front of the head
   (g) The width of the nape

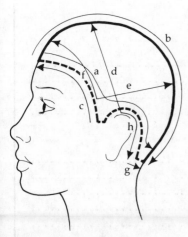

**Fig 19.1 Taking measurements for a wig**

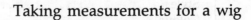

(h) Hairline behind the top of the ear to the corner of the nape.

4 While taking the measurements, look carefully at the scalp and make a note of any abnormalities such as cysts, lumps or an unusually shaped head as these must be taken into consideration by the wig maker.

---

Record card

Name ....................     Telephone no. ..........

Address ................     Reference no ..........

........................

........................

Type of postiche .........

**Measurements** (in centimetres)
1 Circumference .....................................
2 Forehead to nape ..................................
3 Ear to ear across front ...........................
4 Ear to ear across top ............................
5 Temple to temple round back ...................
6 Temple to temple across front .................
7 Nape width ........................................
8 Top of ear to corner nape .......................

Any abnormalities ..................................
........................................................

**Parting details**
Length ...................
Position ...................

**Hair details**
Style .....................................................
Colour ...................................................
Length ...................................................
Curly or straight .......................................

**Other details**
Date required ..........................................
Number required .......................................
Price quoted ...........................................
Name of operator ......................................
Date ordered ...........................................

---

Fig 19.2

5   Complete a record card with all this information and that elicited from the client during the consultation process (*see* Fig 19.2).

6   Make out a detailed order form making sure that the information is accurate. Include in the order any relevant hair cuttings and photographs and inform the wigmaker of the number of wigs required and the date that the client will require the wig.

7   Check the order details with the client then dispatch the order as quickly as possible. Keep a copy of the order for future reference.

# The care and maintenance of postiche

## Preparing postiche before cleaning

The postiche is attached with T-pins to what is known as a malleable block. This block is made in the shape of the head from canvas stuffed with sawdust and can be obtained in various sizes, the average being 56 cm (22″). The hair is combed carefully from the points down to the base (known as the 'foundation') of the postiche. Use a wide-toothed comb to disentangle the hair and hold it at an angle so that there is no possibility of the teeth catching the foundation and tearing it.

## Cleaning synthetic fibre postiche

Postiche made from synthetic fibres may be washed gently in a bowl of lukewarm water with shampoo added.

When cleaning a synthetic fibre wig, turn the wig inside out before immersing in the soapy water then squeeze the postiche gently to assist the cleaning. Rinse thoroughly in lukewarm water then shake out any excess moisture. Allow the postiche to dry naturally without combing. When completely dry it can be brushed into shape as any wave or curl movement in the fibre will return after washing.

It is important to mention that synthetic fibre has a completely different construction to human hair and it will melt and matt together if in contact with too high a temperature. Thus, heated appliances such as hot brushes and curling tongs etc. cannot be used satisfactorily. Because heat should be avoided, it is not possible to curl the synthetic fibres by the usual methods of setting and blowdrying and any client requiring curls or movement in this type of postiche must buy it precurled.

Always follow the manufacturer's instructions on how to care for synthetic postiche. Do not attempt to perm, bleach or colour it and avoid combing it while it is in a wet state as this will cause it to frizz and lose its shape.

## Cleaning human/animal hair postiche

This type of postiche is cleaned with wig cleaner, usually toilet spirit, and must *not* be shampooed as it could matt and tangle the hair. Wigs must be turned inside out before cleaning to ensure that the base is thoroughly cleaned as this is where the grease from the scalp is absorbed when the wig is worn.

Place the wig or hairpiece in a bowl with enough cleaning fluid to completely cover it. Leave the wig to stand in the fluid for a few minutes to loosen the dirt and grease then dip the wig in and out of the bowl to allow the cleaner to work through the lengths of the hair from roots to points.

Use a wax conditioner if the hair is dry or in poor condition, taking care not to wet the foundation when rinsing with water.

Remove any surplus moisture by placing in a towel then leave the wig to dry naturally, preferably on a clothes-line in the open air, for several hours to allow the cleaning fluid to evaporate.

## Setting a human/animal hair wig

The cleaned, dry wig is placed in the correct position on a malleable block which is the same size as the wig. T-pins are placed at the temple, ear peaks and nape of the neck to hold it firm while working then the hair is damped down with warm water (or setting aid if required). To neutralise any yellow discolouration of white hair a blue/mauve rinse may be applied at this stage. Care must be taken throughout the process not to wet the base of the wig as this could make it rot.

Plan the hairstyle in accordance with the client's wishes, referring to the client's record card/wigmaker's form if necessary.

The hair can then be set or blowdried into the required style taking care not to damage the base with any rollers, clips, pins or brushes. If the hair is set, then a net is secured over the finished pli and the wig is placed inside a postiche oven or under a warm dryer and left until completely dry. Long hair which has been chemically treated may take several hours to dry and white hair must be dried naturally or with a cool heat to prevent discolouration. Tissue paper is sometimes placed over a white hair wig while drying to protect it and prevent discolouration.

When dry, allow the hair to cool before removing the rollers, clips and pins then brush the hair to remove any roller, clips or pin marks. Dress in the required style using backcombing/backbrushing if necessary taking care not to damage the wig foundation. Lacquer the finished dressing sparingly and leave a few moments before carefully removing the T-pins. Pad the inside of the wig with tissue paper to keep its shape. If the wig is not to be collected and worn straight away, make sure that it is stored away from a damp atmosphere, in a labelled box prepared with tissue paper or on a malleable block.

## Securing the wig to the head

Comb any existing hair up towards the crown and secure with pins to keep it flat and prevent it from showing underneath the wig. If the finished style has hair combed back from the face, it usually looks more natural if a fine mesh of the client's own hair is left out at the front and then curled back over the false hair to disguise the wig's front hairline.

The wig is secured to the head by placing it in the centre of the front forehead of the client and drawing it back over the crown towards the nape. When the wig is in place make sure that it feels comfortable for the client and check that the balance is correct from all angles. Blend the hair carefully around the hairline so that there are no hard edges and that the wig looks as natural as possible.

If the wig has not been dressed on the head it can often appear too full for the face shape when finally fitted. To alleviate the problem and make sure that the finished style is suitable it may be necessary to flatten the dressing and make other minor adjustments.

Always advise the client on the correct method of brushing, combing and storing the wig to prevent loosening the hair and tearing the foundation, then demonstrate to the client how to attach and remove the wig correctly.

## Securing a toupee to the head

Before placing the toupee on the client's head the scalp should be clean and free of grease to enable the postiche to stick to the scalp. Draw the toupee over the scalp from the front hairline towards the back making sure that it is in the correct position by checking in the mirror. Attach to the client's scalp with double-sided adhesive tape. Clients with some hair on the top may have the toupee clipped into position and there are now various types of postiche which have been designed with snap on clips for rigid fastening.

Gently comb the hair into position, blending in the edges of the toupee with the existing hair, taking care not to snag or pull the base of the postiche. Check that there are no hard edges and that the front hairline is styled to make it appear as natural as possible. This part of the toupee is the most noticeable to others, therefore it is always worthwhile paying it special attention to make sure that it is not combed either too far forward or too far back.

On the first, initial fitting the postiche hair may have to be cut into the shape of the existing hairstyle. If it requires restyling then this *must* be carried out by an expert as mistakes at this stage can be extremely costly.

When the toupee has been fitted, make sure that it feels comfortable and that the client is happy with the result. Demonstrate to the client how to attach and remove the hair piece and give advice on its maintenance. Explain how the hair should be combed to prevent tearing the base and that the base must be kept dry (unless kept dry (unless specially designed otherwise). Stress that the hair does not grow, therefore the colour may fade due to the effect of natural sunlight and that it may be necessary to professionally refresh the colour (or add extra white hairs) in the future. Make sure that the client is aware of the need for professional maintenance of all postiche to prolong its 'life'.

## Adjusting the size of a wig to fit the client

Any alterations or repairs that need to be carried out should always be done from the inside of the wig. The stitching must be done as neatly, evenly and invisibly as possible and the sewing thread to be used must be the same colour as the wig foundation. This also applies when altering or repairing all types of postiche. The two most common types of adjustment are:

1   When the wig is too large from ear to ear, a tuck should be taken vertically behind each ear.

2   When the wig is too deep from front to back then a tuck should be taken across the crown or upper nape area, commencing the tuck at the centre and tapering it down to the side sections. The tuck should be folded *upwards* so that the hair is directed downwards in a natural fall position.

## Measuring the head for a toupee (using a polythene template)

Men can be extremely sensitive about losing their hair and the decision to wear a toupee is usually taken after much thought and deliberation. It is therefore of the utmost importance that the operator allows enough time to be spent making sure that the client has adequate consultation and advice about how the toupee will affect his appearance. It is sometimes a shock to the client to be suddenly confronted with a full head of hair!

It is important to take accurate measurements so that the finished postiche is a perfect fit. Nothing looks more false or attracts the attention more than an ill-fitting toupee, which is just the effect that the client wishes to avoid! As a rule most men wear their hair short which means that there is very little hair with which to blend and disguise the edges of the false hair thus the fit and colour match of the toupee is of paramount importance.

Choosing the colour of the toupee should be done very carefully as the client's existing hair colour could have different shades throughout the head. It will therefore make the finished toupee appear more natural if cuttings of hair are taken from various parts of the head to enable the varying shades to be duplicated in the toupee. This will also help to blend the toupee more easily into the client's own natural hair.

*Procedure*

1  Assemble the equipment and protect the client with a gown.

2  Analyse the client's existing hair and allow adequate consultation to determine exact requirements regarding length, density, texture, amount of curl and finished style of the toupee.

3  Place an oblong piece of polythene (approximately 40 cm by 20 cm/16" by 8") over the bald area of the client's head. For safety reasons the polythene must be kept away from the client's eyes, mouth and nose.

4  Mould the polythene to the head by twisting its ends, then make a firm base by pulling adhesive tape lengthways then across the polythene overlapping the bald area by 2 cm (¾").

5  Mark the bald area by drawing round it carefully with a water-proof marker pen or eyebrow pencil, making sure that it is drawn to the correct size.

6  To outline the front edge, use any stray, wispy hairs that may be visible at the front hairline. If there are none then this will have to be carefully estimated.

7  Indicate with the marker pen the front and back of the template and the direction the hair is to lie on the finished toupee. The length and position of any partings should also be clearly marked on the template.

8  Remove the template from the client's head and wipe the scalp clean of any perspiration caused by the polythene.

9  Cut around the edge of the marked area then check that the completed template fits correctly by replacing it on the client's head.

10  Pad the inside of the template with tissue paper to make sure that it retains its shape, then complete a workroom order in the same manner as a wig. Make sure that all relevant information is included on the order and attach any hair colour samples, indicating their required position on the finished toupee.

11  Dispatch the order to the wigmaker as quickly as possible keeping a record of the transaction for future reference.

# Advertising and sales techniques for postiche and other salon services

Advertising is a means of informing potential clients of the services offered by the salon. To be effective, it must be carefully planned and professionally carried out otherwise it will lose potential clients instead of attracting them.

There are many methods of advertising, some of which are more suitable for the salon than others. Factors which will influence which type of advertising to use are:

- cost
- target population
- product.

## Cost

Any type of advertising must be cost effective and the overall price of the advertising campaign must be measured against the potential profit from selling the goods. A large organisation may have more funds at their disposal than a smaller salon. They may also have a certain amount set aside for advertising which has been built into their yearly budget.

## Target population

This is the category of client that is most likely to be attracted to the product. They may be within a local area or available nationally. The type of potential client and where they live will greatly influence where and how the goods are advertised.

## Product

The **type** of product will also influence the type of advertising necessary. For example, demonstrating toupees at an all women W.I. meeting would not be particularly effective as the target population for toupees is usually men.

## Methods of advertising

Once the factors of cost, target population and product have been decided then it is possible to consider the most appropriate method of advertising to give the best results. The following options are available:

- newspapers and magazines
- direct mail
- posters
- business directories
- local radio and cinema
- transport advertising
- demonstrations
- window display
- personal selling.

## Newspapers and magazines

There are four types of newspapers available: national, regional dailies, local weekly and free newspapers. The cost of advertising in these papers will vary but usually the national press is the most expensive. Any newspaper advertisement should be noticeable but easy to read and understand. The price of the advertisement will depend on the number of words, therefore keep it brief, snappy and to the point! The following points should be considered when selecting which newspaper to use.

(a) A local paper would be the most suitable for a local target population as a national newspaper would not be selective enough.

(b) Local weekly papers have a reading life of one week or more therefore the advertisement will have more chance of being seen.

(c) Advertisers have to pay to advertise in the free papers but research indicates that they are read by a high percentage of the population in each delivery area.

National magazine advertising is usually well out of the price range of most salons, but other magazines such as parish magazines, carnival programmes and cinema, theatre or bingo programmes are worth considering if the target population is local. An advertisement placed in any of these magazines should have visual appeal as this type of literature is usually hastily read.

## Direct mail and leaflets

This can be a good way of informing local people of the services that the salon offers. The literature must be well produced and visually interesting so that it is noticeable and creates a good impression. Care should be taken with the wording to ensure that all the information is clearly stated and precise without being too long winded. If too much information is crammed on to the sheet no one will bother to read it.

There are sometimes offers available for salons using direct mailing for the first time (e.g. free postage on first mail shot). A specialist mailing house will provide a mailing list and will also produce and mail the publicity material for the salon. However, some salons prefer to produce their own material, particularly those with access to word processing or desk-top publishing facilities, in which case the electoral register may be used for the mailing list.

Leaflets can be delivered locally by hand and there are various organisations who are willing to carry out this task for a donation. Sometimes, for a fee, a local newsagent (or local newspaper itself) will slip a leaflet inside each newspaper before it is delivered.

## Posters

These are used to attract local trade and can be displayed at local halls, bus stops, and businesses including the salon. They must look professional and be designed to attract attention. It is often worth enlisting the help of a graphic artist or art student from a local college. Desk-top publishing can also produce professional posters which can be enlarged on a photocopier.

## Business directories

These list businesses together under their specialist areas to enable consumers to easily find the service they require (e.g. *The Yellow*

*Pages*). These are good for long term publicity as they are delivered to all homes within the locality that have a telephone. However, the salon will be listed with other competing salons therefore the entry has to be carefully worded.

## Local radio and cinema

Advertising on the local radio has the advantage that their audiences vary throughout the day therefore it is possible to target potential customers. However, it is cost effective only in areas of high population such as cities or large towns. Advertisements in local cinemas last approximately 15 seconds and the commercial itself is usually a generalised, pre-recorded one on hairdressing which is then personalised with the salon's name, address and services offered. The salon has to enter into a contract with the cinema so this is more of a long term commitment and, unless the cinema is situated near the salon, could have little effect.

## Transport advertising

Advertisements can be displayed on either the inside or outside of buses, trains, taxis, tubes or cars. Commuters do tend to read what is displayed about them while they are sitting immobile during transit. Advertisements appearing on the outside of transport must be visually exciting with a simple message so that they are easy to see and read. However, to be effective, the transport must travel through the salon's area so that it can be easily identified by potential clients.

## Demonstrations

This is an extremely effective way to promote the salon's services and image. It gives potential clients a very clear indication, at first hand, of what the salon can achieve. It also allows the consumer the opportunity to see what is on offer without any obligation or commitment to buy the goods. However, to be successful and to attain the desired result, the demonstration must be carefully planned and professionally executed irrespective of the size of audience or venue. Chapter 21 sets out in detail what to consider and how to carry out a demonstration for promotional use.

## Window display

This is also known as point of sale advertising and can be carried through to the reception area with displays and special offers. Local events, national incidents and seasonal displays (e.g. Christmas) can all be used as a vehicle for the display or promotion. All displays should be changed regularly otherwise they lose their impact and prospective clients fail to notice them. Large stores are extremely conscious of the power of an effective window display and use various devices to entice the consumer into the shop. Next time you walk down the high street, notice how many people are looking in the shop windows and try to see what has attracted them. See Chapter 2, Selling, which explains this in more detail.

## Personal selling

Personal selling is one of the most important forms of advertising but is very reliant on the expertise of the stylist, receptionist and other staff members as sales people. The whole process is far more personal and allows the client to find out more about the product/service by being able to ask questions. However, to be effective the staff must be aware of the importance of their role and must also have adequate product/service knowledge to give informed advice to the client. The staff should be encouraged to wear different forms of false hair themselves if this is the salon's specialism, for example hair extensions, which will enable the client to see a finished product and also enable the staff to discuss and advise the client from first-hand experience. If this is not possible, for example with toupees or specialised wigs which may be only suitable for certain people, then the staff must be given adequate training so that they have the necessary knowledge to carry out the service and advise the client.

## Summary

The collective name for wigs and hairpieces is postiche. Postiche may be made from hair (human or animal) or synthetic fibres. In addition, they may be made by hand, although this is expensive, or by machine. There are a variety of types of postiche for various purposes.

When consulting a client about postiche use it is very important to find out the client's exact requirement, and then to take great care to produce the desired effect. Full records must be kept.

Cleaning wigs and hair pieces is an important operation and there are different techniques for cleaning synthetic fibre and human/animal hair postiche.

Setting an animal/human hair wig involves fixing it to a malleable block, using a coloured rinse if needed and then completing the set or blowdry. Care needs to be taken in dressing the wig.

Securing postiche to the head involves different practical techniques for wigs and for toupees. There is a method for measuring the client's head for a toupee using a polythene sheet.

The advertising and sales techniques for postiche and other salon services can involve a variety of methods and the choice will depend on factors such as cost, target population and product.

The methods of advertising include:

1 Newspapers and magazines – which ones used will depend mainly on cost.
2 Direct mailing – which can be done through the post, possibly by using a specialist firm or leaflets delivered by hand.
3 Posters – which need to be particularly professional looking and striking.
4 Business directories – where careful wording is needed in the entry.
5 Local radio and cinema – this can be effective, though use will depend on cost.
6 Transport advertising – which, as for posters, needs to be professional looking and striking.
7 Demonstrations – these can be very effective at promoting a salon's service and image. Demonstrations need careful planning and professional carrying out.
8 Window display – these need to be changed regularly.
9 Personal selling – one of the most important forms of advertising which needs a high degree of selling skills by the staff involved. This method allows the client to see products in use, particularly so if the salon staff use them themselves.

## Self-assessment questions

1 Give four reasons for wearing a wig.
2 Where is the best quality blond hair obtained from?
3 What can postiche be made from?
4 Name the three main types of wig.
5 When measuring for a wig, what should be looked for on the scalp?
6 What is a malleable block?
7 What is the average size of a malleable block?
8 Why should the comb be held at an angle when disentangling the hair?
9 How do you clean postiche made from synthetic fibre?
10 What happens to synthetic fibre if it is in contact with too high a temperature?
11 Why is it important to use cleaning fluid and not shampoo when cleaning the wig?
12 How can a yellow discolouration of white hair be neutralised when setting the hair?
13 How should a cleaned wig be stored?
14 How is the wig secured to the head?
15 How is a toupee placed on the head?

**Practical assignment – Postiche services** _____

The following task will give you practice in measuring the head for a wig and enable you to feel more confident when completing a record card for the client.

You will need:

- tuition head, clamp and wide-toothed comb
- tape measure
- record card (*see* the example on page 346
- pen
- an illustration or photograph of a hairstyle (not too short).

## Task

(*a*) Set up the tuition head and disentangle the hair.

(*b*) Using the tape measure, take and record the following measurements:

- circumference of the head
- centre front hairline to the nape
- ear peak to ear peak across the front of the head
- ear to ear across the top of the head
- temple peak to temple peak around the back of the head
- temple peak to temple peak across the front of the head
- width across the nape of the neck
- hairline behind the top of the ear to the corner of the nape.

If you are unsure how to take these measurements refer to Fig. 19.1 which shows you in more detail where the measurements are taken.

(*c*) Using your selected illustration/photograph of a hairstyle, complete the remainder of the record card as if ordering a wig to be the same style, length, colour and with the same amount of curl as your illustration.

# MANAGING AND SUPERVISING STAFF

All salons have a hierarchy of staff, each of whom has their own role and responsibilities within the salon organisation. To enable the salon to function as efficiently as possible, these roles and responsibilities must be clearly defined so that each member of staff understands fully what is expected of them. It is impossible for any member of staff to be successful if they do not know what they should be doing in the first place!

Often much time and effort is spent in showing staff how to achieve advanced practical skills but very little time and training is given to salon rules, procedures and responsibilities. Training in these areas, however, will ensure that staff are fully aware of the organisation of the salon and of their own particular place within the structure. This helps to give each staff member a feeling of identity and encourages loyalty, commitment and therefore motivation within the company.

The hierarchy of the salon will depend largely on its size. A large company with a chain of salons will obviously require more managers, supervisors and other specialist staff to organize and oversee their large workforce than a smaller salon which may have to combine a number of roles to create just one manager/supervisor. However, regardless of the salon size, someone within the organisation *must* have overall responsibility for managing the workforce and ensuring that the salon's policies and procedures are carried out. This can be either someone who is specifically employed to carry out this task or it can be the salon owner.

## Role and qualities of a manager

The Occupational Standards branch of the UK Training Agency defines management as the process of 'utilising and facilitating the use of resources to maximum effect'. In other words, the manager's role is to seek to achieve the objectives of an organisation by controlling and organising its resources, including human resources, in the most efficient way possible.

The manager acts as a link between the employer and the workforce and so must be a good communicator and well aware of the salon's rules, procedures and policies and how they affect the workforce.

Managers are not always expected to carry out manual work as their role is to delegate tasks to other people, leaving themselves free to oversee the running of the salon, solve problems and make decisions as and where necessary. In order to delegate effectively, the manager must be fully aware of the abilities of each staff member including both their strengths and their weaknesses. Knowing their strengths enables them to select the most suitable person for each task while knowing their weaknesses allows extra training to be given where it is needed (often called 'staff development').

A manager must ensure that all staff are carefully prepared for their job. They must know the limits of their responsibilities and to whom they are accountable. Supervisors must be trained to set and maintain standards and to ensure that all the staff work as an integrated, well-motivated team with each member knowing what they are supposed to do.

It is important that the manager makes time for meetings to keep everyone informed of what is happening within the organisation and why. A well planned meeting will allow staff the opportunity to air views and offer suggestions, particularly if the agenda, i.e. the list of topics that are to be covered at the meeting, is given in advance to allow them time to consider the issues. Keeping the workforce informed and involving them in decisions will make any changes within the organisation less stressful. If people understand *why* something is happening they will be more likely to implement new policies instead of resisting them.

A manager must also have good administration skills and be able to write reports, keep records of staff attendance and try to ensure that all the salon paperwork is in order. In addition, it is usually the manager's responsibility to listen to the views and problems of both staff and clients. A good manager should identify and solve each problem as it arises, *before* it has a chance to affect the efficiency and goodwill of the salon.

## Role and qualities of a supervisor

According to the Hairdressing Training Board, a supervisor is a 'person responsible for others but also having operative duties with limited formal authority and with responsibility to management'. Thus, a supervisor is a leader who is very much a 'people' person with the ability to communicate effectively between higher management and the work group, acting as a 'go-between' to pass on the objectives and views of each.

The salon must make a profit to enable the staff to remain in employment and the supervisor has a key role in this as it is their responsibility to ensure that the salon runs efficiently with a well motivated team producing work of a high standard. The main duties of a supervisor include:

- inducting new staff
- supervising and monitoring staff
- communicating between management and staff
- counselling staff
- disciplining staff
- dealing with client complaints.

## Inducting new staff

This means giving a new employee all the information they will need and settling them into their new environment as quickly and painlessly as possible. Starting somewhere new can be a bewildering process and a lack of induction can leave the employee feeling confused, anxious and frustrated.

Very often, a large amount of information needs to be taken in at once so an induction programme spread over a period of time is a useful way to ease the learning process. Some salons have a 'probationary' period of about three months during which time the salon and the new staff member can decide whether they are compatible with one another. Any induction programme should be well planned with sessions built in to assess how the new employee is coping with their new environment and whether there are any problems. Solving any initial difficulties quickly prevents problems becoming insurmountable and also helps to create a bond between the employee and the organisation.

The induction programme should include the following:

- general salon rules and procedures
- contracts of employment
- protective clothing and use of equipment
- role and responsibilities of the staff
- training, monitoring and appraisal systems
- reception duties (if applicable).

## General salon rules and procedures

Each salon will have its own rules and procedures and these should be clearly stated at the beginning to prevent misunderstanding at a later date. Issues such as laundry, cleaning rotas, safety precautions, use of hazardous substances and security procedures for handling cash and stock should all be carefully explained to all new members of staff. It is also a good idea to display notices on important procedures, for example what to do in case of fire or accident, in a prominent position in the staff room as a constant reminder that can be easily referred to at any time.

## The contract of employment

This is a signed contract between the employer and the employee which is required by law and is legally binding by both parties. It states the condition of employment and responsibilities of the employee in terms of hours of work, holiday entitlement, grievance procedures, health and safety, codes of conduct, notice of intention to leave employment, equal opportunities, discipline and dismissal procedures, and it usually includes a restraint on working in another salon via a 'radius clause'. Thus it is in the interests of both the employer and employee to ensure that the contract and its contents are fully understood and agreed upon before it is signed.

## Protective clothing and the use of equipment

Some salons provide overalls or uniforms for the staff while others do not, in which case employees either buy their own or wear whatever they wish. However, it should be remembered that the salon must project a professional image and to do so the staff should be dressed accordingly. A salon uniform helps to maintain this professional image and also protect clothing from the effect of strong chemicals such as bleaching and tinting agents.

All new staff should be shown how to safely use and maintain each piece of salon equipment with the emphasis on safety precautions to minimise the risk of any accidents. All staff should be encouraged to report any faulty equipment so that it can be rectified immediately.

## Role and responsibilities

All new staff members must be encouraged to acquire a thorough knowledge of the work of the team, the policies of the organisation and how they themselves fit into the organisation's structure. They must also know what responsibilities they have towards their peers, seniors, clients and the salon. A job description is useful to enable the employee to know their duties exactly and to establish who is responsible for what. If staff do not know what they are supposed to do then it is difficult for them to do it well.

Take time introducing new staff to the other team members and use everyone's names as often as possible. It can be embarrassing at first to try to remember names, particularly in large organisations. Asking a more experienced member of staff to act as a 'mentor' to the new member can sometimes help them to settle in more easily and quickly. This system helps a new person to become part of the team more quickly and to ask questions which they may be reluctant to ask an employer or senior member of staff. Remember that a new team member can be a little disturbing to established relationships so it is important to give existing staff time to adjust.

## Training, monitoring and appraisal systems

Training has been described as the transfer of knowledge/skills from one person to another. It plays an important role in any organisation as it is the mechanism which enables each individual to be effective and produce work of a high standard. A new member of staff must be made aware of the salon's training programme and how it is to be implemented. New senior staff will need to be aware of the mechanisms for updating and extending existing skills to enable them to increase productivity and raise their own standard of work to meet changing demands.

Staff must also be aware of the salon's system of monitoring and assessing their progress and performance to enable them to measure their success and increase their motivation.

Appraisal systems are a useful way of monitoring staff performance. Their aim is to identify strengths and weaknesses and provide a means of setting goals and improving performance standards.

## Reception duties (if applicable)

Larger organisations employ a receptionist who takes over these duties in their entirety. However, in smaller salons the reception duties may be carried out by all members of staff, therefore guidance must be given on the salon's policies and procedures regarding the use of the telephone, booking and cancelling appointments, behaviour towards clients, taking messages and handling cash. Most salons have strict rules regarding these areas and each system should be carefully explained to avoid future mistakes.

## Supervising and monitoring staff

There are numerous areas that the supervisor must take into consideration when supervising and monitoring staff

- leadership
- training
- monitoring and assessing
- record keeping.

## Leadership

A supervisor is very much a 'leader' and to be effective in this role they must take into account not only the needs of the task or job but also those of the team and the individual.

*Team needs* It cannot be stressed too often that to create the right atmosphere within the salon and to work efficiently and effectively, the staff *must* work as an integrated team. Building a team requires special skills of the supervisor as it is never easy to bring together a group of people with different personalities and backgrounds to work together in harmony. However, the following points can be helpful in satisfying the needs of the team and aid cohesion:

- make use of individual talents
- speak up for the team and put their views to management
- consult the team and involve them in the organisation and decision making process
- establish standards and maintain them with the help of the team
- encourage group identity and help the team to give other members mutual support
- book a regular meeting slot and keep the team fully informed of what is happening.

*Individual needs* Various studies have shown that work plays an important role in most people's lives. People do not always work for financial rewards alone although this is obviously an important incentive. Often people also work for other reasons such as personal satisfaction, challenge, status etc. People do *not* work well if there are bad working conditions, fear of redundancy or change, personal worries, lack of incentives or information, lack of importance, boredom or poor relationships with colleagues. The supervisor must therefore take into consideration the needs of the individual and try to provide the right atmosphere and opportunity for personal growth and satisfaction. This can be done in the following ways:

- ensure that the working environment is as pleasant as possible
- understand the organisation's policies and keep staff fully informed of any decisions and changes by holding regular meetings
- be approachable, so that staff feel that they can discuss any problems freely and with confidentiality
- ensure that there is a structured training programme with a system for progression within the organisation
- encourage staff to use and broaden their individual talents and skills
- delegate responsibility and encourage staff to take pride in their work and the salon
- offer incentives to increase productivity and standards.

## Training

A key function of the supervisor is to set standards and to ensure that these standards are maintained. The standards will affect such areas as:

- quality of work
- health and safety
- efficient organisation.

*Quality of work* The type and standard of work that is produced by the salon will obviously present a certain image to prospective clients. The standard of work should be as high as possible. However, standards can be improved by regular training nights for both junior and senior staff. This gives the senior stylists time to experiment with new ideas and fashion trends, and gives the junior staff concentrated training which also enables them to see how new trends and fashions are achieved. Training nights also help to motivate the staff by allowing them time to discuss and air their views and also keeps staff informed of new trends and products and helps them to feel that they are part of a skilled team.

Video tapes of leading stylists demonstrating new techniques are also very useful to keep staff informed of current ideas. The tapes can be viewed time and time again and the tape can be stopped at any stage to clarify any important points. In this way it is often a better training aid than watching a live demonstration.

Attending short courses and demonstrations of new techniques and products improves the standard of work and helps to keep the salon dynamic rather than let it become set in its ways and, ultimately, old fashioned. Most manufacturers have trained technical staff who will come to the salon to demonstrate and instruct staff on any new products. This helps to give encouragement and confidence to try new products and judge their worth. New techniques and skills always generate enthusiasm and therefore help to keep staff motivated (*see* Chapter 21 for detailed information on training).

*Health and safety* A high standard of hygiene and due regard for the health and safety of both staff and clients is absolutely essential in any salon. The supervisor should make routine inspections of equipment and ensure that the salon's policies regarding Health and Safety are fully implemented and that all members of staff are aware of the procedures regarding care and maintenance of electrical equipment, dangerous chemicals, accidents etc.

*Efficient organisation* A smooth running salon not only depends on each staff member knowing what they are supposed to do and how to do it, but it also involves all the individuals working together as a team with common aims and objectives.

## Monitoring and assessing (appraisal)

Each member of staff should have their own individual training programme which matches their particular training needs. To ensure that they are progressing satisfactorily, the supervisor must monitor and assess their performance and keep training records.

Appraisal of staff performance should be against specific criteria. The 'criteria' can be hard to define but one possibility is to use the NVQ statements of competence as defined by the Hairdressing Training Board which is the lead body for hairdressing. Any appraisal should also include the general operation of salon rules, regulations and policies.

To be effective the monitoring and assessment of staff performance must be carried out on a regular basis and if done correctly will give an opportunity to amend the training programme if necessary. Staff should be kept informed of their progress and shown where they are making mistakes and how these can be rectified to enable them to succeed. It is also a good idea to make staff assess their own performance and that of their colleagues. Involving them in the assessment process encourages them to look more critically at their own work which helps them to maintain and raise their own standards.

## Record keeping

Good record keeping is essential to the smooth operation of the salon and enables senior management to acquire any relevant information which it may require as quickly as possible. The supervisor usually has responsibility for keeping the following records accessible and up-to-date.

- recording of work done by each stylist and other staff members to enable any training needs to be quickly identified
- staff attendance and sickness
- staff appraisal, training and assessment so that the progress of each member of staff is monitored
- any disputes, grievances and discipline procedures
- updating of personnel records of employees to ensure that any change in address, circumstances, staff development etc. is duly recorded for future reference
- results of any marketing exercises
- resource allocation including stock control and maintenance of equipment.

# Communicating between management and staff

Communication is the transfer of information from one person to others. It sounds easy but poor communication is the cause of more interpersonal problems than almost anything else in the salon. Communication goes wrong due to a combination of the speaker not being clear about their message and/or the listener picking out (perceiving) things in the message that are not there or taking the wrong emphasis.

The important thing is to be clear as to the key points of the message and relating this to the listener. Good communicators do not have to speak loudly, fast or often. They put the message clearly, simply and make sure the listener understands. This is as true of written as it is of oral information. A supervisor *must* be able to communicate effectively between higher management and the work group. Lack of communication can result in conflict and lack of co-operation between the two parties. Communication can be:

- oral
- by memos
- by meetings
- by being available for discussion.

## Oral

Oral instructions are spoken instructions which need to be kept **clear** and **short**. It is important to identify the **essential** information and concentrate on this. Question the listener to ensure that they have taken in the message you want and that it has no ambiguity. In giving a report or set of instructions to salon personnel, e.g. at a staff meeting, write down and try out (rehearse) what you want to say.

## Memos

A 'memo' is a message and the key points to remember are to keep it clear and short. Use note form and lists as much as possible. The following is an example:

Memo

To    Trainee

From    Manager

Date    1 September 19—

Subject    Stock levels

Please check that the stock levels of shampoo are sufficient for all of next week. Let me know if we need to order more by 4 pm today.

**Fig 20.1**

## Meetings

Meetings are an excellent means of passing on information and receiving staff opinions, ideas and suggestions if they are conducted properly.

Meetings should be held on a regular basis at a regular time slot to ensure that all staff are available. If possible, they should be well planned in advance and staff should be informed of the topics that are to be discussed. To be successful, the meeting should be kept strictly to time and within the limits of the agreed topics on the agenda. If other issues are raised these should be included at the end under 'Any other business' or retained for a future meeting. Make sure that any decisions made are implemented as soon as possible and any tasks allocated to staff are followed up soon after the meeting to ensure that they have been done or are in hand.

## Being available for discussion

During a busy working day this is not always as simple as it seems. However, finding time to talk to staff very often pays dividends as problems are more easily solved and good ideas can be implemented. Being available to staff also enables the supervisor to be aware of the opinions and feelings of their team and therefore in a better position to put their point of view across to higher management when required.

## Counselling staff

Counselling is listening to staff and helping them to find their own solutions to their problems. The need to counsel staff will arise from time to time. The signs that someone may need counselling are behaviour changes, a person who starts looking sad and withdrawn or being irritable etc., or you may get hints from other people.

The key point in counselling is listening, as opposed to solving problems. There is always a natural inclination to try and find solutions for other people's problems. This is not what counselling is about. You need to be a sympathetic ear and, if necessary, a shoulder to cry on. Any 'solutions' need to come from within the person and not from outside.

It is essential to be very careful in the counselling role and refer the person to professional counselling help if appropriate. If you are interested in this type of training contact your local College of Further Education and enquire about courses.

It is important to bear in mind the confidential nature of the conversations. Your staff should feel they can talk to you and be absolutely sure you will not divulge any of what they tell you.

Although this rarely happens it is possible that someone who has told you of various troubles will then use your knowledge of this to attempt to manipulate you over such matters as pace and standard of work. If you feel this is the case, tell the individual concerned that this is not really fair and that at the end of the day, however sympathetic you are, there is a limit to the amount of consideration a person can have in a salon operating as a business in a competitive environment. It is not that you do not care but the salon needs to operate well.

## Disciplining staff

Maintaining discipline in the salon does not necessarily mean 'domination'. If staff are treated fairly and with respect they are more likely to be loyal and hardworking in return. However, it is inevitable that on occasions the supervisor will have to discipline someone about poor or unacceptable performance. These situations include:

• persistent lateness or excessive time off work
• attitude problems shown by being offhand or rude to colleagues and clients
• slovenly or low standards of practical skills.

The disciplinary process should be carried out quietly, objectively and privately away from the other members of staff. Prepare carefully for the disciplinary interview by collecting together all the facts and making sure that they are correct, with dates and times if applicable. Most salons have a book in which to record when staff are off work (it is usual to let the salon know before 9 a.m. when a member of staff needs time off for sickness or other reasons).

During the interview, if appropriate, stress the **positive** aspects of the individual's performance to show you are aware of this, use such phrases as: 'I'm so surprised at this lateness because your general attitude is so good. Is there a problem?'

You must record the matter and what action was taken in accordance with the salon's disciplinary procedure. These procedures are usually contained in the contract of employment and a common system is:

1 two verbal warnings
2 two written warnings (the final one of which is usually the dismissal notice)
3 dismissal.

It is important to ensure that all individuals are aware of these disciplinary procedures.

## Dealing with client complaints

Most clients, if dealt with pleasantly and correctly, are easy to please, but there will always be some who have grievances, whether real or imagined. Tactful dealing with the client is essential to keep their goodwill and create a good impression of the salon. It is very tempting to feel that the salon would be better off without this type of client, but remember that when a client is lost, the salon also loses many more potential clients because the unsatisfied client will almost certainly give a bad impression of the salon's service to others, and if staff are rude to them this will only add truth to their story.

Any complaint by a client must be dealt with immediately, whatever the cause. If it is a complaint against the service, it should be dealt with to their complete satisfaction. For example, in the case of an unsatisfctory perm it is no use trying to persuade the client that it is satisfactory. Instead you should deal with the incident without fuss and re-perm where necessary, giving a quiet explanation as to the cause of failure. This is a far more professional attitude and more acceptable than an argument, which does not solve anything.

If a client is loud in their protests and is embarrassing to you and other clients you should take them quietly to a private part of the salon to rectify the complaint. If it concerns another member of staff it must be rectified with that member of staff present.

Even in the best-run salons, mistakes sometimes happen. A colour does not come up to expectations or a perm may be limp. If this occurs it is often the best policy to tell the client, before they complain, that you are not satisfied with the result and will rectify it immediately. This promotes goodwill and the client will have more trust, feeling that the stylist cares about their hair and will not be satisfied with second-best results. Their recommendations to others could bring many new clients to the salon and are an extremely effective way of advertising.

## Summary

All salons, regardless of size, must have a person with overall responsibility for the managing of staff and organisation of the salon. This person can either be the salon owner (in a small salon) or someone specifically employed as a manager or supervisor.

A manager has more authority and control than a supervisor and is not always expected to work practically in the salon. A supervisor's main duties include: inducting new staff, supervising and monitoring staff, communicating between management and staff, counselling staff, disciplining staff, dealing with client complaints and also working practically alongside their team. Thus a supervisor is a leader, communicator, counsellor, disciplinary, arbitrator and worker.

When inducting new staff into the salon a programme should be devised with information on the general rules and procedures of the salon; contracts of employment; protective clothing and the use of salon equipment; the role and responsibilities of the staff; training, monitoring and appraisal systems and any reception duties that may be required of the new staff member.

The supervisor must take into consideration the following

areas when supervising and monitoring staff: leadership; training; monitoring and assessing; and record keeping. Communication between management and staff can be done orally, through memos, through staff meetings or by the supervisor being available when staff wish to discuss any issues or problems. Counselling may be necessary and this involves listening to staff problems and helping them to find their own solutions. Disciplining of staff may also be necessary on occasions but where this is the case it should be carried out quietly, objectively and privately.

Any disciplinary action is usually recorded and the system operated in most salons is: two verbal warnings followed by two written warnings the final one of which is usually the dismissal notice.

A supervisor must also have the skills and knowledge to be able to deal tactfully with a client if they have a complaint.

## Self-assessment questions

1   Why is it important that all staff are fully aware of the organisation of the salon and their own particular place within the structure?
2   List *three* personal skills necessary for a good manager.
3   What is the definition of a supervisor?
4   List *six* duties of a supervisor.
5   What is meant by 'inducting' a new member of staff?
6   What is a contract of employment?
7   List *seven* reasons why a member of staff may not want to work hard.
8   List *four* ways that a supervisor can communicate between higher management and the workforce.
9   What is counselling?
10  How should the disciplinary process be carried out?

## Practical assignment – Directing and supervising staff job descriptions

Every person employed by the salon should be aware of the tasks that they are expected to carry out during the working day. They should also be aware of their responsibilities towards clients, colleagues and any senior staff/employer.

A job description must give specific guidelines as to the role of the person employed to do that particular job. It should not be in any way ambiguous and consist of clear statements to prevent any misunderstandings or conflict at a future date.

## Task

You are the owner of a small successful hairdressing salon which has just undertaken a restructuring and expansion programme. You will require the following members of staff for a 'Grand Opening' in two months time:

- trainee
- stylist
- manager/supervisor.

1   Decide what duties you consider to be the responsibilities of each of the above members of staff. Information can be obtained from your workplace, careers office, college tutors and textbooks.

2   Make a list of the duties and responsibilities of each and include when and how often these duties should be carried out, e.g. 'Take the towels to the laundry at the end of each day'.

3   Present your work neatly as a job description document which is either typed or word-processed.

# 21 TRAINING STAFF AND DEMONSTRATING SKILLS

Training is an essential part of any working organisation and the ability to organise training programmes and show people a hairdressing procedure are important skills for any supervisor.

## Training salon staff

There are four key areas in successful training:

- planning and preparing for the training session/programme
- carrying out the training, coaching the trainee
- assessing the trainee's performance and progress
- carrying out an overall assessment, and evaluation of the training programme.

Training is a skill and like all skills a good performance is smooth, 'polished' and 'looks easy'. Think of occasions when you would say 'that was really good'. Reflect on *why* this was in terms of the technique and delivery. You will probably find that it involved all of the list above. Experienced trainers often do much of their preparation, responding to trainees during the session and assessment and review of their own performance automatically (almost unconsciously), but to begin with it is necessary to explain these stages.

### Planning and preparing

Planning and preparation are extremely important to the success of a training programme. Care and attention to detail for this is very worthwhile.

The place to start planning is at the **specific objectives** of the programme or session. In other words what is it *exactly* that the trainee should be able to do at the end of the session that they could not do (or not do to a sufficient level of competence) at the start.

The more precise you are about this the easier is the planning of the stages to achieve these objectives. A useful aid in planning to reach a training objective is to bear in mind 'BEEP', a system which can be used for whole programmes, individual sessions or parts of sessions.

**B** – before the training

What is the level of the trainee's existing competence? Are they starting from nothing or do they have previous experience?

**E** – experience

Practice and experimentation must be built into the training programme to enable the trainee to achieve the desired level of competence.

**E** – environment

Where is the training to happen? What equipment and resources will be needed from both within the salon (internal) and/or from outside (external)?

**P** – performance

What are they to be able to do and to what standard, how and in what length of time?

## The training session – coaching the trainee

Having set clear objectives, carefully planned your delivery in terms of content, pace and resources/facilities needed, then organised these resources and facilities, you are now ready to run the session. The best training sessions involve:

- Learning by doing (activity learning)
- Tolerance of mistakes/errors
- Responding positively to individuals.

Plan your session to involve as little 'showing' and as much 'doing' as possible. Use as much time as possible on one-to-one discussions if working with a group. Be active and vigilant and respond positively to *any* request for help or further information. Encourage progress by praise and general positive reinforcement (for example 'that's good!' 'well done', 'you're doing well' etc.). Avoid the negative. If a trainee is not getting much out of the session, try to analyse where the problem is or who is at fault.

## Assessing and recording the trainee performance

If you have clear definitions of your competency goals (such as those used by the National Vocational Qualification) then you have a structure with which to work, both in terms of checking competence (can they do it to the right standard in the required time) as well as a system of recording their achievement.

There are a variety of systems for keeping records. The City and Guilds/Hairdressing Training Board uses a 'tick the box' type based on observation of practical skills and on oral and written assessments. This is a good starting point although you may wish to adapt it to the salon's requirement. The important point is that the system of recording progress is quick, clear and can be modified if required in the future. When a recording system is established it provides a structure for reviewing the training requirements with a trainee.

A review session should be on a one to one basis and in a situation where disturbance and interruptions are minimal. Both the trainee and the supervisor should *prepare* for the review session. If you have a clear set of criteria for competence in an area, the trainee can independently assess their own level of competence and then compare this with the supervisor. This encourages the trainee to feel they have some role in the process and to take it seriously. In addition it concentrates time on the areas of 'mismatch' where the supervisor's and trainee's opinions vary. If both assessments agree then the review can move straight on to producing a plan to achieve the missing or underdeveloped skills.

## Evaluating the training

Evaluation is judging the worth of something (its value). Any evaluation of training hinges on whether it has been 'worthwhile' in that it has achieved its objectives. Even if it has, could it be improved? Perhaps it could be more efficient (using less time and resources) or more effective (with better learning opportunities).

The emphasis throughout this section on 'training' has been the need for clear objectives, careful planning and review with the trainees of their training achievements.

However, much time also needs to be spent on a detailed evaluation as in the planning stage. There is a tendency to 'finish and run', that is, to finish the programme and let that be the end of the supervisor's involvement. This is particularly so if the training has been successful. Post mortems are reserved for the bad ones!

The following notes should help you in planning and preparing training sessions.

1 Specific descriptions of competency levels and how to measure these are given in the Hairdressing Training Board's publication on the National Vocational Qualifications (NVQ) in Hairdressing. NVQ is based on 'Competence statements', and include very useful analyses of what is needed to be 'competent' in the major hairdressing operation.

2 Having identified what you want to achieve, this clarifies and informs you what to do. Your planning should identify the key stages in the learning and concentrate on these. Exactly what these will be will depend on the level of previous experience of the trainee.

3 Having planned what you want to achieve and the steps needed to get there, this then clarifies 'how' you are going to achieve it. What facilities will you need? While the *essential* facilities and equipment will be the usual available in a salon, basic visual aids

could be included such as video, colour slides, wall chart, training manuals, articles cut from magazines and trade journals.

Help can also be obtained from outside the salon from manufacturer's training schools, short courses in your local Further Education College, textbooks, video tapes, demonstrations by manufacturer's technicians, day seminars, and workshops held by leading stylists and private hairdressing schools.

4  Does the trainee receive training from another organisation, such as off-the-job training at college? If so, make sure you are fully aware of the content of the programme. There may be flexibility in these programmes to meet your trainee's needs and it will be worthwhile finding out if their analysis of the training needs of the trainee agree with yours.

In general it is very useful to make contact and co-operate with others providing hairdressing training to your trainees.

5  Will the material you have selected for your training be suitable for a wide range of trainees?; male as well as female?; older people?; people from various ethnic groups? It is very easy to see hairdressers as 'stereotypes', being *young, white and female*. Always bear this in mind, not just because of the desirability (even legal requirement) of 'equal opportunities' but so that your time and effort of planning and preparing the session materials can be used as widely as possible.

Careful, step-by-step review of all parts of the programme using **feedback** from the trainees, management and the supervisor's own feelings and perception can save time in the future and improve even the most successful programmes.

This feedback will arise:

- during the sessions – verbal and non-verbal communication of the level of involvement, employment and learning
- during review – with trainees before and after the programme
- during discussion with salon management on the content and outcomes of the training.

You can also use questionnaires to obtain anonymous feedback from participants, session by session if required. However, if questionnaires are used they should be short and 'tick the box' type responses, with some space allowed for a written comment.

Following the evaluation, ensure that notes on improvement etc., are kept for reference in the future. It is surprising how even the best memories lose the details of evaluation after six busy months. Writing short notes will ensure that lessons learned are taken into consideration and do not have to be re-learnt at a later date.

# Demonstrating practical skills

The ability to demonstrate clearly a hairdressing procedure is very important in both of the following areas:

- demonstrating practical skills to staff
- demonstrating to the public.

## Demonstrating practical skills to staff

This type of demonstration must be carefully planned to ensure that the demonstration clearly illustrates the **key** points you wish to emphasise and the practical skills involved. It is worth remembering that an audience has a limited attention span of 2–3 minutes, so the demonstration should vary in pace and allow time for the trainee to experiment or practise themselves. Learning is more efficient if the trainee is allowed to use all the senses, including those of touch and smell as well as watching and listening.

Good preparation is the key to success when demonstrating and careful planning of the areas, as shown in Fig 21.1.

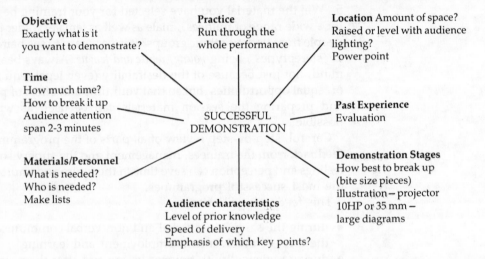

**Objective**
Exactly what is it you want to demonstrate?

**Practice**
Run through the whole performance

**Location** Amount of space?
Raised or level with audience lighting?
Power point

**Time**
How much time?
How to break it up
Audience attention span 2-3 minutes

SUCCESSFUL DEMONSTRATION

**Past Experience**
Evaluation

**Materials/Personnel**
What is needed?
Who is needed?
Make lists

**Demonstration Stages**
How best to break up (bite size pieces)
illustration – projector
10HP or 35 mm –
large diagrams

**Audience characteristics**
Level of prior knowledge
Speed of delivery
Emphasis of which key points?

**Fig 21.1**

There are a number of ways of laying out plans for demonstrations and training. Figure 21.2 is an example of one you may like to use.

| Title ..................... | | Time allowed | |
| --- | --- | --- | --- |
| *Objective* | *Time* | *Method* | *Materials* |
| | | | |

**Fig 21.2**

# Feedback

Feedback is the information you receive from the audience during (and after) your demonstration. During the performance take care to look at the audience, to determine what signals they are sending. Are the signals negative with shifting around, talking or staring into space, or are they positive, with people giving their full attention, everyone sitting still and smiling when you make eye contact? There may be a mixture of both types of signals and it is important to assess the reasons for the differences.

At the end of the demonstration the level of questions and the length of time people linger are signs of their attitudes. Individuals may say flattering (or unflattering) things to you. However, be aware that these are probably people who feel much more strongly than the 'average' audience member.

Formal feedback can be obtained using a short questionnaire on a postcard or small sheet of paper. Keep these short and clear. Try to use 'tick the box' answers for speed but allow some scope for written reactions.

## Evaluation

This is the important stage of reflecting on 'how it has gone'. This review is very important and needs to be taken into consideration when planning the next demonstration. In addition to staff feedback the model and your own evaluation of the session will help you to assess the level of success. In addition, trainee feedback allows you to define 'success' in terms of whether you have reached the training goals with those trainees.

Always find the time to write down a summary of what went well or what did not and any lessons for the future. It may be some time before you do the same thing again and you will then be able to learn from any mistakes as well as the parts of the session which went well.

One final point is that it is essential to stress the importance of safety to both the client and the operator during any demonstrated process. Good hygiene procedures and practices should also be emphasised.

# Staging a demonstration in a promotional context

This is an extremely effective means of improving public relations and promoting the salon. It is also a good way to motivate the entire staff as everyone from the top stylist to the shampooist can be involved. Staging a demonstration is a stimulating experience which reinforces working together 'as a team' and encourages the stylists to give full vent to their creativity.

Hair demonstrations can be linked up with talks on different aspects of haircare or can be used as a showcase to present a specific 'look' which the salon is promoting. Demonstrations can be staged by the salon on its own or as a joint venture with another organisation. For example, Boutiques or In-store Fashion Shows need hairdressers and make-up artists to make the most of their models and show off their fashion clothes to best effect.

The best way to get involved with this type of work is to write or go to see the store/boutique in question, usually in your client catchment area, taking photographs of the salon's work to give an indication of the standard and variety of work the salon can achieve. Invite relevant managers or the public relations officer (PRO) along to your salon to see the work you are doing and offer very competitive rates or, better still, do the show free of charge at first.

The type of audience you wish to attract will make a difference to the type of demonstration you present. Organising a hairdressing demonstration for younger people at a Youth Club will obviously be approached differently from staging a high-profile, expensive demonstration to a mixed audience in a top-class hotel. If the audience has paid a high price for a ticket to attend a top-class venue, then their expectations will differ from the audience that is attending a free demonstration. For this reason, it is extremely important to decide at the beginning what type of demonstration you wish to present and what the target audience will be.

Every hair and fashion demonstration/show *must* be organised to the very last detail and timing needs to be split-second. If not, there can be embarrassing gaps in the programme, misleading information given about the hairstyles and clothes, or the wrong clothes may be worn for that part of the programme.

## Organisation of tasks

Begin by delegating certain tasks and roles to a number of people. Depending on the size and type of demonstration, all or some of the following roles will have to be allocated:

- Co-ordinator
- Compère
- Hairstylists
- Trainee/junior
- Make-up artist
- Wardrobe mistress/dresser
- Disc jockey (DJ)
- Models
- Photographer.

## Co-ordinator

This is the key role as the co-ordinator has overall responsibility for organising and liaising with management on the venue, music, lighting, seating, advertising, and printing and distribution of any necessary tickets. They must also make out a schedule of work and timetable for both the countdown and the actual day of the event to ensure that everyone knows exactly what they are doing and when.

## Compère

This is also an important role, as the person selected will have to speak through a microphone in front of the audience. Therefore, they must have good communication skills and the self-confidence to speak in public.

They must be able to handle interruptions from the audience. Sometimes questions asked during the demonstration can be a useful means of explaining certain processes being carried out on stage, but this really depends on the type of demonstration. Too many questions may sidetrack the commentary and then become an intrusion. It may be necessary to insist that all questions be saved until the end of the session.

The compère must be sensitive at all times to the atmosphere conveyed by the audience and must be able to pitch the commentary at the correct level for the type of audience. Making the commentary too technical may bore the audience, whilst pitching it at too low a level is embarrassing and will make them feel uncomfortable.

If the audience appears restless or uninterested, then the compère must be able to regain the audience's attention by various strategies, e.g. humour; increasing the 'pace' of the demonstration; adding anecdotes; etc.

For demonstrations linked to hair care it may be possible to contact leading manufacturers to see if any of their senior sales staff would be willing to take on this role.

## Hairstylists

They must be quick and efficient. If dressing the hair in public they must be confident working in front of an audience. When styling the hair for a Fashion Show, they often have to work in very cramped, backstage quarters. They must be able to create and convert hairstyles on long or short hair quickly, using temporary methods of curling, such as heated rollers, hot sticks, or curling tongs, as it may not be possible to wet the hair.

## Trainee/juniors

They are needed to carry out any of the preliminary tasks on the hair or to help the stylists before, during and after the performance. They must make sure that everywhere is cleaned and tidied after use and check that all equipment is cleaned and returned to the salon. Often it is useful to allow the trainee to help the stylist at the demonstration, as it gives them valuable experience of working in front of an audience, boosts their confidence and makes them feel an important member of the team.

## Make-up artist

They must be fully briefed about the clothes and hairstyles that the models will be wearing and should be given a full list of who is wearing what, so they can make sure that the hair, clothes, colours and make-up styles all match.

If you do not know a freelance beautician, try the local press, *Yellow Pages,* or final year students on a Beauty Therapy course at a local college. However, always check the standard of the make-up artist's work first before engaging them, and remember that stage make-up needs to be slightly darker and heavier than normal, to counteract the strong lighting.

## Wardrobe mistress/dresser

A person is needed to take charge of the clothing and accessories and to make sure that they are co-ordinated with the hair and make-up. Before a Hair and Fashion Show, the clothing must be clean, pressed and placed in the correct order, usually on a rail in the changing room. The Wardrobe Mistress must then make sure that the correct outfit is worn by the correct person during the show/demonstration. All clothing should be checked and then safely returned after the event. A useful tip when having a lot of costume changes is to list (or sketch) all clothes, accessories and shoes on a piece of paper and pin this to the outside of a black plastic bag which contains all the parts of the particular outfit.

## Disc jockey

The DJ must be carefully briefed on the format of the demonstration or show and should be given a list with the order of any scenes, e.g. sports, bridal, together with who will be appearing and what music is required for each particular part. Very specific instructions should also be given as to the volume of the music, and when it needs to be faded out completely – for example, whilst the compère is talking.

The music should not be an intrusion but should complement the 'looks' that are being portrayed. It must also be on cue, as any unwanted silent gaps are embarrassing to both the audience and the people involved. Always go through the music carefully with the DJ and rectify any misunderstandings or problems at the rehearsal stage.

## Models

Depending on the type of demonstration or show, the models should be chosen to show off the hair and clothes to best effect. If they will be only sitting having their hair done on stage and standing at the end, then attractive clients from the salon will probably be suitable as models. However, many girls are shy and find it difficult to walk down a catwalk correctly to music; therefore, it is often better to use professional models. If this is too expensive ask at the local college, polytechnic or private modelling school to see if any of their final year modelling or fashion students would be willing to model. Often they are delighted to gain the experience and the photographs of them in action are very useful when they re creating their portfolio for use after their training.

## Photographer

Local newspapers can be contacted to cover the event. For added marketing impact, the event could be linked to a special offer advertisement giving discounts to those members of the public who attend the demonstration.

Always have your *own* photographer, in addition to the press, as news photographers do not always take the shots you would wish and sometimes do not even attend.

Decide on the general effect you want from the finished photographs and then, if possible, give the photographer a list of the shots you require. Remember that any good pictures can be blown up and displayed in the salon or sent to various newspapers and magazines with a short report of the event as an interest story. If it is published, this is an excellent way of promoting the salon.

A video taken of the event is a good training and evaluating aid for both present and future staff, as it can show any mistakes and where improvements can be made. If it is edited, it can be used as a marketing tool to show the standard and variety of work that can be achieved by the salon.

## Planning the event

Careful planning is absolutely essential to your succes; therefore make a checklist of all the things that must be done before you start. You will need to include in your checklist:

## Venue

The location will depend on the type of demonstration and the funds available. If the salon is servicing an In-store Fashion Show, then obviously there will be no charge. If, however, the venue is to be in a hotel or community centre, there may be a fee. So, before committing yourself, compare the prices and *facilities* of a variety of places.

Consider carefully the lighting, seating space, staging, access to water, electric sockets, changing area and fire precautions. Check what car parking facilities are available and whether the venue is easily accessible by public transport.

These issues are important as they will affect your final choice of venue. They will determine the size of your audience (fire precautions also often limit numbers) and the type of presentation it is possible to stage. For example, a big fund-raising event will require a central location, good car parking facilities, enough seating space, and adequate lighting to give good visual impact to the whole audience. Sometimes it is necessary to bring additional spot lighting and, if this is the case, always make sure that the electrical systems can withstand the additional load.

## Date

This may be dependent on the venue, which could have only certain dates available. If there is a free choice, then decide on the type of audience you wish to target and check local newspapers, libraries, etc., to make sure that the date you have chosen will not clash with any other events.

Consider also any holidays, such as annual or bank holidays, and the time of year. During busy summer months will your staff have *time* to put in the necessary preparation before the demonstration? In winter will the weather be too bad for people to attend?

## Printing/publicity

If tickets and programmes are required, enquire into sponsorship by manufacturers or local business firms. They may be willing to print the tickets and/or programmes free of charge in return for publicity. Asking local businesses to advertise in the programme for a small fee will often offset the printing costs. Always acknowledge any sponsorship, advertising or other help received.

Publicise the event well in advance in the local press and place posters in local shops (including your own salon), local colleges, libraries and community centres. Remember that people can only attend if they know all about it well in advance.

It may also be worth while sending free tickets to local dignitaries and VIPs, as this gives added interest to the press.

After the event send photographs and a short report to your local newspaper and trade journals.

## Costings

Make a list of all the 'outgoings' for the demonstration. This list could include: hire of venue; printing, publicity, flowers; maaterials used on the hair such as mousse, lacquer, gels, etc.; laundering of gowns and towels; refreshments; helpers' fees (e.g. make-up artist); and any other sundry expenses. Add together the outgoings and then divide this figure by the number of people you expect to attend. This will give you the *minimum* price required for each ticket. Remember that there may not be a full attendance and therefore it may be necessary to charge more, and donate any profit to charity.

Some salons prefer to stage a demonstration free of charge and offset the expenses as advertising or promotion of the salon.

## Refreshments

These can be anything from coffee or cheese and wine to a full buffet, depending on the type of event, the budget allowance and when it is to be held, i.e. during the day or in the evening.

Refreshments can be served in the middle of the presentation as an interval, or at the end so that staff and models can mingle with the audience to answer any questions and talk about the hair salon. This part of the event can be especially good for the salon's public relations!

## Schedule of work

Make out a list of the people needed to help with the demonstration and then make out a detailed timetable for practice sessions and rehearsals, ensuring that everyone attends.

Work out a 'countdown' timesheet and then a timetable for the actual day of the demonstration. Everyone involved in the demonstration *must* know not only their own role but also where they fit into the programme as a whole. So, to keep the event under control, write down each production number in order, together with the following information:

- Music for the scene.
- Name of models.
- What clothes they will be wearing.
- What accessories, e.g. shoes, hair ornaments.
- What hairstyle for each model.
- Prices, if necessary.

Give a copy of this information to the compère, DJ, hairstylists, make-up artist, wardrobe mistress and models. Pin another copy next to the door in the changing room for communal reference so that everyone knows the schedule and exactly what is going on.

If the event has been carefully prepared beforehand, there will be less chance of mistakes and excessive stress on the day.

## Evaluation and feedback

This can be both during and after the event. During the demonstration the audience will express either positive or negative reactions. Positive reactions can be determined by the way in which the audience listens attentively, asks relevant questions when appropriate, and can also be felt in the general atmosphere. Negative reactions can be very noticeable – if the audience fidgets in their seats, lacks concentration and attention, talks together or walks out either during the demonstration or at the interval.

Walking amongst the audience after the demonstration will also give a good indication as to whether the event has been successful or not. If the audience is enthusiastic and wanting to know more about the hairstyles, the clothes and the salon, then this is usually an indication of a successful event. If, however, the audience is non-committal, unwilling to give an opinion or avoids eye contact, this could be an indication that they have not enjoyed themselves.

It is *very* important to have a debriefing session with the entire staff as soon after the event as possible to find out what worked well and what problems there were.

Write down all the important points to use for future reference and give an indication of how to improve future performance. Keep a record of all transactions and costings to evaluate if your predictions were accurate. Make notes on any improvements or savings that could be made.

Feedback from clients may take a period of time. Regular clients are usually delighted that 'their' salon has a high profile. However, other members of the audience may have been perfectly happy with their current salon, but may become a new client much later. Staff should be encouraged to ask any new clients whether they attended the event, in order to determine its impact on the local community.

## Sample timesheet for a hair and fashion show

*Night before:*
Collect clothes, accessories and any props. Check that all equipment, tools and materials needed for the hair are clean and ready.

*8.00 a.m.:*
Arrive at venue. Divide clothes into production numbers or 'looks' and place *in order* on the rail. Pin up the schedule on the wall.

*8.30 a.m.:*
Models, hairstylists and make-up artist arrive.

*9.00–10.45 a.m.:*
Rehearsals. Make sure that everything is in the correct order and that the compère and DJ have been fully briefed.

Anything that goes wrong or missing can be rectified at this stage.

*10.45–12.00:*
Dress models, hairstylists and make-up artist. Do hair and make-up. Check that programmes are laid out on the audience's seats.

Make sure that the photographer and local press are positioned where they can see. Also check that the compère's script has the details about any VIPs or sponsorship, and all credits for make-up artists, boutique or fashion house, and hair salon.

*12.00–12.45 p.m.:*
The Presentation.

*12.45 p.m. onwards:*
Refreshments. Models and stylists mingle with the audience, answering any questions on the hair and salon. Make a note of all comments made by the audience for the future debriefing session.

*3.00 p.m.:*
Collect all clothes and equipment and check that nothing is missing.

## Summary

**Successful training requires careful organisation, the key areas being: planning and preparation of the training session/programme, coaching of the trainee, assessment of trainee performance and progress and an overall assessment of the training programme.**

**Review of all parts of the programme can be obtained by feedback from the trainees, supervisors and managers during the sessions, during the review and by the use of questionnaires.**

**When planning and preparing the training session, make use of training manuals such as the Hairdressing Training Board's NVQ Levels I, II and III in hairdressing. Plan what needs to be achieved, how to achieve it and what resources will be needed. Make sure that you are aware of the content of any 'off-the-job' training which may be carried out at a college or training centre and that your training materials are suitable for all types of people to ensure equal opportunities for all.**

**Demonstration of practical skills can be either to trainees during training sessions or to the public as a marketing exercise for the salon. Both types of demonstration require careful planning and should be evaluated to assess how effective they have been. The main difference between the two types of demonstration is that the 'marketing' type needs to be highly polished with the emphasis on presentation rather than technical detail.**

## Self-assessment questions

1 Give a definition of 'Training'.
2 What does BEEP stand for?
3 How should a 'review session' be carried out?
4 What is 'evaluation'?
5 What is 'feedback'?
6 List *four* ways of obtaining feedback from a training programme.
7 What is the best way to get involved in outside hair demonstrations?

8 What could happen if a hair demonstration was not organised down to the very last detail?

9 List the tasks and roles that should be delegated to people when organising an outside demonstration.

10 List *seven* areas that need to be carefully considered when planning a demonstration of the salon's hairdressing skills to an outside audience.

**Practical assignment – Training staff and demonstrating practical skills** _____

Careful planning and organisation of a training session can be very time consuming and requires systematic preparation.

## Task

For this practical assignment you are required to *plan* a training session on *shampooing* for a new trainee who has just joined your salon.

Lay out your plan in the format shown on p. 376. To help you to organise your training session answer the following questions which will take you step-by-step through the planning process.

(a) Make a list of what you want the trainee to know at the end of the session e.g. what type of shampoo to select for greasy, limp, dry or fine hair etc.

(b) What do you want to demonstrate and what is the most interesting way that you can do this?

(c) What resources will you need with regard to consumables, personnel and location etc.

(d) How much time will be needed and how can you vary the 'pace' of the demonstration?

(e) Have you any available back-up literature such as diagrams, photographs, illustrations etc.?

(f) What key points need to be emphasised and why?

(g) How much past experience or prior knowledge has the trainee? Can it be used to help the trainee to understand? (e.g. shampooing their own hair)

(h) Have you included all the Health and Safety aspects in your demonstration?

(i) How are you going to test what and how much the trainee has learnt?

(j) How are you going to assess the success or weak areas of the training session?

# GLOSSARY

**Abundant** sometimes referred to as the density of the hair. It is a term used in hairdressing to describe a plentiful amount of hair per square inch/cm and is of significance when assessing the hair before a treatment.

**Acid** any substance which when dissolved in water gives off hydrogen ions. It produces a solution with a pH value below 7.

**Acid conditioners** conditioners which help to restore the hair to an acid state.

**Acid mantle** idea that natural oil (sebum) and sweat produce a slightly acid condition on the skin.

**Activators** *see* boosters.

**Aerosol** strictly speaking means droplets of liquid in air, but has come to mean the pressurised canisters that produce a spray of droplets, e.g. lacquer.

**Aesculap scissors** scissors which have one (or both) blades serrated.

**Afro comb** a comb with thick, large prongs usually made from vulcanite that can be used to create volume without frizz on Afro-Caribbean or extremely curly hair.

**Afro hair** Afro-Caribbean hair which is usually extremely curly and brittle.

**AIDS** stands for Auto-Immune Deficiency Syndrome. This very dangerous disease could possibly be transmitted from one person to another in the salon by blood contamination. For example, when someone is cut by a razor and the razor is not cleaned, and then it is used again and cuts another person. There is some risk but there have been no recorded cases of transmission in this way in the hairdressing salon.

**Alkali** *see* base.

**Allergic dermatitis** *see* dermatitis.

**Allergy** when the body 'over-reacts' to something called the primary irritant. Often requires a number of exposures to the irritant to produce a body reaction, i.e. a period of sensitisation. When sensitised the body reacts each time the irritant is present.

**Allergy test** *see* skin test.

**Alopecia** the general name for hair loss or balding. There are a number of different types including:

   **alopecia areata** hair loss in patches, cause not known.

**alopecia diffusa** general thinning of hair, can be due to a number of causes, e.g. some drugs.

**traction alopecia** hair is pulled out by tension applied to the hair, e.g. some hairstyles.

**Amino acids** building blocks of protein. They make up polypeptide chains.

**Ammonium carbonate** an ingredient often used in powder bleaches to increase the alkalinity of the mixture.

**Ammonium sulphite** used in some hair straighteners (relaxers).

**Ammonium thioglycollate** active ingredient in traditional alkaline (pH 9.5) perm lotions. Acid perms contain glycerol thioglycollate.

**Anagen** actively growing phase of the hair growth cycle.

**Antibiotics** chemicals which can destroy bacteria.

**Antibodies** chemicals in the blood which help to destroy germs.

**Antiseptics** chemicals which inhibit the growth of micro-organisms, e.g. bacteria, in which case they are called bacteriostatic.

**Arrector pili muscle** a small muscle in the skin which is connected to the hair follicle. When it contracts it pulls the follicle upright and produces 'goose pimples' (goose flesh) and causes the hair to rise.

**Assessment (of client)** judging a client's requirements in terms of their face, shape, lifestyle, hair types and condition before a treatment.

**Assessment (of staff)** often called **appraisal**. This should be done against specific criteria and is a positive process of finding out what staff can or cannot do well.

**Auxiliary detergent** weaker cleaners added to shampoo to improve its properties, e.g. these can thicken, help condition hair or give a rich lather.

**Backbrushing** pushing the hair back on itself using a brush to create volume to the hairstyle when dressing hair.

**Backcombing** pushing the hair back on itself at the roots to produce a padded effect which gives volume to the hairstyle. Backcombing on top of the hair mesh to blend the hair is termed 'teasing'.

**Bacteria** type of micro-organism which can be neutral or useful or harmful (pathogenic) and cause disease.

**Bacteriostatic** of chemicals that inhibit the growth of bacteria; the basis of most antiseptics.

**Balance** term used in hairdressing to refer to the shape of the final hairstyle in relation to the client's face, head, neck and body. The silhouette of a hairstyle helps to show up any defects in its balance.

**Balding/baldness** *see* alopecia.

**Barber's itch (sycosis barbae)** caused by staphylococci bacteria which cause inflammation of the beard hair follicles.

**Barrier cream** a cream used to protect the client's skin when carrying out processes which could cause skin irritation or staining, e.g. when perming, tinting or bleaching.

**Basal** layer of the skin which produces new cells sometimes referred to as germinativium or malpighian layer.

**Base** any substance which can react with an acid to form a substance called a salt and water. Soluble bases are called alkalis and have pH values above 7.

**Benzol alcohol** used as a solvent in semi-permanent dyes to allow the dye to penetrate the hair shaft more efficiently.

**Bevel cutting** club cutting the hair on a curve. The hair is held between the fingers and then bent up and in towards the scalp; when this hair is then cut straight across, graduation is created on the ends of the hair.

**Bimetallic (bimetal) strips** often used in thermostats. Consist of two different metals fixed together which expand and contract differently, making the strip bend when heated or cooled. The movement can be used to, e.g. switch electricity on and off.

**Blackheads** caused by a skin pore becoming blocked by a plug of grease and dirt, often the first stage of a spot.

**Bleach** chemicals used to lighten or decolourise the colouring pigment of the hair. Types include simple, oil, powder (or paste) and emulsion bleaches.

**Blepharitis** *see* styes.

**Block colouring** a fashion colouring technique usually used to emphasise the shape of a short hairstyle by graduating various colours in 'blocks' through the hair from the nape through to the front of the head.

**Blowdrying** a method of drying the hair with the aid of brushes, combs and/or hands to create a natural, soft effect which can be either curly or smooth depending upon the desired result.

**Blow waving** a method of waving the hair with the aid of a comb or brush and the heated air from a hand dryer.

**Boil (furuncle)** caused by staphylococci bacteria. Symptoms are red, round area which is very sensitive with a central core containing pus.

**Boosters (activators)** oxidising agents which add to the action of the main oxidiser (often hydrogen peroxide).

**Brighteners (brightening shampoos)** mild bleaches which lift the hair base colour shade slightly.

**Camomile** the flower of this plant produces a golden-yellow dye when dried then infused in water.

**Canities** technical name for hair growing without pigment. Produces 'white' hair.

**Carbuncle** a group of boils.

**Catagen** a stage in the hair growth cycle where old hair is replaced.

**Catalyst** substance which speeds up (accelerates) a chemical reaction.

**Cell division** process which produces the new cells that the body needs for growth and repair. The cells divide into two which grow and then can divide again.

**Cells** tiny units making up the body.

**Chipping in** haircutting technique used to remove bulk or weight from the ends of the hair and for softening the outline shape of the haircut.

**Chopsticks** a perming rod which produces a considerable volume with uniform angular curl.

**Circuit breakers (earth leakage devices)** automatic switches which switch the electrical supply off in the event of overloading or a fault.

**Citric acid** technical term for lemon juice.

**Club cutting** cutting the hair straight across to remove length but not bulk.

**Cohesive set (wet setting)** hair that is wet then moulded and dried in the moulded position, e.g. setting, blowdrying.

**Cold sores (herpes)** caused by a virus. The symptoms are cracking and oozing of skin around the mouth.

**Collagen**   an elastic protein found in the skin (dermis). It gives skin its elasticity, i.e. the ability to stretch and return to shape.

**Colour flashes**   fashion tinting technique of lightening a band of hair around the front hairline.

**Colour reducer**   used to remove unwanted artificial colour pigments from the hair.

**Compounds**   substances made up of different types of atoms joined together.

**Compound henna**   an inorganic dye which is a mixture of vegetable henna and a metallic dye. It reacts with hydrogen peroxide and is therefore not used in salons any more as the chemical processes available to the client are severely restricted if the hair has been treated with metallic salts.

**Concave cutting**   *see* inversion

**Concave mirror**   surface of the mirror goes in slightly and reflects an enlarged image.

**Condition**   an overall summary of the client's hair type, damage (if any) to the hair and amount of oil present etc.

**Conditioner**   a product designed to leave the hair in good condition. Types include: oil-based (emollients), substantive and mild acid rehabilitating rinses.

**Conduction**   energy, e.g. electricity or heat, passing through a material (conductor).

**Conjunctivitis**   eye infection which causes a general inflammation and weeping of the front of the eye.

**Contact dermatitis**   *see* dermatitis.

**Contagious**   disease spread by direct or indirect contact, e.g. touch.

**Contraction**   the way in which many materials get smaller (contract) when cooled.

**Contra-indications**   things to look for which would prevent hairdressing operations.

**Convection**   heat transfer by moving air or water carrying heat with it.

**Convex mirror**   surface of the mirror bulges out slightly and reflects a reduced image.

**Corynebacterium acne**   *see* acne.

**Cornified layer**   dead, protective outermost layer of the skin.

**Cortex**   *see* hair cortex.

**Covering dyes**   dyes which tint hair darker or a similar shade (tone) to the natural, base colour shade of the hair.

**Croquignole**   a term used for winding the hair from the hair points down towards the roots.

**Cross-checking**   a procedure to check that a hairdressing treatment, e.g. cutting, tinting, bleaching, has been thoroughly and correctly carried out.

**Cross-linkages (cross-links)**   hold the polypeptide chains in place in the hair cortex.

**Cuticle**   *see* hair cuticle.

**Cutting comb**   a pliable comb that is smaller and thinner than most other combs to enable the hair to be cut nearer to the scalp when using the 'scissor-over-comb' method of cutting hair.

**Dandruff**  *see* pityriasis.

**Decolourising**  removal of colour from a pigment by either oxidation, e.g. bleaching or reduction.

**Decomposition**  breakdown. Often used to describe the breakdown of hydrogen peroxide into water and oxygen.

**Delivery note**  a document that is usually received with an order. The contents of each should be checked not only against one another but also against the original order to ensure that the correct stock has been delivered in good condition.

**Depilatory**  a product used to remove hair. Generally works by breaking down the hair structure so that the hair disintegrates.

**Demonstrations**  are very effective if properly planned. They can be used to show staff techniques and to promote/publicise the salon.

**Density**  *see* abundance.

**Dermal papilla**  a bundle of blood vessels and fat cells in the centre of the hair bulb. It provides the chemicals for hair growth.

**Dermatitis**  inflammation, swelling and cracking of the skin: contact dermatitis is a response to a substance (called the primary irritant) which may need previous exposure until body 'over-reacts' to it, i.e. a period of sensitisation.

**Dermis**  inner layer of the skin which gives it its elasticity.

**Development (developing)**  producing the final colour of hair tints and bleaches or the transition from straight to curled hair during the softening and moulding stages of perming.

**Diagnostics**  means looking at the client's hair and scalp. Recognising skin and scalp condition and knowing what to do about them. Particularly important is knowing which conditions prevent hairdressing operations and which do not.

**Dilate**  to widen or expand. The blood vessels 'dilate' during scalp massage allowing the blood to pass more freely through them.

**Disinfectant**  chemicals which kill micro-organisms, e.g. bacteria, in which case they are described as bacteriocidal.

**Distilled water**  purified water which is free from dissolved salts. Used in the salon for diluting hydrogen peroxide and it is also recommended for use in steamer reservoirs.

**Dressing comb**  a comb (usually made of vulcanite) with a fine end and a rake end that is used for disentangling and dressing the hair.

**Dressing hair**  the final stage of the hairdressing process when the hair is arranged into the finished style using a variety of techniques (brushing, combing, teasing etc.), tools (brushes, combs, fingers), and dressing aids (dressing creams, sprays etc.).

**Droplet infection**  one way germs can be spread in the air, in the tiny droplets blown when someone coughs or sneezes.

**Earthing**  a part on an electrical system that provides an 'easy' route for electricity into the ground. It helps to prevent electric shock.

**Eczema**  similar to dermatitis, words are often used interchangeably. The general distinction is weeping of the skin and eczema is caused by internal factors.

**Eddy currents**   small ripples of electricity produced in the skin by the high-frequency machine.

**Effleurage**   hand massage involving slow, stroking movements. Used at the beginning and end of every massage treatment.

**Elasticity**   refers to stretching, i.e. the ability of a material to lengthen under tension and then return to its original length when the tension is removed.

**Electrode**   used in conjunction with the high-frequency machine. The electrodes used on the scalp are usually the rake, used for general thinning, the bulb for spot baldness or the saturator for general thinning or as a 'tonic' to aid hair condition.

**Emollients**   *see* conditioners.

**Emulsions**   droplets of one liquid suspended in another. **Emulsifying agents** help this process.

**Epidermis**   the upper layer of the skin which has an outer horny layer of dead, flattened cells that are constantly flaking off to be replaced by cells that have been produced in the basal, the lowest layer of the epidermis.

**Evaporation**   the conversion of a liquid into a gas. When this happens (e.g. sweating) it produces a cooling effect.

**Fibrils**   small thread-like fibres. Protofibrils, microfibrils, and macrofibrils are found in the cortex.

**Film former**   a thin coating on the hair, e.g. PVP in hair spray forms a thin plastic coating on the hair after the alcohol has evaporated.

**Fish-hook ends**   hair points which are bent back on themselves. Creates a 'frizzed' look on the ends of the hair which can be removed by wetting when caused during setting but can only be removed by cutting if the hair has been permed in this position.

**Finger waving**   setting the hair using 'S' shaped movements formed with the fingers and a comb.

**Flammable**   will burn when set alight.

**Flea (pulex irritans)**   a blood sucking parasite on the body, in clothing, bedding etc. Moves by jumping.

**Fluoresce (fluorescent)**   to glow. This happens in fluorescent lighting (strip lighting) tubes.

**Flying colours**   *see* painted lights.

**Follicle**   *see* hair follicle.

**Folliculitis**   swelling and reddening of the hair follicle often with pus formation.

**Fragilitis crinum (split ends)**   where the points of the hair fray and split. No 'cure': they must be cut off.

**Fresh air**   air which is usually cool, dry and free from contamination.

**Fungi (tinea)**   are plants made up of tiny threads called hyphae, some of which are parasites on humans, e.g. ringworm.

**Furuncle**   *see* boil.

**Fuse**   deliberate 'weak link' in an electrical system. Designed to melt and break the circuit if there is a fault.

**Fuse size**   the thickness of fuse wire used in a fuse. Measured in amps (short for amperes).

**Gel**   a thickened liquid (technically, a liquid with high viscosity).

**Germinative layer**   growing layer of the skin epidermis (*see* basal).

**Glimmering (polishing)** adding colour to the hair using tin foil painted with tint in a polishing motion.

**Graduation** a hair cutting term used to describe the effect created when the top layers of the hair lie above the underneath layers. A steeply graduated haircut is referred to as high layering, while very little graduation in a haircut is referred to as low layering.

**Hair bulb** bulge on lower part of the hair root. The area from which hair grows.

**Hair colour restorer** metallic dye containing lead acetate and sodium thiosulphate.

**Hair cortex** inner bulk of hair made up of fibres.

**Hair cuticle** the outer layer of the hair, made of overlapping scales.

**Hair cuttings** cuttings of hair taken from various parts of the head to enable certain tests to be carried out, e.g. incompatibility, porosity, elasticity etc.

**Hair fixing sprays** developed from plastic polymers dissolved in alcohol which coat the hair with a plastic film.

**Hair fly** when hair tends to lift away from the scalp due to static electricity.

**Hair follicle** tiny pit in the skin from which hair grows.

**Hair growth cycle** consists of three phases (stages): anagen – active growth; telogen – resting; catagen – hair replaced by new one.

**Hair growth pattern** the growth direction of the hair due to the angle of the follicle in the scalp.

**Hair lacquer** *see* hair fixing sprays.

**Hair medulla** possible third, central area of hair.

**Hair mesh** a section of hair gathered together in some way for a hairdressing operation.

**Hair root** the part of the hair which is buried in the skin.

**Hair shaft** the part of the hair which is visible beyond the skin surface.

**Hardness of water** where particular mineral salts present in water react with soap to produce soap scum. Temporary hard water is removed by boiling and causes lime scale; permanent hard water cannot be removed by boiling but can be removed by other methods (*see* soft water).

**Head louse** *see* lice.

**Henna (Lawsone)** an orange/red vegetable dye obtained from the dried leaves of the Egyptian privet (Lawsonia).

**Hepatitis** a very dangerous disease which can be transmitted in the salon.

**Herpes simplex** *see* cold sores.

**High-frequency treatment** uses a high voltage machine (apparatus) which produces a warming of the skin and encourages blood flow.

**Highlighting** technique of lightening fine strands of hair using bleach and/or tint.

**Hirsutism** literally means 'very hairy'. What happens in practice is that the areas which usually have the fine vellus hair grow darker, thicker secondary hair.

**Hone** to sharpen, e.g. a razor, before shaving.

**Horny layer** *see* cornified layer.

**Humidity** the amount of water vapour (moisture) present in the air.

**Hydrogen ions** hydrogen atoms which have lost an electron. The number of hydrogen ions in a solution is the basis of the pH scale.

**Hydrogen peroxide** an effective oxidising agent which decomposes to produce water and oxygen. Used for oxidising permanent waves, para dyes and bleaches.

**Hydrometer** used for measuring the density of liquids. One type, a peroxometer can be used for direct measurement of the strength (concentration) of hydrogen peroxide solutions.

**Hygiene** practices likely to reduce the chances of infection or infestation.

**Hygrometer** device for measuring the amount of water vapour (humidity) in the air.

**Hygroscopic** ability of some materials (including hair) to absorb water vapour (moisture) from the air.

**Hyperaemia** increased flow of blood to the skin. Can cause the skin to redden. The most common form of this phenomenon is a 'blush'.

**Hypertrichosis** the growing in specific place of thick pigmented hair in areas where usually only fine vellus hair grow.

**Impetigo** caused by staphylococci bacteria. Characteristics include blisters and weeping, formation of yellow crusts. Common as a secondary infection.

**Incompatible** means 'will not go together'.

**Incompatibility test** a test to determine whether the hair has been previously treated with an incompatible chemical, (e.g. metallic dye); if positive, hairdressing treatments should be avoided.

**Infectious** of a disease spread by air or water.

**Infection** invasion of the body by pathogens (germs).

**Infestation** animal parasites living on the body. Sometimes used to refer to premises, e.g. a house 'infested' with mice.

**Inorganic dye** a dye containing metallic salts. These metallic salts react with hydrogen peroxide; therefore perming, bleaching and para tinting should be avoided on hair coated with this type of dye.

**Insulation** material which slows down (or stops) energy, e.g. electricity, heat, passing through it.

**Inversion (concave)** refers to a rounded inwards shape that is cut into the hair.

**Invoice** a document which lists and gives the price of the various products contained in an order. It should be checked against the delivery note to ensure that the order is correct before paying for the goods.

**Ion exchange resin** *see* soft water.

**Itchmite (sarcoptes scabiei)** causes scabies (or the itch). Very small parasites which are almost invisible to the unaided eye. The females burrow into the skin and lay eggs which causes intense itching (usually at night). Scratching often leads to secondary infections, e.g. impetigo.

**Karaya gum** an Indian gum used in some setting agents. Requires a preservative to prevent it going mouldy.

**Keratin** hard, fibrous protein found in hair, skin and nails.

**Keratinisation** process by which skin, hair, and nail cells become filled with keratin.

**Lanolin** a wax which is obtained from sheep's wool, and is often used in traditional conditioning agents, shampoos and hand creams.

**Lanugo hair** the first hair produced by babies, often while in the womb.

**Lacquer** weak adhesive which helps to hold the hairstyle in place. They are generally non-sticky and water soluble (*see* hair fixing sprays).

**Lawsone** *see* henna.

**Layering** a form of graduation. **High layering** has steep graduation. **Low layering** has very little graduation.

**Lead acetate** an ingredient in some hair colour restorers.

**Leuco-compounds** breakdown products produced by decolourising (removing colour) from a developed para tint.

**Lice** parasitic insects (all have six legs, none can fly). Headlouse (pediculus capitis) produces an infestation called pediculosis. The adults are small and lay pearl coloured eggs (nits) which are cemented to the hair shafts particularly in the nape and behind the ears. Other types of lice include the body louse (pediculus corporis) and pubic louse (phthirus pubis).

**Lightening dyes** para dyes which tint the hair lighter than the hair's natural colour.

**Line and balance** the relationship between the finished hairstyle and the shape of the client's face, facial features and body size.

**Live (or 'line')** cable bringing electricity into a circuit or piece of electrical apparatus. Such cables are colour-coded brown.

**Lowlights** adding small strands of colour to the hair either throughout the head or where necessary to emphasise and enhance the finished hairstyle.

**Macrofibrils** largest of the tiny fibres making up the hair cortex.

**Male pattern baldness** an inherited condition that affects approximately 40% of males by the age of 40.

**Malpighian layer** *see* basal.

**Massage** the general name for rubbing and kneading actions. It generally increases blood flow to the massaged area.

**Matter** anything having a physical form. 'States' of matter are: solid, liquid and gas.

**Melanin** black/brown natural pigment in the hair and skin.

**Melanocytes** cells which produce and lay down natural pigments in the hair and skin.

**Membrane** the very thin, outer covering on cells.

**Meniscus** the surface of a liquid.

**Mesh (or section)** *see* hair mesh.

**Microfibrils** small bundles of fibres making up macrofibrils in the hair cortex.

**Micro-organisms** tiny living animals or plants.

**Mineral salts** substances needed in the diet. Commonly dissolved in tap water.

**Mirror** usually of glass with reflecting 'silver' backing. Types include: concave mirror – the surface of which goes in slightly producing an enlarged image; convex mirror – the surface of which bulges out slightly producing a reduced image; plane mirror – the surface of which is flat, reflecting an image the same actual size.

**Monilethrix** a rare condition where there are bead-like swellings along the hair shaft.

**Mousses**  foams produced by a propellant gas blowing through a liquid.

**Muscles**  help to bring about movement of the body and maintain 'posture'.

**Nascent oxygen**  single atoms of oxygen (unlike oxygen gas which has two atoms, $O_2$). Highly reactive and responsible for developing tints, bleaches and oxidising ('neutralising') perms.

**Neutral**  cable taking electricity away from a circuit or appliance. Such cables are colour-coded blue.

**Neutralisation**  an acid and a base reacting together to make a compound (or salt) and water.

**Nichrome wire**  often used in heating elements in electrical appliances. High resistance to the flow of electricity produces heat in the wire.

**Nitro dyes**  dyes which are similar to para dyes in structure but with a low solubility. They are washed out of the hair after six to eight shampoos.

**Nits**  eggs of the parasitic louse (*see* lice).

**Non-verbal communication**  the very powerful transfer of information by body movements, eye contact, facial expression and tone of voice.

**Normalisation**  a term sometimes used in perming to mean 'oxidisation'.

**Normaliser**  another name for the 'oxidiser' (often called 'neutraliser') used in perming.

**Oral communication**  spoken words, often less important than **non-verbal communication**.

**Oxidation**  the addition of oxygen or the removal of hydrogen from a substance. Chemicals that can do this are called oxidising agents or oxidisers.

**Ozone**  a gas ($O_3$) produced by high frequency which can destroy micro-organisms.

**Painted lights (flying colours)**  the technique of tinting fine strands of hair using a 'vent' brush, wide-toothed comb or fine artist's brush to emphasise the shape of a hairstyle.

**Papova virus**  *see* wart.

**Para dye (aniline dye)**  permanent, semi-permanent, synthetic, organic dye. Must be mixed with hydrogen peroxide to be effective.

**Parasite**  a living thing that lives on or in another living thing (called the parasite's host).

**Patch test**  *see* skin test.

**Pathogenic**  disease causing. Pathogenic micro-organisms (pathogens) are germs.

**Pediculus**  *see* lice.

**Pediculus capitis**  infestation of the scalp by head lice (*see* lice).

**Percentage strength (%)**  a way of expressing strength (concentration) of hydrogen peroxide solutions (*see* volume strength). Based on parts per hundred (%) of 'pure' peroxide in a solution.

**Peroxometer**  *see* hydrometer.

**Petrissage**  massage movements involving kneading actions.

**pH scale**  a scale of acidity or alkalinity. Has 14 points; 7 is neutral (neither acid nor alkaline), below 7 is acid and above 7 is alkaline.

**Pheomelanin**  red/yellow natural pigment in the hair and skin.

**Pin curls**  type of setting where the hair is wound flat. Types are: clockspring, barrel spring, stem and sculptured curls.

**Pityriasis (full name pityriasis simplex)**  the technical name for dandruff (scurf) due to the flaking of the scalp skin.

**Pityriasis steatoides**  greasy dandruff. An over-production of sebum causes flakes of skin to stick to the scalp which may then lead to seborrhoeic dermatitis.

**Plane mirror**  mirror with a flat surface that reflects the image the same size as the object.

**Plane wart**  a small, smooth topped wart.

**Plantar wart**  inward growing wart usually on the feet (verrucae).

**Pli**  the name often used for the finished 'set' when setting the hair.

**Pointing**  *see* chipping in.

**Polypeptide chains**  the smallest chains in the hair cortex made up of amino acids.

**Post-damping**  applying perm reagent to the curlers after they have been wound.

**Posture**  the way in which someone stands.

**Predisposition test**  *see* skin test.

**Prepigmentation**  tinting bleached hair to its original colour.

**Presaturation**  applying perm reagent to the hair mesh as it is wound.

**Primary colours**  the three colours, yellow, red and blue, from which all others can be made.

**Primary irritant**  *see* allergy and dermatitis.

**Propellent**  gas which forces spray or foam from a pressurised container, e.g. lacquer or mousse.

**Protofibrils**  tiny chains making up microfibrils in the hair cortex.

**Psoriasis**  a non-infectious skin condition. Often seen as silvery scales with red skin underneath; the silvery scales flake off when rubbed.

**Pulex irritans**  human flea. It has long back legs which allow it to jump from one person to another.

**Pull-burn**  a burn on the skin caused by winding the hair too tightly when perming.

**Pus**  liquid collecting in infections, e.g. spots. It is a mixture of dead body cells and bacteria.

**Pustule**  raised 'head' of a spot containing pus.

**Reagent**  substance that is used to produce a chemical reaction.

**Reduction**  the opposite of oxidation. It involves removal of oxygen or addition of hydrogen to a substance. Chemicals that do this are reducing agents.

**Reduction dye**  a metallic dye which uses pyrogallol as a reducing agent.

**Regrowth**  the hair nearest the scalp which has grown since the last hairdressing treatment, therefore has natural colour and wave.

**Rehabilitating rinse**  *see* conditioners.

**Relative humidity**  *see* humidity.

**Relaxer cream**  reagent for straightening hair.

**Relaxing hair**  *see* straightening.

**Resistance**  electrical resistance refers to how easy it is for electricity to pass through a material. High resistance often produces heat, e.g. in heating elements.

**Restructurant** type of conditioner which is substantive, 'adds to' the hair shaft. Makes hair less porous.

**Retouch** applying a chemical treatment to a regrowth.

**Reverse graduation** a haircutting term used to describe the effect created when the top layers of the hair lie below the underneath layers.

**Ringworm (tinea)** caused by a parasitic fungus. When present on the scalp it produces reddened, round patches with a stubble of hair. Types include: **tinea capitis** – fungal infection of the scalp; **tinea corporis** – fungal infection of the body; **tinea pedis** – fungal infection of the feet, commonly known as 'athlete's foot'.

**Root sheath** *see* hair root sheath.

**Root** *see* hair root.

**Salt** *see* neutralisation.

**Saponification** technical name for soap making process.

**Saprophyte** bacteria which feeds on and causes the decay of dead, organic material.

**Sarcoptes scabiei** *see* itchmite.

**Scrunching** when used in relation to fashion colouring it is a method of lightening the ends of the hair using either tint, bleach or a combination of both.

**Scurf** *see* pityriasis.

**Sebaceous cyst (wen)** a raised lump on the skin caused by a blockage of the sebaceous gland.

**Sebaceous gland** produces natural oil sebum which coats the hair and the skin. A blocked gland can lead to a build up of sebum in a wen (sebaceous cyst).

**Seborrhea** is an overproduction of sebum. Causes oily hair and skin, it can be triggered by hormone changes at puberty. It may also cause swelling, itching and reddening on the scalp, called seborrhoeic dermatitis.

**Sebum** natural oil made by sebaceous gland in hair follicles. It waterproofs and conditions the hair and skin.

**Secondary hair** sometimes called terminal hair. It is the thick, usually darker hair on the scalp and body.

**Secondary infection** it occurs where an earlier infection produces conditions which encourage a second type of pathogen to invade the body, e.g. impetigo is a common secondary infection of scabies caused when the skin is broken through scratching.

**Selenium sulphide** a substance used in shampoo to combat dandruff. It reduces the activities of the germinative layer of the skin thus reducing flaking.

**Sensitisation** *see* allergy and dermatitis.

**Sensitivity test** *see* skin test.

**Setting** various methods both wet and dry, used to give hair a temporary style. Setting aids help to produce and prolong the set.

**Shampoo** a solution for cleaning hair. Usually a soapless base containing a mixture of ingredients to remove dirt and oil from the hair.

**Shimmer lights** a tinting technique that produces a similar effect to painted lights. The hair is combed into position with a gel, then the raised part of the ridges has tint applied to it with a fine brush.

**Shingle**  a graduated hair cut where the nape hair is cut extremely short, usually with the clippers or scissors over comb.

**Skin epidermis**  the outer part of the skin, made up of layers. The bottom layer (germinative) grows and moves towards the surface, eventually producing the dead outer layer of the skin (cornified).

**Skin test**  a test taken to see if a person has an allergy to a substance. The material to be tested is placed on the skin and checked to see if a 'rash' develops. If such a reaction takes place the person is probably allergic to that substance.

**Slicing (tramming)**  a method of tinting whereby slices of colour are placed in the hair where required.

**Slither cutting**  *see* tapering.

**Soap**  an emulsifying agent commonly made by reacting fat and/or oil with an alkali (a process called saponification). The soap emulsifies (makes into droplets) the oil and dirt on the skin.

**Soap scum**  grey/white deposits formed when soap reacts with 'hard' water. The main ingredient in scum is calcium stearate.

**Sodium chloride**  the technical name for common salt.

**Sodium hydroxide**  an alkali used in the production of hard soap.

**Soft water (water softening)**  unlike hard water, soft water does not contain those mineral salts which form soap scum with soap. Water softening involves making the hard water soft. This is done by removing the mineral salts from the water. A common commercial method uses an ion exchange resin, e.g. zeolite.

**Spot tinting/bleaching**  tinting or bleaching the hair where required to correct uneven colour faults.

**Stale air**  air which can be over-moist, warm and contaminated by smells and/or micro-organisms.

**Staphylococci**  bacteria which cause skin infections, e.g. spots.

**Static electricity**  produced by rubbing (friction) between certain materials, e.g. plastic and hair. Causes hair fly.

**Steamer**  apparatus which produces moist heat. Used to aid the development of some hairdressing processes.

**Sterilisation**  a process which kills all micro-organisms.

**Straightening (relaxing) hair**  methods used to remove curl/wave from the hair.

**Streptococci**  bacteria which cause infections, e.g. sore throat. Divide to form chains.

**Strop**  a leather strap used to sharpen open, cut-throat razors.

**Styes (blepharitis)**  caused by bacteria invading the hair follicle of eye lashes (commonly of the lower eye-lid) causing reddening and swelling.

**Substantive**  something which joins with or enters the hair shaft. *See* conditioners.

**Sulphide dye**  an inorganic metallic dye.

**Sulphonation**  process used in the manufacture of soapless detergents.

**Sulphur bonds**  cross linkages that hold the polypeptide chains, sometimes referred to as 'S' bonds', disulphide bonds, cystine linkages or sulphur bridges.

**Surface tension** tendency for water to form a film on the surface when in contact with something.

**Sycosis barbae** *see* barber's itch.

**Symptoms** the characteristic 'signs' of a disease.

**Tail comb** a comb used for sectioning, lifting or weaving the hair. It has a fine end and a tail end. A variation of the tail comb is the pin-tail comb which has a thin, metal, stiletto tail end.

**Tapering (slither cutting)** a method of cutting hair using a 'slithering' movement which removes bulk and length.

**Tension** effect produced by pulling.

**Telogen** the stage in the hair growth cycle where hair growth stops; a resting stage.

**Tempering** hardening a metal, e.g. styling iron.

**Tensile strength** how much tension is needed to break, often expressed as a weight.

**Terminal hair** *see* secondary hair.

**Test cutting** taken before a hairdressing process to ensure the best choice, and to determine the effects of the products to be used on the hair.

**Texture** the texture of the hair refers to its diameter. Fine hair is narrow in diameter while thick hair has a much larger diameter.

**Thermostat** a device used to control temperature.

**Thinning** a haircutting method that removes weight and bulk from the hair.

**Thixotropic** a thickened liquid (gel) which changes to a liquid when stirred or brushed.

**Tinea** *see* ringworm *and* fungi.

**Tints** dyes used to colour the hair. They can be lightening or covering, temporary, semi-permanent or permanent.

**Tissue** a number of body cells working together.

**Toners** tints used to 'mask' unwanted colour tones.

**Tortoiseshell highlights** woven strands of hair which are then tinted with three or four different colours throughout the head or where required.

**Toxins** poisonous substances.

**Traction alopecia** *see* alopecia.

**Tragacanth gum** white powder obtained from the bark of a shrub grown in Turkey, which can be used in setting agents.

**Tramming** *see* slicing.

**Translucent** allows light to pass through, and scatters (diffuses) it.

**Transparent** allows light to pass through.

**Triethanolamine lauryl sulphate** an organic salt which is the basis of most soapless shampoos as it is mild to the hair.

**Trichloroethane** commonly used as a solvent to dry clean hair wigs or hair-pieces (postiche).

**Trichorphexis nodosa** condition where hair splits and frays at swellings along the length.

**Ultra violet radiation** part of electromagnetic spectrum not visible to the eye, which is used in UV sterilisers and triggers melanocytes in the skin, producing a sun-tan.

**Vegetable dye**   a dye obtained from plants, e.g. camomile.

**Vellus hair**   the fine, often unpigmented (or slightly pigmented) downy hair, e.g. present on the female face.

**Verrucae**   *see* warts.

**Vibro machine**   a mechanical form of massage. The machine has various attachments, the most common of which are the spiked applicator, the sponge applicator and the bell-shaped applicator. It is used in conjunction with hair/scalp treatments to stimulate blood flow, and promote healthy hair.

**Virus**   the smallest type of micro-organism; it cannot survive long outside the body. It causes colds, 'flu, 'cold sores' (herpes) and some types of wart.

**Viscous**   a 'gel-like' consistency, the state between a liquid and a solid.

**Visible spectrum**   light that can be seen by the eye. It makes up the 'colours of the rainbow'.

**Volatile**   a liquid which evaporates quickly.

**Voltage**   the electrical 'pressure' behind the flow of electricity.

**Volume strength (vol strength; 'vols')**   a way of expressing strength (concentration) of hydrogen peroxide solutions. It means the number of volumes of oxygen gas given off by one volume of peroxide. For example, when completely broken down 1 cm$^3$ 20 vol hydrogen peroxide would give off 20 cm$^3$ of oxygen gas.

**Warts (verrucae)**   some warts are caused by a virus (papova virus) which makes the skin produce raised lumps. On the feet, the pressure of the body weight can cause the wart to grow inwards creating a verruca (plantar wart).

**Water vapour**   water that has changed from its liquid state to a gas. When there is a lot of water vapour present in the air the atmosphere is known as humid.

**Wen**   *see* sebaceous cyst.

**Wet setting**   *see* cohesive set.

**Winding**   term for insertion and rolling up of rollers, curlers etc., in the hair.

**Yeast**   associated with (but *not* the cause of) dandruff (*see* pityriasis).

**Zinc pyrithione**   substance found in medicated or anti-dandruff shampoos.

# INDEX